WORKBOOK for

Mechanical Ventilation:

Physiological and Clinical Applications

Fourth Edition

evolve

To access your Instructor Resources, visit:

http://evolve.elsevier.com/Pilbeam/ventilation

Evolve ® Resources for **Mechanical Ventilation: Physiological and Clinical Applications, 4th edition**, offers the following features:

- **Additional Content**
  "Special Techniques in Mechanical Ventilation" provides additional information on this important topic.

- **WebLinks**
  Links to places of interest on the web specific to respiratory care.

- **Links to Related Products**
  See what else Elsevier has to offer in a specific field of interest.

WORKBOOK for

Mechanical Ventilation:

Physiological and Clinical Applications

Fourth Edition

Sindee Kalminson Karpel, MPA, RRT, AE-C

Clinical Coordinator
Respiratory Care Program
Edison College
Fort Myers, Florida

Neil Rodia, MS, RRT

Professor
Department of Allied Health Sciences
Borough of Manhattan Community College
The City University of New York
New York, New York

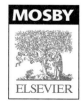

MOSBY

ELSEVIER

MOSBY
ELSEVIER

11830 Westline Industrial Drive
St. Louis, Missouri 63146

WORKBOOK FOR MECHANICAL VENTILATION: PHYSIOLOGICAL
AND CLINICAL APPLICATIONS, FOURTH EDITION
Copyright © 2006, Mosby, Inc., an affiliate of Elsevier, Inc.

ISBN-13: 978-0-323-03296-4
ISBN-10: 0-323-03296-6

Previous edition copyrighted 1999

ISBN-13: 978-0-323-03296-4
ISBN-10: 0-323-03296-6

Managing Editor: Mindy Hutchinson
Senior Developmental Editor: Melissa K. Boyle
Publishing Services Manager: Melissa Lastarria
Project Manager: Gail Michaels
Designer: Amy Buxton

**Working together to grow
libraries in developing countries**

www.elsevier.com | www.bookaid.org | www.sabre.org

ELSEVIER   BOOK AID
            International   Sabre Foundation

Printed in the United States of America

Last digit is the print number: 9 8 7 6 5 4

Contents

To my husband, Larry Karpel, for his unwavering support and encouragement, and to my sons, Brad and Jordan, for providing me with daily challenges.

SKK

To my mother, Beatrice, and to the memory of my father, Julio Rodia. I also wish to thank my colleagues, Professors Everett Flannery and Michael Nazzaro for their friendship and encouragement. And special thanks to my long-time friend, mentor, and co-author, Sindee Karpel, for her support and guidance throughout this project.

NR

WORKBOOK for
Mechanical Ventilation:

Physiological and Clinical Applications

Fourth Edition

Preface

The goal of this workbook is to assist the respiratory care student in the mastery of the information presented in *Mechanical Ventilation: Physiological and Clinical Applications*, fourth edition, by Susan P. Pilbeam and J.M. Cairo.

Reading a textbook like this requires active reading, which is very different from passive reading for pleasure. The student should expect to read more slowly and carefully when reading material that he or she will be expected to understand and remember. Comprehension is not an automatic response to the movement of the eyes across a line of print. To make the reading process active, the reader must focus attention on what information is needed from the material. Reading with a purpose (e.g., to answer questions) increases concentration, comprehension, retention, and interest in the subject matter.

We would like to suggest that the student use the text and workbook in the following manner:

First, preview or survey the text chapter by reading the chapter title, outline, objectives, and key terms. Remember, the chapter learning objectives indicate what the author intends for the reader to know after finishing with the chapter. Skim the chapter headings and subheadings. Read the chapter summary. This highlights the structure of the chapter and emphasizes important concepts.

Next, turn the chapter title into a question. The idea here is that asking a question focuses your reading on finding information that will answer the question. It makes reading a more active search for meaning. Use the review questions in the workbook to help you focus on important points in the chapter. Read carefully (in manageable chunks) to answer these questions. Note important details and relationships of ideas. The review questions in this workbook are based on the author's learning objectives for each chapter. Pay particular attention to charts, graphs, tables, boxes, and figures because they are included to help learn the material.

Then review the workbook chapter review questions and their answers. Be able to answer all of the questions. Use the answers as a guide for highlighting the textbook. This will ensure that highlighting is being done efficiently.

After this, answer the critical thinking questions and the case study questions in the workbook. This will help with analysis and application type questions seen on the board exams. Then attempt the NBRC-type questions. Once the chapter has been completed, test your critical vocabulary by trying the key terms crossword puzzle.

Sindee K. Karpel, MPA, RRT, AE-C
Neil Rodia, MS, RRT

Oxygenation and Acid-Base Evaluation

Learning Objectives

Upon completion of this chapter the reader will be able to do the following:

1. List the normal values for arterial and mixed venous blood gas measurements.
2. Estimate normal PaO_2 based on age.
3. Interpret PaO_2 values at varying altitudes.
4. Assess the $P(A-a)O_2$ value, the PaO_2/P_AO_2 ratio, and the PaO_2/F_IO_2 ratio to determine oxygenation status.
5. Compare the P_{50} value to normal to determine any shifts of the oxyhemoglobin dissociation curve.
6. Evaluate the CaO_2 (given Hb, PaO_2, and SaO_2) to determine oxygenation status.
7. Interpret an arterial blood gas measurement.
8. Calculate a change in pH based on a change in $PaCO_2$.
9. Differentiate the bicarbonate from the pH (hydrogen ion content) and the $PaCO_2$.
10. Estimate a $PaCO_2$ value based on a change in a patient's alveolar ventilation and CO_2 production.
11. Calculate changes in bicarbonate based on changes in pH or $PaCO_2$.

Key Terms Crossword Puzzle

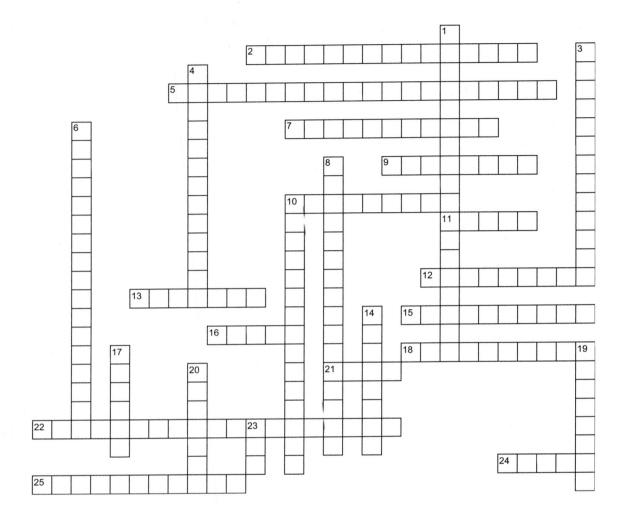

Across

2 Inability of oxygen to move through the alveolar-capillary (A-C) membrane

5 High pH and low $PaCO_2$ (two words)

7 Hypoxia caused by reduced cardiac output

9 Tendency of oxygen to combine with hemoglobin

10 Low arterial oxygen pressure

11 Primary organ for the removal of carbon dioxide

12 High pH

13 Organ that compensates for too much or too little carbon dioxide

15 Difference between the normal buffer base and the actual buffer base

16 Perfusion without ventilation

18 Hypoxia caused by cyanide poisoning

21 Syndrome that results in a PaO_2/F_IO_2 ratio of 200 or lower

22 Low pH and high $PaCO_2$ (two words)

24 Condition in which ABG values show no compensation

25 Buffer for carbon dioxide

Down

1 High pH and high bicarbonate (two words)

3 PaO_2 of 60 to 79 mm Hg (two words)

4 Type of hemoglobin that causes a left shift in the OHDC

6 Low pH and low bicarbonate (two words)

8 Cause of decreased blood carbon dioxide level

10 Cause of elevated blood carbon dioxide level

14 Low pH

17 Hypoxia caused by a lower than normal red blood cell (RBC) count

19 Condition in which ABG results show kidneys and lungs causing the same pH change

20 Indicated by a PaO_2/F_IO_2 ratio of 200 to 300

23 Abbreviation for a condition indicated by a PaO_2 to F_IO_2 ratio between 200 and 300

Review Questions

1. Arterial blood normally carries _____ millimoles (mmol) of dissolved CO_2.

2. Venous blood normally carries _____ mmol of dissolved CO_2.

3. The normal amount of combined CO_2 carried in arterial blood is _____ mmol/L; in venous blood, it is _____ mmol/L.

4. The normal total CO_2 in arterial blood is _____ mmol/L; in venous blood, it is _____ mmol/L.

5. The normal PCO_2 for arterial blood is _____ mm Hg; for venous blood, it is _____ mm Hg.

6. Normal arterial pH is _____, and normal venous pH is _____.

7. The normal value for HCO_3^- in arterial blood is _____ mEq/L; in venous blood, it is _____ mEq/L.

8. Base excess for both arterial and venous blood normally is _____.

9. The normal PaO_2 is _____ mm Hg, and the normal P_vO_2 is _____ mm Hg.

10. Hemoglobin in arterial blood is normally _____% saturated; in venous blood, it normally is _____% saturated.

11. The normal amount of dissolved O_2 in arterial blood is _____ vol%; in venous blood, it is _____ vol%.

12. In normal arterial blood, _____ vol% of O_2 is combined with hemoglobin.

13. In normal venous blood, _____ vol% of O_2 is combined with hemoglobin.

14. Total O_2 content for arterial blood is _____ vol%; for venous blood, it is _____ vol%.

15. In the spaces provided, give the clinical estimate of PaO_2 based on age.

Age	Estimated PaO_2 (mm Hg)
24	_____
32	_____
40	_____
48	_____
56	_____
60	_____
68	_____
76	_____
84	_____

Use Table 1-4 in the text for questions 16 through 20.

16. How does altitude affect PaO_2?

_____

_____

_____

_____

_____

17. For a normal individual, what is the expected P_AO_2 at 10,000 feet?

_____

18. What is the expected PaO_2 at 15,000 feet without supplemental oxygen when the $PaCO_2$ is 40 mm Hg?

_____

19. At an altitude of 10,000 feet, what is the expected PaO_2 when the $PaCO_2$ is 30 mm Hg?

_____

20. Which type of hypoxia occurs at high altitudes?

_____

21. Define the terms *hypoxia* and *hypoxemia*.

_____

_____

_____

_____

22. Match the causes of hypoxia with the appropriate term.

    Type of Hypoxia

    ___ Affinity hypoxia
    ___ Circulatory hypoxia
    ___ Histotoxic hypoxia
    ___ Hypoxemic hypoxia
    ___ Anemic hypoxia

    Cause

    (a) Decreased tissue perfusion from decreased cardiac output
    (b) Cyanide poisoning
    (c) Reduced release of oxygen from hemoglobin to tissues
    (d) Decreased RBC count
    (e) Lower than normal PaO_2

23. Identify the severity of hypoxemia for each of the following oxygen values for a 24-year-old adult breathing room air.

    (a) $PaO_2 = 84$ mm Hg _____

    (b) $SaO_2 = 92\%$ _____

    (c) $PaO_2 = 78$ mm Hg _____

    (d) $SaO_2 = 88\%$ _____

    (e) $PaO_2 = 47$ mm Hg _____

    (f) $SaO_2 = 72\%$ _____

    (g) $PaO_2 = 35$ mm Hg _____

24. The ability of the lungs to bring in and transfer oxygen to the alveolar capillaries can be assessed by what three formulas?

    _____

    _____

    _____

25. What are the normal values for the three formulas listed in question 24?

    _____

    _____

    _____

26. Assess the oxygenation status for a patient with the following values (barometric pressure [PB] = 760 mm Hg):

    $PaO_2 = 155$ mm Hg, $P_AO_2 = 235$ mm Hg, $F_IO_2 = 0.40$, $PaCO_2 = 40$ mm Hg.

    _____

    _____

    _____

    _____

27. Assess the oxygenation status for a patient with the following values (PB = 760 mm Hg): $PaO_2 = 58$ mm Hg, $P_AO_2 = 67$ mm Hg, $F_IO_2 = 0.21$, $PaCO_2 = 66$ mm Hg.

    _____

    _____

    _____

    _____

28. Assess the oxygenation status for a patient with the following values (PB = 760 mm Hg): $PaO_2 = 99$ mm Hg, $P_AO_2 = 183$ mm Hg, $F_IO_2 = 0.30$, $PaCO_2 = 25$ mm Hg.

    _____

    _____

    _____

    _____

29. Assess the oxygenation status for a patient with the following values (PB = 760 mm Hg): $PaO_2 = 98$ mm Hg, $P_AO_2 = 673$ mm Hg, $F_IO_2 = 1.00$, $PaCO_2 = 40$ mm Hg.

    _____

    _____

    _____

    _____

30. Assess the oxygenation status for a patient with the following values (PB = 760 mm Hg): $PaO_2 = 84$ mm Hg, $P_AO_2 = 282$ mm Hg, $F_IO_2 = 0.50$, $PaCO_2 = 60$ mm Hg.

    _____

    _____

    _____

    _____

31. Name five factors that can reduce the attraction of hemoglobin and oxygen and promote the unloading of oxygen at the cellular level.

    _____

    _____

    _____

    _____

    _____

32. Name six factors that can increase the attraction of hemoglobin and oxygen and promote the binding of oxygen to hemoglobin.

_____

_____

_____

_____

_____

_____

33. Define the acronym P_{50}.

_____

_____

34. Assess the following P_{50} values for a right or left shift in the OHDC.

P_{50}	Type of OHDC shift
(a) 0 mm Hg	_____
(b) 29 mm Hg	_____
(c) 34 mm Hg	_____
(d) 37 mm Hg	_____
(e) 18 mm Hg	_____

35. Calculate the total arterial oxygen content for a patient with a PaO_2 of 95 mm Hg, a SaO_2 of 98%, and an Hb of 9 g/dL.

_____

_____

36. Calculate the total arterial oxygen content for a patient with a PaO_2 of 78 mm Hg, a SaO_2 of 92%, and an Hb of 15 g/dL.

_____

_____

_____

37. Calculate the total arterial oxygen content for a patient with a PaO_2 of 52 mm Hg, a SaO_2 of 90%, and an Hb of 18 g/dL.

_____

_____

_____

38. Calculate the total arterial oxygen content for a patient with a PaO_2 of 45 mm Hg, a SaO_2 of 70%, and an Hb of 11 g/dL.

_____

_____

_____

39. Explain how cardiac output affects tissue oxygenation.

_____

_____

_____

_____

_____

40. What is pulmonary shunt?

_____

_____

_____

41. Calculate the % shunt using the following information (see Table 1-3 of the text): Hb = 12 g/dL, P_AO_2 = 673 mm Hg, S_AO_2 = 100%, PaO_2 = 98 mm Hg, SaO_2 = 99%, $P_{\bar{v}}O_2$ = 35 mm Hg, $S_{\bar{v}}O_2$ = 73%.

_____

_____

42. What effect does a low total oxygen content have on % shunt?

_____

_____

43. Name five disorders that can increase percent shunt and cause severe hypoxemia.

_____

_____

_____

44. Under normal circumstances, how much alveolar ventilation is required to maintain ABG values within normal limits?

_____

_____

Refer to Figure 1-3 in the text for questions 45 and 46.

45. What would happen to the P_AO_2 and P_ACO_2 if alveolar ventilation dropped to 2 L/min?

_____

_____

_____

46. Why do changes in P_ACO_2 affect PaO_2?

_____

_____

_____

47. For a healthy individual breathing room air at sea level, regardless of the level of alveolar ventilation, the sum of P_AO_2 and P_ACO_2 is _____ mm Hg.

48. What are the plateau values for P_AO_2 and P_ACO_2 for a healthy individual severely hyperventilating on room air at sea level?

_____

_____

49. Estimate the expected $PaCO_2$ for the following alveolar ventilation and CO_2 production values.

Alveolar Ventilation	CO_2 Production	Expected $PaCO_2$
3 L/min	100 L/min	(a) _____
3.5 L/min	175 L/min	(b) _____
5 L/min	200 L/min	(c) _____
5.5 L/min	275 L/min	(d) _____

50. Interpret the following ABG values (R/A = Room air).

pH	$PaCO_2$ (mm Hg)	PaO_2 (mm Hg)	SaO_2 (%)	HCO_3^- (mEq/L)	F_IO_2	Acid/base balance (acute or chronic)	Oxygenation status
(a) 7.45	25	58	95	17	R/A	_____	_____
(b) 7.55	27	105	100	23	R/A	_____	_____
(c) 7.25	90	34	58	38	R/A	_____	_____
(d) 7.52	30	45	86	24	40%	_____	_____
(e) 7.32	39	82	94	16	30%	_____	_____
(f) 7.44	25	65	91	17	30%	_____	_____
(g) 7.31	26	95	96	14	R/A	_____	_____
(h) 7.38	59	64	91	39	50%	_____	_____

51. Using the simplified Henderson-Hasselbalch equation and Table 1-7 in the text, calculate the [H+] and estimate the pH for the following situations.

$PaCO_2$ (mm Hg)	HCO_3^- (mEq/L)	[H+]	Approximate pH
(a) 25	19	_____	_____
(b) 15	10	_____	_____
(c) 35	17	_____	_____
(d) 48	26	_____	_____
(e) 55	33	_____	_____
(f) 65	31	_____	_____
(g) 55	21	_____	_____
(h) 20	5	_____	_____

52. What is the HCO_3^- when the pH is 7.4 and the $PaCO_2$ is 70 mm Hg, 50 mm Hg, and 30 mm Hg, respectively?

_____

_____

_____

53. During acute alveolar hyperventilation, as the $PaCO_2$ decreases by _____, the HCO_3^- decreases by about _____.

54. During acute alveolar hypoventilation, as the $PaCO_2$ increases by _____, the HCO_3^- increases by about _____.

55. What should the HCO_3^- change to when the $PaCO_2$ acutely rises to 60 mm Hg?

_____

56. What should the HCO_3^- change to when the $PaCO_2$ acutely decreases to 30 mm Hg?

_____

57. What should happen to the pH when the $PaCO_2$ falls from 40 to 20 mm Hg?

_____

58. What should happen to the pH when the $PaCO_2$ rises from 40 to 60 mm Hg?

_____

59. What change in pH should occur when the $PaCO_2$ rises from 60 to 80 mm Hg?

_____

60. What value should the respiratory therapist anticipate for HCO_3^- if the patient acutely hypoventilates and is found to have a $PaCO_2$ of 80 mm Hg through ABG analysis?

_____

_____

_____

Critical Thinking Questions

1. Why is it important for a respiratory therapist to look at the patient's hemoglobin level when assessing the patient's oxygenation status?

_____

_____

_____

2. Will supplemental oxygen reverse hypoxemia caused by low hemoglobin levels? Explain your answer.

_____

_____

3. Patients with chronic obstructive pulmonary disease can live with very low PaO_2 levels. How do their bodies compensate for this chronic hypoxemia?

_____

_____

_____

4. What $P\bar{v}O_2$ should you expect in a patient who has circulatory hypoxemia?

_____

_____

_____

_____

_____

5. What would you expect the P_{50} of a healthy newborn to be?

_____

Case Studies

Case Study #1

A respiratory therapist working in the emergency department encounters a 28-year-old female with Kussmaul breathing. Her room air ABG values are as follows: pH = 7.06, $PaCO_2$ = 12 mm Hg, PaO_2 = 106 mm Hg, SaO_2 = 97%, HCO_3^- = 5 mEq/L.

1. What acid-base imbalance is present?

_____

2. What oxygen therapy is appropriate at this time?

_____

3. What is the most likely cause of this patient's condition?

_____

Case Study #2

An 11-year-old boy is brought to the emergency department with audible wheezing. His mother states that he has not slept in 2 days. The boy is sitting up and using all accessory muscles. ABG analysis at this time shows the following: pH = 7.41, $PaCO_2$ = 25 mm Hg, PaO_2 = 38 mm Hg, SaO_2 = 64%, HCO_3^- = 15 mEq/L.

1. What is the acid-base status?

_____

2. What is the oxygenation status?

_____

3. Is this an acute or a chronic problem?

_____

4. What therapies are most appropriate at this time?

_____

After treatment another ABG analysis is done, with the following results: pH = 7.44, $PaCO_2$ = 30 mm Hg, PaO_2 = 58 mm Hg, SaO_2 = 94%, HCO_3^- = 19 mEq/L.

5. What are the most notable changes in these ABG results compared with the previous values?

_____

_____

_____

Case Study #3

A patient who had abdominal surgery 4 days ago has the following ABG values: pH = 7.48, $PaCO_2$ = 28 mm Hg, PaO_2 = 95 mm Hg, SaO_2 = 98%, HCO_3^- = 21 mEq/L.

1. What is this patient's acid-base status?

_____

2. What is this patient's oxygenation status?

_____

The patient's current hemoglobin content is 6 gm%.

3. Does this change the patient's acid-base balance and/or oxygen status? Explain.

_____

_____

_____

_____

NBRC–Style Questions

1. A patient's ABG results are as follows: pH = 7.34, $PaCO_2$ = 53 mm Hg, PaO_2 = 68 mm Hg, HCO_3^- = 27 mEq/L. Which of the following interpretations correlates with these results?
   a. Partially compensated respiratory alkalosis
   b. Uncompensated metabolic alkalosis
   c. Compensated metabolic acidosis
   d. Partially compensated respiratory acidosis

2. A patient's ABG results on room air are as follows: pH = 7.61, $PaCO_2$ = 70 mm Hg, PaO_2 = 62 mm Hg, HCO_3^- = 38 mEq/L. Based on these data, which of the following is the most likely interpretation of the patient's acid-base status?
   a. Overcompensated respiratory acidosis
   b. Partially compensated metabolic alkalosis
   c. Blood gas analyzer error
   d. Fully compensated metabolic alkalosis

3. An unconscious victim of a fire who is suspected of having carbon monoxide poisoning arrives at the emergency department. The patient is intubated and placed on a mechanical ventilator with an F_IO_2 of 100%. ABG and co-oximetry results show the following: pH = 7.37, $PaCO_2$ = 37 mm Hg, PaO_2 = 487 mm Hg, HCO_3^- = 18 mEq/L, HbCO = 30%, Hb = 15 g/dL. Which of the following is the amount of oxygen dissolved in this patient's plasma?
   a. 0.1 vol%
   b. 0.5 vol%
   c. 1.5 vol%
   d. 4.5 vol%

4. What is the $P(A-a)O_2$ for a patient receiving 30% oxygen from an air entrainment mask with the following ABG values (PB = 760 mm Hg): pH = 7.41, $PaCO_2$ = 37 mm Hg, HCO_3^- = 26 mEq/L, PaO_2 = 103 mm Hg?
   a. 65 mm Hg
   b. 111 mm Hg
   c. 125 mm Hg
   d. 182 mm Hg

5. Calculate the arterial oxygen content for a patient breathing 40% supplemental oxygen whose records show the following clinical data: PaO_2 = 38 mm Hg, $PaCO_2$ = 83 mm Hg, pH = 7.21, SaO_2 = 54%, Hb = 10 g/dL.
   a. 7.4 vol%
   b. 8.4 vol%
   c. 13.5 vol%
   d. 20.5 vol%

6. A 62-year-old patient in the emergency department is in respiratory distress. His ABG values on room air are as follows: pH = 7.45, $PaCO_2$ = 52 mm Hg, PaO_2 = 49 mm Hg, SaO_2 = 82%, HCO_3^- = 34 mEq/L. Based on these data, which of the following is the most likely interpretation of this patient's acid-base status and oxygenation status?
    I. Moderate hypoxemia
    II. Severe hypoxemia
    III. Compensated metabolic alkalosis
    IV. Partially compensated respiratory acidosis
   a. I and III
   b. I and IV
   c. II and III
   d. II and IV

7. A patient's ABG values are as follows: pH = 7.11, $PaCO_2$ = 98 mm Hg, PaO_2 = 33 mm Hg. This patient's hypoxemia is most likely due to which of the following?
   a. Shunt from pneumonia
   b. Diffusion defect from pulmonary fibrosis
   c. Reduced inspired oxygen because of high altitude
   d. Hypoventilation from respiratory center depression

8. A 74-year-old male is admitted to the intensive care unit (ICU) with a history of increasing dyspnea, cough, and sputum production. He has a 120 pack-year smoking history, although he quit 5 years ago. On examination he has decreased chest expansion despite use of the accessory muscles of respiration. His nail beds are cyanotic. ABG analysis reveals the following: pH = 7.21, $PaCO_2$ = 75 mm Hg, PaO_2 = 41 mm Hg. The most likely cause of this patient's hypoxemia is which of the following?
   a. Shunt from pneumonia
   b. Diffusion defect from emphysema
   c. Increased dead space from pulmonary embolism
   d. Hypoventilation from chronic obstructive pulmonary disease

9. Which of the following patients is the most hypoxemic?
   a. Patient A: PaO_2 = 85 mm Hg, SaO_2 = 95%, Hb = 7 gm%
   b. Patient B: PaO_2 = 55 mm Hg, SaO_2 = 85%, Hb = 15 gm%
   c. Patient C: PaO_2 = 95 mm Hg, SaO_2 = 98%, Hb = 6 gm%
   d. Patient D: PaO_2 = 50 mm Hg, SaO_2 = 91%, Hb = 19 gm%

10. PaO_2 declines to some extent in which of the following situations?
    I. Anemia
    II. High altitude climbing
    III. Hypoventilation on room air
    IV. Carbon monoxide poisoning
   a. I and II
   b. II and III
   c. III and IV
   d. I and IV

11. A 25-year-old patient arrives at the emergency department complaining of pleuritic chest pain of 5 to 6 hours' duration. He is a nonsmoker. The chest radiograph and physical examination are otherwise normal. ABG results on room air are as follows: pH = 7.46, $PaCO_2$ = 31 mm Hg, PaO_2 = 83 mm Hg, SaO_2 = 98%, HCO_3^- = 21 m Eq/L. Interpretation of this patient's oxygenation status reveals which of the following?
   a. Mild hypoxemia
   b. No abnormal conditions
   c. Blood gas analyzer error
   d. Ventilation/perfusion abnormality

12. A patient in the emergency department has the following ABG values: pH = 7.20, $PaCO_2$ = 80 mm Hg, PaO_2 = 37 mm Hg. Which of the following is the clinical condition that could produce these results?
   a. Diabetic ketoacidosis
   b. Pulmonary emboli
   c. Severe infection
   d. Drug overdose

13. A patient's ABG results are as follows: pH = 7.43, $PaCO_2$ = 30 mm Hg, PaO_2 = 92 mm Hg, SaO_2 = 97%, HCO_3^- = 19 m Eq/L. Which of the following is the best interpretation of these results?
   a. Acute respiratory acidosis
   b. Chronic respiratory alkalosis
   c. Acute metabolic acidosis
   d. Chronic metabolic alkalosis

14. Calculate the alveolar-arterial oxygen tension difference for a 50-year-old patient breathing supplemental oxygen from a 40% air entrainment mask. The patient's ABG values are as follows: pH = 7.38, $PaCO_2$ = 48 mm Hg, PaO_2 = 79 mm Hg, HCO_3^- = 26 mEq/L. The barometric pressure is normal.
   a. 44 mm Hg
   b. 146 mm Hg
   c. 186 mm Hg
   d. 225 mm Hg

15. Salicylate overdose causes which of the following conditions, as demonstrated by ABG results?
    a. Acute respiratory acidosis
    b. Acute respiratory alkalosis
    c. Acute metabolic acidosis
    d. Acute metabolic alkalosis

Helpful Internet Sites

- Johnson NF: Clinical arterial blood gas analysis. Available at www.boardprep.com/pdfs/abgs.pdf
- Grogono AW: Acid-base tutorial, Tulane University School of Medicine, Department of Anesthesiology. Available at www.acid-base.com/
- Queensland Anaesthesia Education Website: *An on-line book on acid-base physiology*. Available at www.qldanaesthesia.com/AcidBaseBook/ABindex.htm
- Siggaard-Andersen O: Acid-base website with useful definitions and link to strong ion difference editorial. Available at www.osa.suite.dk/

CHAPTER 2

Basic Terms and Concepts of Mechanical Ventilation

Learning Objectives

Upon completion of this chapter the reader will be able to do the following:

1. Draw a graph showing changes in pleural and alveolar (intrapulmonary) pressure that occur during spontaneous ventilation and during a positive pressure breath.
2. Convert mm Hg to cm H_2O.
3. Calculate a time constant.
4. Compare several time constants and explain which will receive more volume during inspiration.
5. From a figure showing abnormal compliance or airway resistance, determine which lung unit will fill more quickly or fill with a greater volume.
6. Define the terms *transpulmonary pressure, transrespiratory pressure, transairway pressure, transthoracic pressure, elastance, compliance,* and *resistance*.
7. Explain how changes in lung compliance affect the peak pressure measured on the manometer during inspiration with a mechanical ventilator.
8. Write the formulas for calculating of compliance and resistance.
9. Identify three terms that mean the same as mouth pressure.
10. Provide the value for intraalveolar pressure during normal, quiet breathing during the phases of inspiration and exhalation.
11. Describe the airway conditions required to increase resistance.
12. Identify three advantages of negative pressure ventilation.
13. Define peak inspiratory pressure, baseline pressure, and plateau pressure.
14. Describe the measurement of plateau pressure.
15. Give the percentage of passive filling (or emptying) for 1, 2, 3, and 5 time constants.
16. Calculate the transairway pressure, given the peak inspiratory pressure, a plateau pressure of 20 cm H_2O, and the flow rate.

Key Terms Crossword Puzzle

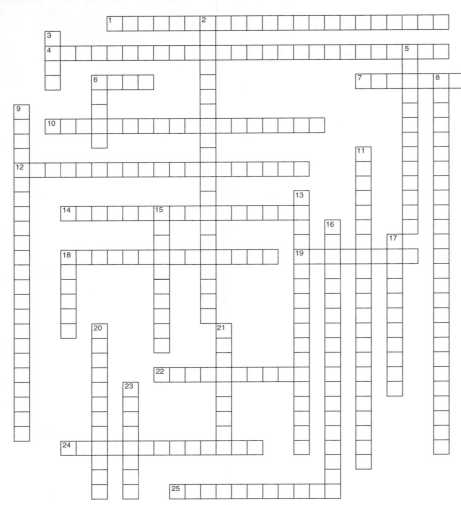

Down

2 Pressure measured at the mouth (three words)
3 Abbreviation for ventilation using small pulses of pressurized gas at rates of 100 to 400 breaths/min
5 A complication of positive pressure ventilation that causes an inadvertent buildup of positive pressure in the alveoli (two words)
6 Abbreviation for type of ventilation that uses lower than normal tidal volumes and respiratory rates of 60 to 100 breaths/min
8 The pressure between the alveolus and the pleural space responsible for maintaining alveolar inflation (three words)
9 Another term for the highest pressure recorded at the end of inspiration (three words)
11 Airway communication between the lung and pleural space (two words)
13 The highest pressure recorded at the end of inspiration (three words)
15 The ease with which the lungs distend
16 The movement of oxygen into the bloodstream and of carbon dioxide out of the bloodstream (two words)
17 The movement of air into the lungs for gas exchange and out of the lungs for carbon dioxide removal
18 A functional unit of the lung
20 A mathematical expression used to describe the filling and emptying of lung units (two words)
21 The tendency of the lungs to return to their original form after being stretched
23 The difference between an area of high pressure and an area of low pressure

Across

1 An alternate term for pressure in the airways of the lungs (three words)
4 The total amount of gas remaining in the lungs after a resting expiration (three words)
6 Abbreviation for a form of ventilatory support characterized by respiratory rates up to 4000 breaths/min
7 The pressure measurement when there is no gas flow
10 Pressure measured in the esophagus that is used to represent intrapleural pressure (two words)
12 The movement of oxygen into cells and the movement of carbon dioxide out of cells (two words)
14 The measurement of elastic forces that oppose lung inflation (two words)
18 Pressure in the airways of the lungs (two words)
19 Another term for intrinsic PEEP (hyphenated word)
22 The impedance of gas flow through the conductive airways
24 A deliberate increase in the ventilator's baseline pressure (two words)
25 The movement of gas molecules across a membrane

Review Questions

1. Explain the difference between ventilation and respiration.

   _____

   _____

   _____

2. The movement of oxygen and carbon dioxide into and out of the alveolar capillaries is known as _____; the movement of oxygen and carbon dioxide into and out of body tissues is called _____.

3. Describe the conditions necessary for air to flow from Point A to Point B in the following figure.

   Point A   Point B

   _____

   _____

4. Convert the measurements in column 1 into the units in column 2.

Column 1	Column 2
(a) 25 cm H_2O	_____ mm Hg
(b) 40 cm H_2O	_____ mm Hg
(c) 15 mm Hg	_____ cm H_2O
(d) 47 mm Hg	_____ cm H_2O
(e) 40 mm Hg	_____ kPa
(f) 95 mm Hg	_____ kPa
(g) 2 ATM	_____ mm Hg
(h) 1 ATM	_____ kPa
(i) 15 kPa	_____ cm H_2O
(j) 2068 cm H_2O	_____ ATM

5. The pressure in the potential space between the parietal and visceral pleurae is known as _____. At the end of exhalation during spontaneous breathing, this pressure is approximately _____; at the end of inspiration, it is about _____.

6. Use the following figure to answer (a) and (b).

   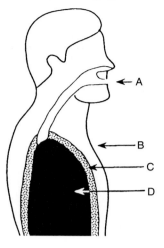

   (a) Identify the various pressures in the respiratory system.

   _____

   (b) Give at least three other names for pressure A.

   _____

   _____

   _____

7. How is intrapleural pressure (P_{pl}) estimated?

   _____

   _____

   _____

8. The pressure gradient between airway pressure and alveolar pressure is known as _____. This pressure is responsible for the movement of air in the _____. This gradient is calculated by the formula _____.

9. The pressure needed to expand or contract the lungs and the chest wall at the same time is _____. This pressure gradient is calculated by the formula _____.

10. The pressure that maintains alveolar inflation is known as _____ and is calculated by the formula _____.

11. The pressure required for inflation of the lungs and airways during positive pressure ventilation is called _____ and is calculated by the formula _____.

12. Use the following figure to answer (a) through (d).

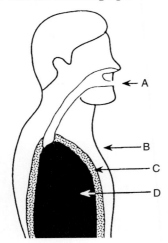

(a) What pressure gradient is represented by Point A–Point B?

_____

(b) What pressure gradient is represented by Point D–Point B?

_____

(c) What pressure gradient is represented by Point D–Point C?

_____

(d) What pressure gradient is represented by Point A–Point D?

_____

13. On the following graph, label the x axis and the y axis, draw the changes in intraalveolar pressure that occur during a spontaneous breath, and label inspiration and expiration.

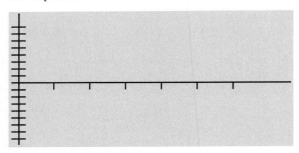

14. Explain how a negative pressure ventilator causes air to move into an individual's lungs.

_____

_____

_____

15. List three advantages of using negative pressure ventilators.

_____

_____

_____

16. What is the transairway pressure when the P_M is +25 cm H_2O and the P_{alv} is +5 cm H_2O?

_____

17. On the following graph, draw and label the changes in intrapulmonary pressure that occur during a positive pressure breath with a PIP of 30 cm H_2O, a $P_{plateau}$ of 20 cm H_2O, a PEEP of 5 cm H_2O, an inspiratory time of 2 seconds, and an expiratory time of 4 seconds.

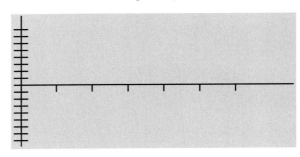

18. On the following graph, draw and label the changes in intrapulmonary pressure that occur during a positive pressure breath with a PIP of 45 cm H_2O, a $P_{plateau}$ of 25 cm H_2O, a PEEP of 10 cm H_2O, an inspiratory time of 1 second, and an expiratory time of 2 seconds, followed by a spontaneous breath with the same baseline.

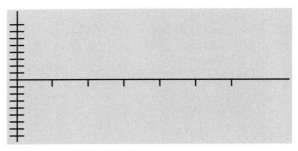

19. The highest pressure recorded at the end of inspiration is called _____ or _____.

20. The pressure at which expiration ends is called _____.

21. When end-expiratory pressure is higher than atmospheric pressure, this is called _____.

22. The pressure required to overcome the elastic recoil of the lungs is known as _____ and is measured in a mechanically ventilated person by _____

_____.

23. What two types of forces oppose inflation of the lungs?

_____ and _____.

24. The relative ease with which a structure distends is known as _____, and the tendency of a structure to return to its original form after being stretched is known as _____.

25. Pulmonary compliance is defined as _____

_____

and is written as a formula as _____.

26. Normally, total compliance of the lungs and thorax is about _____ but can range from _____ to _____.

27. While the individual is mechanically ventilated, what is the compliance value for a male with normal lungs? _____ For a female with normal lungs? _____

28. What is the formula for calculating static compliance?
_____

29. When more pressure is required to deliver a specific volume, what is happening to compliance?

_____

30. Calculate static compliance when $P_{plateau}$ is 27 cm H_2O, baseline pressure is 10 cm H_2O, and tidal volume is 750 mL.

_____

31. Calculate static compliance when $P_{plateau}$ is 35 cm H_2O, baseline pressure is 5 cm H_2O, and tidal volume is 575 mL.

_____

32. Calculate static compliance when $P_{plateau}$ is 18 cm H_2O, baseline pressure is 0, and tidal volume is 650 mL.

_____

33. What happens to PIP as the lungs become harder to ventilate? What happens to lung compliance?

_____

_____

34. Define _resistance_.

_____

_____

35. What is the formula for Raw?

_____

36. What is the normal resistance range for flow rates of 0.5 L/sec?

_____

37. What lung disease causes both Raw and static compliance to increase?

_____

38. Calculate the P_{TA} when PIP is 27 cm H_2O and $P_{plateau}$ is 20 cm H_2O.

_____

_____

39. How much pressure is needed to overcome Raw when PIP is 30 cm H_2O and $P_{plateau}$ is 20 cm H_2O?

_____

40. What is the normal amount of pressure lost to Raw when a patient has a proper-size ET tube?

_____

41. Calculate Raw for a ventilated patient with the following data: PIP = 48 cm H_2O, $P_{plateau}$ = 30 cm H_2O, set flow rate = 40 L/min.

_____

_____

_____

_____

42. Calculate Raw for a ventilated patient with the following data: PIP = 25 cm H_2O, $P_{plateau}$ = 15 cm H_2O, set flow rate = 60 L/min.

_____

_____

_____

43. Why are the characteristics of the lung not homogenous?

_____

_____

44. Compare the filling time and volume for a normal lung unit, a low-compliance unit, and a unit with high Raw using the same driving pressure.

_____

_____

_____

_____

45. What factors contribute to resistance to breathing?

_____

_____

_____

_____

46. What clinical factors can increase Raw by reducing the radius of the airways?

_____

_____

_____

47. How many seconds will it take to allow 86% of the tidal volume to be exhaled when compliance is 25 mL/cm H_2O and resistance is 30 cm H_2O/L/sec?

_____

_____

_____

48. Calculate the time constant for a mechanically ventilated patient when the tidal volume is 600 mL, PIP is 30 cm H_2O, $P_{plateau}$ is 24 cm H_2O, flow rate is 60 L/min, and there is no PEEP.

_____

_____

_____

_____

49. What percentage of passive filling occurs for 1, 2, 3, 4, and 5 time constants?

_____

50. The time constant for patient #1 is 0.05 second; for patient #2 it is 3 seconds; and for patient #3 it is 0.5 second. If the same filling pressure is used for each, which patient receives the most volume during inspiration? Why?

_____

_____

_____

_____

51. Calculate the time constant for a compliance of 55 mL/cm H_2O and resistance of 6 cm H_2O/L/sec.

_____

52. What inspiratory time setting allows 95% volume emptying for a patient with the time constant calculated in question 51?

_____

53. Why do patients with increased Raw develop air trapping with high set ventilator rates?

_____

_____

_____

54. Calculate the time constant for a mechanically ventilated patient when the tidal volume is 700 mL, PIP is 45cm H_2O, $P_{plateau}$ is 18 cm H_2O, the flow rate is 60 L/min, and PEEP is 5 cm H_2O.

_____

_____

55. Which of the two lung units in the following figure receives more volume given the same amount of time for inspiration? Explain your answer.

_____

_____

56. Which of the two lung units in the following figure fills more quickly? Explain your answer.

_____

_____

_____

Critical Thinking Questions

1. When PIP is 43 cm H_2O and $P_{plateau}$ is 18 cm H_2O, how much pressure is required to overcome Raw?

_____

_____

2. What would you expect the time constants to be for a patient with adult respiratory distress syndrome?

_____

3. Explain why the lung units of patients with emphysema have long time constants.

_____

_____

4. What would you expect the time constants to be for a 30-week (gestational age) premature infant?

_____

Case Studies

Case Study #1

A respiratory therapist reviews the following information about an intubated patient receiving mechanical ventilation:

Time	PIP	$P_{plateau}$	V_T	Set Flow Rate	PEEP
0800	18 cm H_2O	10 cm H_2O	600 mL	45 L/min	5 cm H_2O
1000	24 cm H_2O	12 cm H_2O	600 mL	45 L/min	5 cm H_2O
1200	35 cm H_2O	11 cm H_2O	600 mL	45 L/min	5 cm H_2O

1. What is the P_{TA} at 0800, 1000, and 1200?

_____

_____

2. What is the Raw at 0800, 1000, and 1200?

_____

_____

3. What is the static compliance at 0800, 1000, and 1200?

_____

_____

4. Calculate 1 time constant at 0800, 1000, and 1200.

_____

_____

_____

5. What caused the PIP to rise between 0800 and 1200? What problems will this cause with ventilating the patient?

_____

_____

_____

Case Study #2

The following information is obtained from the flow sheet of an intubated patient receiving mechanical ventilation:

Time	PIP	$P_{plateau}$	V_T	Set Flow Rate	PEEP
1000	40 cm H_2O	28 cm H_2O	550 mL	40 L/min	0
1200	47 cm H_2O	37 cm H_2O	550 mL	40 L/min	5 cm H_2O
1400	54 cm H_2O	43 cm H_2O	550 mL	40 L/min	7 cm H_2O
1600	45 cm H_2O	33 cm H_2O	450 mL	60 L/min	12 cm H_2O

1. Complete the table below. Show all calculations.

Time	P_{TA}	Raw	C_S	Time Constant
1000				
1200				
1400				
1600				

2. What is the cause of the increase in PIP between 1000 and 1400?

_____

3. What would be the minimum inspiratory time for this patient at 1600 hours?

_____

NBRC–Style Questions

1. Calculate the static effective compliance during the delivery of a ventilator breath at a tidal volume of 650 mL with a $P_{plateau}$ of 28 cm H_2O.
   a. 0.04 cm H_2O/L
   b. 0.23 L/cm H_2O
   c. 23 mL/cm H_2O
   d. Not enough information is given

2. A patient receiving mechanical ventilation has a set tidal volume of 825 mL and a set peak flow of 50 L/min. The PIP is 46 cm H_2O, and the $P_{plateau}$ is 22 cm H_2O. The Raw is equal to _____ cm H_2O/L/sec.
   a. 13.7
   b. 26.5
   c. 28.9
   d. 38.2

3. Calculate the ventilation time constant for the following data:
   PIP = 29 cm H_2O
   $P_{plateau}$ = 23 cm H_2O
   Tidal volume = 600 mL
   PEEP = 5 cm H_2O
   Inspiratory flow rate = 45 L/min
   a. 0.017 second
   b. 0.021 second
   c. 0.21 second
   d. 0.27 second

4. Which of the following can cause a mechanically ventilated patient's PIP to increase from 20 to 40 cm H_2O while C_S remains relatively unchanged?
   a. Removal of mucous plugs
   b. Increased Raw
   c. Tension pneumothorax
   d. Decreased elastance

5. An increase in PIP and $P_{plateau}$ with a stable P_{TA} may be caused by which of the following?
   a. Acute respiratory distress syndrome
   b. Acute asthma exacerbation
   c. Retained secretions in the airways
   d. ET tube that is too small

6. Which of the following occurs when a patient's lung-thoracic compliance improves?
   I. $P_{plateau}$ decreases.
   II. PIP decreases.
   III. $P_{plateau}$ increases.
   IV. P_{TA} increases.
   a. I and II
   b. I and IV
   c. II and III
   d. III and IV

7. Over the course of several hours, a respiratory therapist has detected an increase in the P_{TA} of a mechanically ventilated patient. The patient's $P_{plateau}$ has remained stable. Which of the following may be the cause of this increase?
   a. Improving lung-thoracic compliance
   b. Acute respiratory distress syndrome
   c. Fluid buildup in the peritoneal cavity
   d. Removal of airway secretions

8. A patient's P_{TA} is rising while the $P_{plateau}$ remains unchanged. Which of the following courses of action should be taken to correct this problem?
   I. Administer a bronchodilator
   II. Insert a large-bore needle into the third intercostal space
   III. Measure auto-PEEP
   IV. Suction airway secretions
   a. II
   b. III and IV
   c. I and IV
   d. I and III

9. Calculate the C_S for a mechanically ventilated patient who has an exhaled tidal volume of 825 mL, a $P_{plateau}$ of 47 cm H_2O, and PEEP of 8 cm H_2O.
   a. 15 mL/cm H_2O
   b. 18 mL/cm H_2O
   c. 21 mL/cm H_2O
   d. 47 mL/cm H_2O

10. Which of the following situations demonstrates the highest Raw?
    a. PIP = 65 cm H_2O, $P_{plateau}$ = 55 cm H_2O, flow rate = 60 L/min
    b. PIP = 52 cm H_2O, $P_{plateau}$ = 18 cm H_2O, flow rate = 45 L/min
    c. PIP = 45 cm H_2O, $P_{plateau}$ = 30 cm H_2O, flow rate = 50 L/min
    d. PIP = 30 cm H_2O, $P_{plateau}$ = 10 cm H_2O, flow rate = 40 L/min

Helpful Internet Sites

- Johns Hopkins School of Medicine's Interactive Respiratory Physiology: Air flow. Available at http://oac.med.jhmi.edu/res_phys/Encyclopedia/AirFlow/AirFlow.html
- Johns Hopkins School of Medicine's Interactive Respiratory Physiology: Airway resistance. Available at http://oac.med.jhmi.edu/res_phys/Encyclopedia/AirwayResistance/AirwayResistance.html
- Johns Hopkins School of Medicine's Interactive Respiratory Physiology: Alveolar pressure. Available at http://oac.med.jhmi.edu/res_phys/Encyclopedia/AlveolarPressure/AlveolarPressure.html
- Johns Hopkins School of Medicine's Interactive Respiratory Physiology: Chest wall. Available at http://oac.med.jhmi.edu/res_phys/Encyclopedia/ChestWall/ChestWall.html
- Johns Hopkins School of Medicine's Interactive Respiratory Physiology: Compliance. Available at http://oac.med.jhmi.edu/res_phys/Encyclopedia/Compliance/Compliance.html
- Modell HI, Modell TW: *Simulations in physiology: the respiratory system* (free downloadable software). Available at http://www.physiologyeducation.org/index.html

CHAPTER 3

How Ventilators Work

Learning Objectives

Upon completion of this chapter the reader will be able to do the following:

1. List the basic types of power sources used for mechanical ventilators.
2. Name a ventilator that uses a specified power source.
3. Distinguish between a closed loop and an open loop system.
4. Explain the difference in function between positive pressure and negative pressure ventilators.
5. Define *user interface*.
6. Describe a ventilator's internal and external pneumatic circuits.
7. Recognize from a description a single circuit and a double circuit ventilator.
8. Identify the components of an external circuit (patient circuit).
9. Explain the function of an externally mounted exhalation valve.
10. Compare the functions of the three different types of volume displacement drive mechanisms.
11. Describe the function of the proportional solenoid valve.

Key Terms Crossword Puzzle

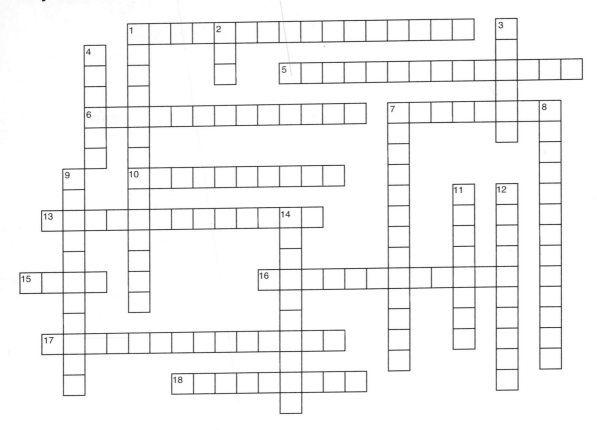

Across

1 Pathway of tubes inside the ventilator is an internal _____ (two words)
5 Single chip made of integrated circuits
6 Another name for the control panel (two words)
7 Pneumatic valve that uses an electromagnetic field and is controlled by a microprocessor
10 Device with an internal volume that can be changed
13 What's inside the black box
15 Type of controller
16 Stepper motor that controls a hinged clamp device (two words)
17 Mechanical device that causes gas to flow to the patient (two words)
18 Uses 50 psi as a power source

Down

1 Connects to the patient (two words)
2 Ventilator mode in which the operator sets a minimum minute ventilation (abbreviation)
3 Mechanism for changing internal volume
4 A type of controller
7 A ventilator whose source gas powers the machine and is delivered to the patient's airway
8 Type of ventilator with two internal pneumatic circuits (two words)
9 Type of valve that controls gas flow (two words)
11 Unintelligent system (two words)
12 Intelligent system (two words)
14 Uses AC or DC as a power source

Review Questions

1. Name the three types of power sources used by ventilators to provide the energy to perform the work of ventilating the patient.

   _____

   _____

   _____

In questions 2 through 7, what specific power source does each of the following ventilators use?

2. Bird Mark 7 _____

3. VIASYS Health Care Intermed Bear 33

   _____

4. Lifecare PLV-102 _____

5. Servo^i_____

6. LTV 800, 900, and 1000 _____

7. Bio-Med MVP-10 _____

8. Describe an open loop system.

   _____

   _____

   _____

9. Describe a closed loop system.

   _____

   _____

   _____

10. How do ventilators cause air to move into the lungs?

    _____

    _____

11. Explain the difference in function between positive pressure ventilators and negative pressure ventilators.

    _____

    _____

    _____

    _____

    _____

12. The place on the ventilator where the operator inputs the desired ventilator parameters is known as the

    _____.

13. Inside a ventilator, gas flow passes through what type of circuit?

    _____

14. After leaving the ventilator, gas flow passes through the _____ on its way to the patient.

15. The gas flow from the ventilator's power source goes directly to the patient. This is known as what type of internal pneumatic circuit?

    _____

16. The ventilator's primary power source generates a gas flow that compresses another device, such as a bellows or bag. The gas inside this device goes to the patient. This is a description of what type of internal pneumatic circuit?

    _____

17. List the four basic elements of a patient circuit.

    _____

    _____

    _____

    _____

18. Identify the labeled parts of the external pneumatic circuit of a ventilator in the following figure.

    A _____

    B _____

    C _____

    D _____

19. Explain how an external exhalation valve operates.

    _____

    _____

    _____

    _____

    _____

    _____

    _____

    _____

20. Name the three types of flow control valves available on current ventilators.

_____

_____

_____

21. Explain how each of the flow control valves operates.

_____

_____

_____

_____

_____

_____

_____

_____

22. The internal hardware that converts electrical or pneumatic energy into a system that provides a breath to a patient is called the _____.

23. Name four types of compressors used in ventilators.

_____

_____

24. Explain how a spring-loaded bellows functions.

_____

_____

_____

25. What type of ventilator uses the spring-loaded bellows as its volume displacement device?

_____

26. Explain how a linear drive piston functions.

_____

_____

_____

_____

27. What type of ventilator uses the linear drive piston as its volume displacement device?

_____

28. Explain how a rotary drive piston functions.

_____

_____

_____

_____

29. What type of ventilator uses the rotary drive piston as its volume displacement device?

_____

30. Current ICU ventilators have what type of internal functions?

_____

_____

31. What type of ventilator uses the Coanda effect as the basis for its internal control system?

_____

Critical Thinking Questions

1. A patient ventilated in the SIMV mode becomes apneic. Explain how both a closed loop system and an open loop system might respond to this circumstance.

_____

_____

_____

_____

2. If the exhalation valve malfunctions, what happens to the inspiratory gas flow?

_____

_____

3. What type of ventilator could be used during a magnetic resonance imaging (MRI) procedure?

_____

Case Studies

Case Study #1

A patient receiving mechanical ventilation needs to be transported to another medical center for treatment. What type of power source would be appropriate during patient transport?

_____

Case Study #2

A patient becomes apneic while mechanically ventilated in a mode that allows spontaneous breathing. The ventilator automatically activates an alarm and switches to full ventilatory support. Is this an open loop system or a closed loop system? Explain.

_____

_____

_____

NBRC–Style Questions

1. The power used by a mechanical ventilator to perform the work of ventilating the patient is known as which of the following?
   a. Force
   b. Pressure
   c. Input power
   d. Output power

2. Which of the following statement(s) is true concerning combined power ventilators?
   I. They must have an electrical power source and two 50 psi gas sources.
   II. They often have RAM and ROM for data and preprogrammed modes.
   III. The electrical power provides the energy to deliver the breath.
   IV. The pneumatic power controls the internal function of the machine.
   a. II
   b. I and III
   c. III and IV
   d. I, II, and IV

3. The internal circuit of a ventilator routes the gas directly from its power source to the patient. This is known as which of the following?
   a. External circuit
   b. Internal circuit
   c. Single circuit
   d. Double circuit

4. Which of the following is one of the functions of the exhalation valve?
   a. Regulate pressure
   b. Ensure adequate humidification
   c. Ensure gas delivery on inspiration
   d. Determine the patient's tidal volume

5. A closed loop system is used to guarantee minute ventilation to a patient. The minute volume delivered to the patient differs significantly from the set minute volume. The ventilator will do which of the following?
   a. Activate an alarm and shut off
   b. Switch to 100% oxygen
   c. Double the minute volume
   d. Alter the volume delivered

6. The mechanical device that causes gas to flow to the patient is known as which of the following?
   a. Drive mechanism
   b. Power transmission
   c. Exhalation valve
   d. Solenoid valve

7. Volume displacement devices include which of the following?
   I. Pistons
   II. Stepper motors
   III. Concertina bags
   IV. Proportional solenoids
   a. I and IV
   b. I and III
   c. II and III
   d. II and IV

8. Which of the following is the flow control valve that uses an electromagnetic field?
   a. Digital valve
   b. Stepper motor
   c. Solenoid valve
   d. Rotating blade

9. The operation of which type of ventilator is based on the wall attachment phenomenon, or Coanda effect?
   a. Fluidic ventilator
   b. Electrically powered ventilator
   c. Pneumatically powered ventilator
   d. Microprocessor controlled ventilator

10. Which of the following is the volume displacement device that creates a sinusoidal flow wave pattern during inspiration?
    a. Spring-loaded bellows
    b. Linear drive piston
    c. Rotary drive piston
    d. Concertina bag

Helpful Internet Sites

- Negligan P: Critical Care Medicine: Brief history and modes of ventilation. University of Pennsylvania. Available at www.ccmtutorials.com/rs/mv/page4.htm
- Maquet: *Technical comments for managing a Servo ventilator.* Available at www.maquet.com/criticalcare/goldenmoments/default.aspx

CHAPTER 4

How a Breath Is Delivered

Learning Objectives

Upon completion of this chapter the reader will be able to do the following:

1. Write the equation of motion and define each term in the equation.
2. Give two other names for pressure ventilation and volume ventilation.
3. Compare pressure, volume, and flow delivery in volume-controlled breaths and pressure-controlled breaths.
4. Name the two main patient-trigger variables.
5. Identify the patient-trigger variable that requires the least work of breathing for a patient receiving mechanical ventilation.
6. Explain the effect on the volume delivered and the inspiratory time if a ventilator reaches the preset maximum pressure limit during volume ventilation.
7. Classify a given breath (e.g., patient-triggered, volume-limited, or time-cycled) as mandatory, or spontaneous.
8. Describe the pressure-time and flow-time waveforms that occur with pressure-support ventilation.
9. Recognize the effects of a critical leak (e.g., a patient disconnect) on pressure readings and volume measurements.
10. Define *inflation hold* and explain its effects on inspiratory time.
11. Give an example of a current ventilator that provides negative pressure during part of the expiratory phase.
12. From a clinical example of ventilator settings, provide the triggering, limiting, and cycling mechanisms.
13. Based on the description of a pressure-time curve, identify a clinical situation in which expiratory resistance is increased.
14. Compare use of the terms *time cycling, volume cycling,* and *flow cycling* as they might be applied to a microprocessor-controlled ventilator in a volume-controlled mode using a set machine rate and flow.
15. Define the following terms and explain how these factors affect a breath: *expiratory retard, positive end-expiratory pressure, continuous positive airway pressure,* and *bilevel positive airway pressure.*

Key Terms Crossword Puzzle

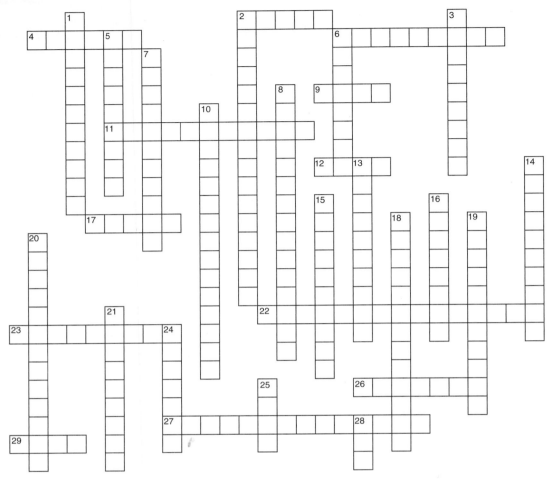

Across

2 Variable that ends inspiration
4 A specific amount that begins inspiration
6 Gas law that governs tubing compressibility (two words)
9 Applying positive pressure during expiration with mechanical ventilation (abbreviation)
11 Ventilator begins inspiration (two words)
12 Applying negative pressure during expiration (abbreviation)
17 Maximum value a variable can attain.
22 Primary variable used by the ventilator to cause inspiration (two words)
23 Gas speed reaches a maximum amount (two words)
26 Pressure reading during an inspiratory pause
27 Maneuver performed to measure auto-PEEP (two words)
29 Baseline pressure at zero (abbreviation)

Down

1 Gas speed begins inspiration (two words)
2 The way a ventilator marks the end of inspiration (two words)
3 Most common mechanism for ending inspiration in the pressure support mode (two words)
5 A breath initiated by the ventilator is a _____ breath
6 Pressure level from which a ventilator breath begins
7 Sets a maximum deliverable volume on a ventilator (two words)
8 Pressure-targeted ventilator mode in which the patient breathes spontaneously (two words)
10 Ventilator mode in which the set limit is pressure (two words)
13 Breathing out
14 The patient is making no effort; ventilation is being _____ by the ventilator
15 Breathing in
16 A variable that begins inspiration
18 Variable controlling a certain phase of a breath (two words)
19 Breath controlled by the patient
20 Breath begun by the operator (two words)
21 Ventilator ends inspiration (two words)
24 Variable that begins inspiration
25 Method of applying above ambient pressure to a spontaneously breathing patient (abbreviation)
28 Type of ventilation that assists both inspiration and expiration (abbreviation)

Review Questions

1. What two pressures act on the respiratory system during either spontaneous breathing or mechanical ventilation?

   _____

   _____

2. The motion caused by the interaction of these two pressures is known as _____.

3. Write out the equation of motion.

   _____

4. Explain both sides of the equation of motion.

   _____

   _____

   _____

   _____

5. List three synonyms for *volume ventilation*.

   _____

   _____

6. List three synonyms for *pressure ventilation*.

   _____

   _____

7. What three variables can the ventilator control?

   _____

8. The primary variable used by a ventilator to cause inspiration is called _____.

9. During pressure-controlled breaths, the compliance and resistance of a patient's lungs change; what happens to volume and flow?

   _____

   _____

10. During volume-controlled breaths, the compliance and resistance of a patient's lungs change; what happens to the pressure?

    _____

    _____

11. During flow-controlled breaths, the compliance and resistance of a patient's lungs change, what happens to volume and pressure?

    _____

    _____

12. Both pressure and volume waveforms can be affected by changes in lung characteristics when what type of control variable is used?

    _____

13. Name the two types of ventilators that are time controllers.

    _____

    _____

14. Describe the relationship between flow and volume in the form of a formula.

    _____

15. When the operator selects a volume waveform, what happens to the flow waveform?

    _____

16. List the three places where ventilators measure pressure.

    _____

    _____

    _____

17. A breath initiated by the patient but ended by the ventilator is what type of breath?

    _____

18. A breath initiated by the ventilator is known as a _____ breath.

19. A breath initiated by the patient and ended by the patient is a _____ breath.

20. List the four phases of a breath.

    _____

    _____

    _____

21. The phase variable that begins inspiration is known as the _____.

22. The ventilator has measured an elapsed amount of time and delivers a breath; this describes what type of breath?

    _____

23. The type of breath described in question 22 is sometimes called _____.

24. A paralyzed patient who makes no effort to breathe is said to be in this mode: _____.

25. At what pressure should pressure sensitivity be set? _____.

26. Explain autotriggering.

    _____

    _____

27. If the flow sensitivity is set at 2 L/min and the baseline flow is 8 L/min, at what flow will the ventilator be triggered to give a breath?

    _____

    _____

28. Describe volume triggering.

    _____

    _____

For questions 29 through 31, refer to the following pressure-time curve.

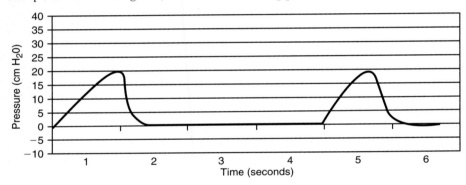

29. What mode of ventilation is shown on this graph? _____

30. What is the expiratory time? _____

31. What is the inspiratory time? _____

For questions 32 through 35, refer to the following pressure-time curve.

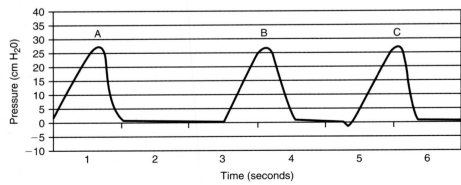

32. What type of trigger does wave A have? _____

33. What type of trigger does wave *B* have?

    _____

34. What type of trigger does wave *C* have?

    _____

35. What mode does this graph show?

    _____

36. Name the three types of patient triggers.

    _____

37. The type of trigger involved when a patient inhales a specific volume that begins inspiration is called

    _____.

38. The maximum value a variable can attain is known as a _____.

In questions 39 through 43, classify the breaths described as mandatory, assisted, or spontaneous.

39. Pressure triggered, pressure limited, time cycled:

    _____

40. Flow triggered, volume limited, time cycled:

    _____

41. Time triggered, pressure limited, time cycled:

    _____

42. Flow triggered, pressure limited, flow cycled:

    _____

43. Pressure triggered, flow limited, volume limited, volume cycled:

    _____

44. In setting up flow triggering, the higher the flow trigger setting, the _____ sensitive the ventilator is to the patient.

45. Which type of patient triggering requires less work of breathing? _____

46. How should the maximum safety pressure be set?

    _____

    _____

47. What happens when the maximum safety pressure setting is reached during inspiration?

    _____

    _____

48. How do most ICU ventilators achieve volume cycling?

    _____

    _____

    _____

49. What is the tubing compressibility factor for most adult ventilator circuits? _____

50. Give two reasons exhaled tidal volume may not equal the set tidal volume when a breath is volume cycled.

    _____

    _____

51. A large leak is detected in the ventilator system during pressure support ventilation. How will the ventilator end inspiration?

    _____

    _____

52. The ventilator cycles to expiration when the patient's exhaled gas flow drops to a certain percentage of the peak inspiratory flow rate. This describes what type of end to inspiration?

    _____

53. When could a pressure-cycled ventilator be used?

    _____

    _____

54. What happens to the inspiratory and expiratory times during an inflation hold?

    _____

55. Air trapping can occur with insufficient

    _____.

56. The pressure level from which a ventilator breath begins is called the _____.

57. The addition of positive pressure to exhalation is called _____.

58. What type of ventilator assists both inspiration and expiration by pushing air into the lungs and pulling it back out at extremely high frequencies?

    _____

59. A patient on mechanical ventilation is allowed to exhale. The ventilator then closes both the expiratory and inspiratory valves. This maneuver, known as _____, measures the amount of

    _____.

60. The presence of air trapping may be observed on what type of graph?

_____

61. What are the three methods of detecting air trapping on a ventilator?

_____

_____

_____

62. Increased resistance to exhalation may be caused by what devices?

_____

63. Accumulation of moisture in an expiratory filter causes _____.

64. What ventilator mode involves breathing spontaneously at pressures above ambient pressure?

_____

65. Increasing the baseline during mechanical ventilation with intermittent mandatory breaths is known as

_____.

66. Sleep apnea may be treated with either _____

or _____.

67. How does flow cycling occur with pressure-support ventilation?

_____

_____

_____

_____

_____

Critical Thinking Questions

For questions 1 through 4, refer to graphs A and B (simultaneous graphs of two breaths).

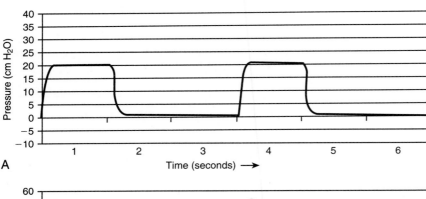

A   Time (seconds) →

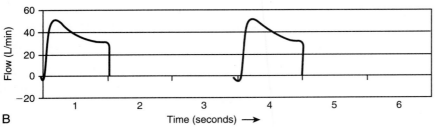

B   Time (seconds) →

1. What is the limiting mechanism for these breaths? _____

2. Name the two possible modes these graphs represent. _____

3. What is the trigger mechanism for the breaths shown? _____

4. What is the cycling mechanism for the breaths shown? _____

For questions 5 through 8, refer to the following pressure-time curve.

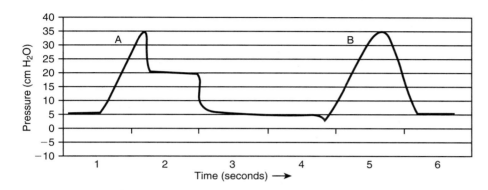

5. What is the trigger variable for waveform A? _____

6. What is the trigger variable for waveform B? _____

7. The transairway pressure is _____

8. What is the baseline? _____

Case Studies

Case Study #1

You are a respiratory therapist assigned to the ICU of a local hospital, and you have been called to assess a patient who may require mechanical ventilation. The physical examination reveals the following: respiratory rate = 25 breaths/min, BP = 145/90 mm Hg, pulse = 115 beats/min; breath sounds are bilaterally decreased, especially in the bases. The results of ABG analysis are as follows: pH = 7.44, $PaCO_2$ = 36 mm Hg, PaO_2 = 42 mm Hg, SaO_2 = 70%, HCO_3^- = 22 mEq/L on a nonrebreathing mask. Other parameters include these: MIP = −75 cm H_2O, VC = 70 mL/kg, V_T = 7 mL/kg.

1. Explain the primary area of concern for this patient.

_____

_____

_____

2. What is the most appropriate type of ventilatory support for this patient at this time?

_____

The next day the respiratory therapist returns to the ICU and finds the patient receiving mechanical ventilation. The graphic display is shown in the following figure.

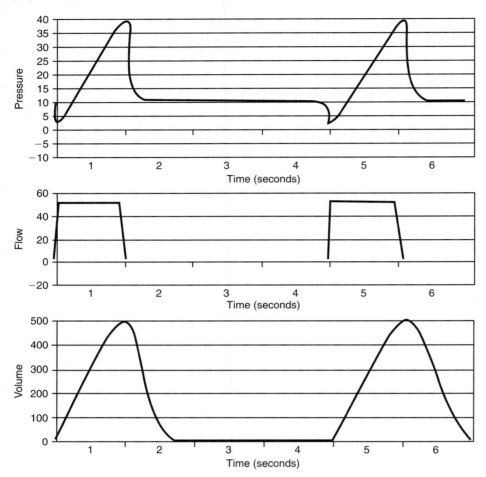

3. What type of ventilation is this patient receiving? _____

4. What is (are) the limiting variable(s)? _____

5. What trigger variable is used at this time? _____

The respiratory therapist also notes that the patient is diaphoretic and using accessory muscles while assisting the ventilator.

6. Do any of the graphic displays give clues to the source of this patient's problem? If so, which one(s)?

_____

7. What is the source of this patient's problem?

_____

_____

_____

8. What must the respiratory therapist do to resolve this problem?

_____

_____

Case Study #2

A mechanical ventilator is set up to provide volume assist/control ventilation to a postoperative patient.

1. What parameters does the respiratory therapist need to set?

   _____

   _____

2. During ventilation the patient's peak inspiratory pressure reaches approximately 28 cm H_2O. What should the respiratory therapist set as the maximum safety pressure?

   _____

   _____

3. What is the purpose of the maximum safety pressure?

   _____

   _____

While assessing the patient and checking the ventilator, the respiratory therapist notices that although a volume of 500 mL has been set, the patient exhales only 400 mL, and the maximum safety pressure is reached on each breath.

4. What is the most likely cause of the low volume return? Explain your answer.

   _____

   _____

   _____

   _____

5. If the maximum safety pressure was not reached on each breath and the exhaled volume was 100 mL less than the set volume, what could be the possible causes?

   _____

   _____

NBRC–Style Questions

1. A breath that is triggered, limited, and cycled by the mechanical ventilator is which of the following?
   a. Assisted breath
   b. Mandatory breath
   c. Spontaneous breath
   d. Synchronized breath

2. A breath that is triggered, controlled, and ended by the patient is which of the following?
   a. Assisted breath
   b. Controlled breath
   c. Spontaneous breath
   d. Synchronized breath

3. A breath that is patient triggered, ventilator controlled, and ventilator cycled is which of the following?
   a. Assisted breath
   b. Controlled breath
   c. Spontaneous breath
   d. Pressure-supported breath

4. During pressure-controlled ventilation, the patient's airway resistance increases; this causes which of the following to occur?
   a. Peak pressure increases.
   b. Peak pressure decreases.
   c. Tidal volume increases.
   d. Tidal volume decreases.

5. During volume-controlled ventilation, the patient's lung compliance improves; this causes which of the following to occur?
   a. Peak pressure increases.
   b. Peak pressure decreases.
   c. Tidal volume increases.
   d. Tidal volume decreases.

6. During volume-controlled ventilation, which waveform remains unchanged despite changes in lung characteristics?
   I. Volume-time curve
   II. Pressure-time curve
   III. Flow-time curve
   a. I
   b. II
   c. I and III
   d. II and III

7. When both pressure and volume waveforms are affected by changes in lung characteristics, which of the following variables is controlled?
   a. Time
   b. Flow
   c. Volume
   d. Pressure

8. A high-frequency oscillator controls which of the following variables?
   a. Flow
   b. Time
   c. Volume
   d. Pressure

9. When the ventilator is time triggering and the rate has been set at 20 breaths/min, the interval between breaths is which of the following?
   a. 2 seconds
   b. 3 seconds
   c. 4 seconds
   d. 5 seconds

10. During flow triggering, the base flow is set at 5 L/min and the ventilator triggers when it senses 3 L/min returning to its flow-measuring device. The flow sensitivity setting is which of the following?
    a. 2 L/min
    b. 3 L/min
    c. 5 L/min
    d. 8 L/min

11. During pressure-support ventilation, the patient triggers the ventilator, the set pressure is reached, and the ventilator cycles at 5 seconds. What is the cause of this time cycle?
    a. A leak in the system
    b. This is the normal setting.
    c. Increased lung compliance
    d. Change in airway resistance

12. The most common cycling mechanism used for pressure support ventilation is which of the following?
    a. Time
    b. Flow
    c. Volume
    d. Pressure

13. The maneuver that is used to measure plateau pressure is which of the following?
    a. Flow limiting
    b. Expiratory hold
    c. Inspiratory hold
    d. Pressure limiting

Helpful Internet Sites

- The Worldwide Anaesthetist Journal Club: New approaches to ventilation. Available at www.anaesthetist.com/anaes/vent/newvent.htm#recruit
- Pulmonetics Systems: Breath types and ventilator modes. Available at www.smallsitebuilder.com/downloads/Chapter3.pdf

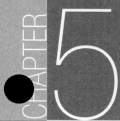

Establishing the Need for Mechanical Ventilation

Learning Objectives

Upon completion of this chapter the reader will be able to do the following:

1. Define acute respiratory failure and respiratory insufficiency.
2. Identify goals and objectives of mechanical ventilation.
3. List respiratory, cardiovascular, and neurological findings in mild to moderate hypercapnia and severe hypercapnia.
4. Recognize from clinical cases the three categories of disorders that may lead to respiratory insufficiency or acute respiratory failure.
5. Compare normal values with abnormal critical values that indicate the need for ventilatory support for the following: vital capacity, maximum inspiratory force, peak expiratory pressure, FEV_1, peak expiratory flow rate, V_D/V_T ratio, $P(A-a)O_2$, and PaO_2/P_AO_2 ratio.
6. Recommend the appropriate respiratory therapy for specific patient cases, including oxygen therapy, continuous positive airway pressure, noninvasive positive pressure ventilation, and invasive ventilation.
7. Differentiate among patients who need oxygen therapy, bronchodilator therapy, continuous positive airway pressure, or mechanical ventilation.
8. Discuss situations in which mechanical ventilation would not be appropriate even though the patient meets the criteria for ventilation.

Key Terms Crossword Puzzle

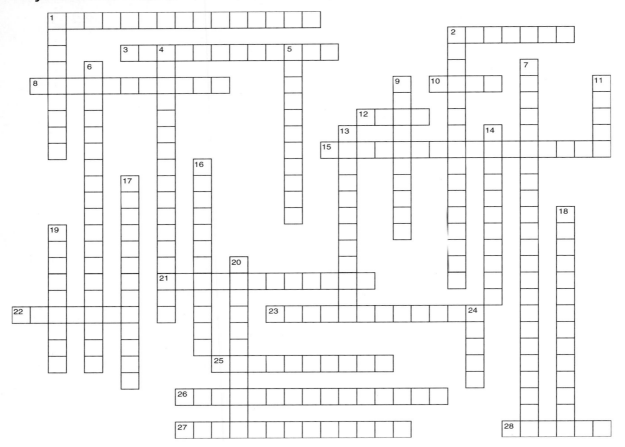

Across

1 Area of the body above the collar bone
2 Type of respiratory failure also referred to as *lung failure*
3 A simple device used to measure volumes at the bedside
8 Normal respiratory balance
10 Abbreviation for an indicator of airway obstruction
12 State of unconsciousness
15 Neuromuscular disorder that leads to weakness of the skeletal muscles, especially those of the face, throat, and respiratory system (two words)
21 Type of abnormal respiration characterized by alternating progressive hypopnea and hypoventilation ending in brief apnea (two words)
22 Pus in the pleural space
23 Type of breathing pattern in which the rib cage and abdomen do not move outward together
25 Sleepiness
26 Condition characterized by alveolar flooding caused by an acute insult (three words)
27 Neuromuscular syndrome characterized by lower extremity weakness that progresses to the upper extremities and face (two words)
28 Toxic condition arising from infection

Down

1 State of lethargy and immobility with diminished responsiveness to stimulation
2 Controversial treatment for a closed head injury
4 Latin for acute, severe asthma (two words)
5 Early indicator of hypoxia
6 Abnormal deficiency of oxygen in the arterial blood that is resistant to treatment (two words)
7 Absent or inadequate respiratory activity (three words)
9 Blood in the pleural space
11 Type of respiration characterized by irregular periods of apnea alternating with periods of deep breathing
13 Type of respiratory failure also referred to as *pump failure*
14 Breathing pattern characterized by abnormal movement of the thorax and abdomen
16 Above the sternum
17 Common measurement of ventilatory mechanics (two words)
18 Abnormal condition characterized by an anteroposterior and lateral curvature of the spine
19 Rapid breathing
20 Pertaining to the space between two ribs
24 Condition in which perfusion of vital organs is inadequate to meet their metabolic needs

Review Questions

1. Ventilation is responsible for maintaining the homeostasis of what three factors?

   _____

   _____

   _____

2. What are the basic physiological objectives of mechanical ventilation?

   _____

   _____

   _____

3. Name five clinical objectives of mechanical ventilation.

   _____

   _____

   _____

   _____

   _____

4. List 10 physical signs of respiratory distress.

   _____

   _____

   _____

   _____

5. Respiratory activity that is inadequate to maintain carbon dioxide clearance and oxygen uptake is known as _____.

6. Acute life-threatening or vital organ–threatening tissue hypoxia is known as _____ or _____.

7. Basic treatment for lung failure includes _____, possibly in combination with _____.

8. The inability of the body to maintain a normal $PaCO_2$ is known as _____ or _____.

9. The ventilatory pump consists of _____, _____, and _____.

10. List five disorders that reduce the drive to breathe.

    _____

    _____

    _____

    _____

11. List five disorders associated with neuromuscular function that can cause hypoventilation and possibly respiratory failure.

    _____

    _____

    _____

12. Chest wall deformities that result in increased work of breathing include

    _____

    _____

    _____

13. What pulmonary diseases cause increased airway resistance and result in increased work of breathing?

    _____

    _____

14. Initial rapid assessment of a patient with possible respiratory failure includes what components?

    _____

    _____

    _____

15. What are the two early signs of hypoxia?

    _____

16. Which two breathing patterns might patients with central nervous system dysfunctions have?

    _____

17. How often should a patient with a neuromuscular disorder and respiratory fatigue be monitored for changes in respiratory status?

    _____

18. In a patient with a neuromuscular disorder and respiratory fatigue, which two measurements should be made to test for muscle strength? What are their cutoff points?

    _____

    _____

19. What limits tolerance of an increase in the work of breathing?

_____

20. List three signs of increased work of breathing.

_____

_____

_____

21. Up to how many seconds does it take to obtain the most negative maximum inspiratory pressure?

_____

22. What is a normal maximum inspiratory pressure?

_____

23. What is the normal range for vital capacity?

_____

24. Acute respiratory failure is most likely present when minute ventilation exceeds _____.

25. What ventilatory maneuver is used to indicate increased airway resistance? What measurement is considered critical?

_____

_____

26. Adequate airway patency can be determined by measuring _____.

Values of _____ indicate severe airflow obstruction.

27. What laboratory value reflects adequacy of ventilation? _____

28. The normal range for the V_D/V_T ratio is _____ to _____ at normal tidal volumes. The critical value for this measurement is _____.

29. Complete the following table for oxygen status assessment.

Measurement	Normal Range	Critical Value
$P(A\text{-}a)O_2$	_____	_____
PaO_2/P_AO_2	_____	_____
PaO_2/F_IO_2	_____	_____

30. Noninvasive positive pressure ventilation is the treatment of choice for what type of patient?

_____

_____

31. A patient develops congestive heart failure during NPPV; what action should be taken at this time?

_____

_____

32. What is the most appropriate action for a spontaneously breathing patient with refractory hypoxemia?

_____

_____

33. A patient has a PaO_2/P_AO_2 ratio of 0.28. Therefore, of all the oxygen available in the alveoli, what percentage is reaching the patient's arteries? _____

34. List the four standard criteria for mechanical ventilation.

_____

_____

_____

_____

35. In what type of situation would intubation be contraindicated?

_____

_____

36. List five absolute contraindications to NPPV in an adult.

_____

_____

_____

_____

_____

37. A 48-year-old woman with a past medical history of congestive heart failure and hypertension is brought to the emergency department with acute onset of dyspnea. The patient has frothy pink sputum, her pulse is 120 and irregular, and respirations are 26 breaths/min and labored. Breath sounds reveal bilateral crackles and rhonchi. ABG results are as follows: pH = 7.31, $PaCO_2$ = 48 mm Hg, PaO_2 = 50 mm Hg, SaO_2 = 72% on a nonrebreathing mask. What respiratory therapy modalities should be recommended for this patient?

_____

_____

_____

_____

_____

38. A 79-year-old male with inoperable lung cancer develops acute, severe dyspnea. The patient's pulse is 104 and regular; respirations are 24 breaths/min with use of accessory muscles. Breath sounds are decreased bilaterally in the bases. What treatment should the respiratory therapist recommend for this patient?

_____

_____

_____

39. A 51-year-old woman arrives in the emergency department complaining that she has had shortness of breath and chest tightness for 2 days. Physical examination reveals that the pulse is 122, and respirations are 35 breaths/min with use of accessory muscles. Breath sounds reveal bilateral inspiratory and expiratory wheezing and are diminished in the bases. The patient is alert and oriented but extremely anxious. ABG results are as follows: pH = 7.22, $PaCO_2$ = 55 mm Hg, PaO_2 = 51 mm Hg on room air. What course of treatment is most appropriate for this patient?

_____

_____

_____

_____

_____

40. A 65-year-old man was admitted this morning to the ICU with an exacerbation of COPD. Currently, the physical examination findings are as follows: pulse = 107 and regular, respirations = 24 breaths/min and slightly labored, T = 38.5° C, BP = 141/90 mm Hg. Breath sounds are considerably diminished, especially in the bases. ABG results are these: pH = 7.44, $PaCO_2$ = 33 mm Hg, PaO_2 = 52 mm Hg. What recommendations should the respiratory therapist make for this patient?

_____

_____

_____

_____

41. A 23-year-old male is brought to the emergency department by ambulance after a bicycle accident in which he suffered head trauma. The patient is unresponsive; his pulse is 112 and regular; respirations are 40 breaths/min and shallow; and breath sounds are decreased throughout. ABG results are as follows: pH = 7.21, $PaCO_2$ = 59 mm Hg, PaO_2 = 50 mm Hg on a nasal cannula at 6 L/min. What recommendations should the respiratory therapist make for this patient?

_____

_____

_____

_____

_____

_____

_____

42. Calculate the arterial oxygen content for a patient with the following ABG results: pH = 7.44, $PaCO_2$ = 44 mm Hg, PaO_2 = 59 mm Hg, SaO_2 = 91%, F_IO_2 = 0.21, Hb = 12 g/dL. Show all your work.

_____

_____

_____

43. Calculate the arterial oxygen content for a patient with the following ABG results: pH = 7.34, $PaCO_2$ = 22 mm Hg, PaO_2 = 58 mm Hg, SaO_2 = 90%, Hb = 8 g/dL. Show all your work.

_____

_____

_____

44. Calculate the arterial oxygen content for a patient with the following ABG results: pH = 7.36, $PaCO_2$ = 59 mm Hg, PaO_2 = 48 mm Hg, SaO_2 = 79%, Hb = 18 g/dL. Show all your work.

_____

_____

_____

_____

45. Calculate the P(A-a)O$_2$ for the patient in question 37 (assume the nonrebreathing mask is delivering approximately 70% oxygen). Show all your work.

_____

_____

_____

_____

_____

46. Calculate the PaO$_2$/P$_A$O$_2$ ratio for the patient in question 37 (show all your work). What does this mean, and is this a critical value? Show all your work.

_____

_____

_____

47. Calculate the PaO$_2$/F$_I$O$_2$ ratio for the patient in question 37. Is this a critical value? Show all your work.

_____

_____

_____

48. Calculate the P(A-a)O$_2$ for the patient in question 39. Is this value an indication for mechanical ventilation? Show all your work.

_____

_____

_____

_____

49. Calculate the PaO$_2$/P$_A$O$_2$ ratio for the patient in question 39. Is this a critical value? Show all your work.

_____

_____

50. Calculate the PaO$_2$/F$_I$O$_2$ for the patient in question 39. Is this a critical value? Show all your work.

_____

_____

Critical Thinking Questions

1. You are called to the emergency department to perform a cardiopulmonary assessment of a newly arrived patient who had been involved in a motor vehicle accident. What components would you include in your rapid physical assessment?

_____

_____

_____

_____

2. After your initial physical assessment of the patient in question 1, what diagnostic evaluations should be performed to assess the need for mechanical ventilation?

_____

_____

3. Describe how a patient in respiratory distress might look.

_____

_____

_____

4. Discuss the difference in clinical presentation between a patient who needs oxygen therapy only and one who needs mechanical ventilation.

_____

_____

_____

_____

_____

_____

Case Studies

Case Study #1

A 35-year-old male with a history of asthma is admitted to the ICU from the emergency department. The patient is alert and oriented but extremely anxious. He is sitting up and leaning on the bedside tray table. Physical examination reveals the following: pulse = 142, BP = 178/86 mm Hg, T = 37.9° C, respirations = 33 breaths/min and labored. Chest auscultation reveals significantly decreased breath sounds throughout with slight wheezing on exhalation. ABG results on a 40% air via entrainment mask are as follows: pH = 7.33, $PaCO_2$ = 44 mm Hg, PaO_2 = 48 mm Hg, SaO_2 = 79%, HCO_3^- = 22 mEq/L, Hb = 14.8 g/dL. The peak expiratory flow reading is 70 L/min after three consecutive bronchodilator treatments.

1. What is the cause of the patient's tachycardia?

2. Using the four oxygenation indicators, explain the oxygenation status of this patient (assume PB is 760 mm Hg).

3. Although this patient's $PaCO_2$ is within normal limits, why is it significant in this case?

4. What respiratory care treatment should be suggested for this patient?

Case Study #2

A 46-year-old female was admitted to the ICU a few hours ago with an acute exacerbation of myasthenia gravis. She is alert and oriented, her pulse is 102 and regular, BP is 140/75 mm Hg, temperature is 37.4° C, and respirations are 30 breaths/min and very shallow. Breath sounds are decreased throughout. There is no cough. The patient complains of weakness and trouble swallowing. ABG results on room air are as follows: pH = 7.36, $PaCO_2$ = 38 mm Hg, PaO_2 = 60 mm Hg, SaO_2 = 90%, HCO_3^- = 20 mEq/L, Hb = 12.6 g/dL. The maximum inspiratory pressure is 30 cm H_2O.

1. What is this patient's oxygenation status? Explain your answer.

2. Evaluate this patient's ventilatory status.

3. What treatment or monitoring recommendations should be made for this patient?

Case Study #3

A 76-year-old female arrives in the emergency department in severe respiratory failure caused by COPD. Her ABG results are as follows: pH = 7.15, $PaCO_2$ = 90 mm Hg, PaO_2 = 43 mm Hg, HCO_3^- = 24 mEq/L, SaO_2 = 52% with an F_IO_2 of 0.5. CPAP is 5 cm H_2O. The patient is drowsy.

1. What is this patient's oxygenation status? Explain your answer.

2. Evaluate this patient's ventilatory status.

3. What treatment or monitoring recommendations should be made for this patient?

NBRC–Style Questions

1. A 43-year-old male was admitted to the hospital last night with a stab wound to the right anterior thorax. The wound was repaired in surgery. Currently the patient is alert and somewhat belligerent. He is in the ICU and has a chest tube in the right hemithorax. Vital signs are as follows: pulse = 120, respirations = 32 breaths/min and shallow, BP = 148/90 mm Hg, T = 38° C. Breath sounds are considerably diminished over the right base, and chest expansion is decreased over the right side. The patient is not coughing. ABG results are as follows: pH = 7.48, $PaCO_2$ = 26 mm Hg, PaO_2 = 66 mm Hg, SaO_2 = 94%, HCO_3^- = 19 mEq/L, F_IO_2 = 0.35 (via air entrainment mask), Hb = 11.4 g/dL. Which of the following is the most appropriate action to take at this time?
   a. Increase the F_IO_2 to 0.5
   b. Place the patient on bilevel positive airway pressure
   c. Administer albuterol via a small-volume nebulizer
   d. Intubate and mechanically ventilate the patient at an F_IO_2 of 1

2. Hypercapnic respiratory failure is characterized by which of the following?
   I. Lower than normal PaO_2
   II. Alveolar hypoventilation
   III. Higher than normal $PaCO_2$
   IV. Increased $P(A-a)O_2$
   a. I and IV
   b. I, II, and III
   c. II, III, and IV
   d. I, II, III, and IV

3. Which of the following is the underlying physiological process that leads to pure hypercapnic respiratory failure?
   a. Low $\dot{V}/\dot{Q}$ ratio
   b. Diffusion impairment
   c. Intrapulmonary shunting
   d. Alveolar hypoventilation

4. A 65-year-old male comes to the emergency department complaining of increasing shortness of breath over the past 3 days. He appears to be in moderate respiratory distress. He has a 100 pack-year smoking history. His vital signs are as follows: HR = 115 beats/min; RR = 28 breaths/min; BP = 170/95 mm Hg; T = 38° C oral. ABG results on nasal cannula (1 L/min) are as follows: pH = 7.3, $PaCO_2$ = 70 mm Hg, PaO_2 = 48 mm Hg, SaO_2 = 67%, HCO_3^- = 35 mEq/L. The most appropriate treatment at this time is to initiate which of the following?
   a. Bronchodilator therapy
   b. Air entrainment mask at F_IO_2 0.35
   c. Intubation and mechanical ventilation
   d. Noninvasive positive pressure ventilation

5. A 55-year-old female with a history of chronic congestive heart failure and extreme obesity comes to the emergency department. She is alert but disoriented. Vital signs are as follows: pulse = 133 beats/min, BP = 145/94 mm Hg, T = 37° C, respirations = 28 breaths/min (shallow and labored). She has no cough. Breath sounds are decreased throughout with bilateral inspiratory coarse crackles. ECG shows sinus tachycardia with a widened QRS complex and an occasional premature ventricular contraction. ABG results on a 50% air entrainment mask are these: pH = 7.34, $PaCO_2$ = 47 mm Hg, PaO_2 = 55 mm Hg, SaO_2 = 87%, HCO_3^- = 24 mEq/L. The respiratory therapist should recommend which of the following at this time?
   a. Use of a nonrebreathing mask
   b. Continuous positive airway pressure
   c. Intubation and mechanical ventilation
   d. Noninvasive positive pressure ventilation

6. An 18-year-old man is brought to the emergency department via ambulance after a bicycle accident. The patient is unconscious, and his Glasgow Coma Score is 6. Vital signs are as follows: pulse = 110 and regular, BP = 96/55 mm Hg, T = 36.6° C, respirations = 38 breaths/min and shallow. No cough is present. Chest auscultation reveals decreased breath sounds throughout. ABG results on a simple mask at 6 L/min are these: pH = 7.22, $PaCO_2$ = 58 mm Hg, PaO_2 = 52 mm Hg, SaO_2 = 76%, HCO_3^- = 22 mEq/L. Based on these findings, the respiratory therapist should initiate which of the following?
   a. Nonrebreathing mask
   b. Continuous positive airway pressure
   c. Intubation and mechanical ventilation
   d. Noninvasive positive pressure ventilation

7. A 135-lb patient with Guillain-Barré syndrome has been monitored by the ICU respiratory therapist over the past 6 hours. The maximum inspiratory pressure and the vital capacity have been recorded as follows:

Time	MIP	VC
0700	-40 cm H_2O	3.1 L
0915	-35 cm H_2O	2.8 L
1125	-25 cm H_2O	1.5 L
1310	-15 cm H_2O	0.64 L

After the last entry, what therapeutic intervention should the respiratory therapist recommend?
a. 50% air entrainment mask
b. Continuous positive airway pressure
c. Intubation and mechanical ventilation
d. Noninvasive positive pressure ventilation

8. A 40-year-old woman comes to the emergency department with a 2-day history of dyspnea; productive cough with thick, green sputum; fever; and chills. The respiratory therapist's assessment reveals the following: pulse = 105, respirations = 30 breaths/min, T = 39° C. Chest excursion is diminished on the right, and dull percussion is noted over the right base. Chest auscultation reveals coarse crackles and wheezes over the right base. ABG results on room air are as follows: pH = 7.35, $PaCO_2$ = 31 mm Hg, PaO_2 = 72 mm Hg, SaO_2 = 88%, HCO_3^- = 24 mEq/L. The respiratory therapist should recommend which of the following?
a. Oxygen via nasal cannula at 4 L/min
b. Continuous aerosol with F_IO_2 0.3
c. Continuous positive airway pressure
d. Noninvasive positive pressure ventilation

9. Which of the following demonstrates the need for intubation and mechanical ventilation?
a. Refractory hypoxemia
b. Acute respiratory failure
c. Chronic respiratory failure
d. Hypoxic respiratory failure

10. Which of the following is a disorder that may cause hypercapnic respiratory failure as a result of increased work of breathing?
a. Asthma
b. Botulism
c. Metabolic acidosis
d. Cerebral hemorrhage

Helpful Internet Sites

- Lyager S, Steffensen B, Juhl B: Indicators of need for mechanical ventilation in Duchenne muscular dystrophy and spinal muscular atrophy. Available at www.chestjournal.org/cgi/content/abstract/108/3/779
- Hornick D: Acute respiratory failure. Virtual Hospital. Available at www.vh.org/adult/provider/emergencymedicine/ARF/AcuteRespiratoryFailure.html
- Criner GJ: Respiratory failure. Available at www.temple.edu/pulmonary/profess/facultypresentations/Respiratory%20failure/index.htm
- Snow V, Lascher S, Mottur-Pilson C: Evidence base for management of acute exacerbations of chronic obstructive pulmonary disease. Available at www.annals.org/ cgi/reprint/134/7/595.pdf

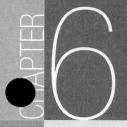

Selecting the Ventilator and the Mode

Learning Objectives

Upon completion of this chapter the reader will be able to do the following:

1. Based on a patient's history and assessment, select from the following methods of therapeutic intervention: positive or negative pressure ventilation, invasive or noninvasive ventilation, volume or pressure ventilation, and full or partial ventilatory support.

2. Compare the advantages and disadvantages of volume and pressure ventilation.

3. Explain the differences in function among continuous mandatory ventilation (also called assist/control ventilation), synchronized intermittent mandatory ventilation, and spontaneous ventilation.

4. Use the terms *trigger*, *cycle*, and *limit* to define the following modes and to graph pressure/time to show the pressure delivered with each mode: volume-targeted continuous mandatory ventilation, pressure-targeted continuous mandatory ventilation, volume-targeted synchronized intermittent ventilation, pressure-targeted synchronized intermittent mandatory ventilation, and pressure support ventilation.

5. Define each of the following terms: *pressure augmentation, pressure regulated volume control, volume support, mandatory minute ventilation, airway pressure release ventilation, bilevel positive airway-pressure,* and *proportional assist ventilation.*

6. For each presented mode of ventilation, name the type of patient who would most benefit from that mode.

Key Terms Crossword Puzzle

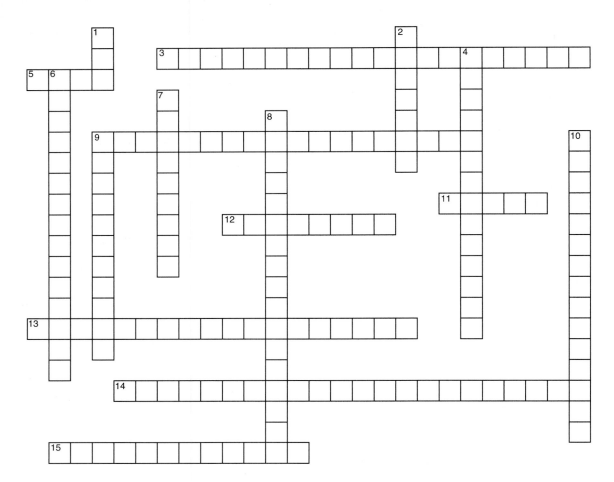

Across

3 Overventilation in the CMV mode causes this condition (two words)
5 Abbreviation for a mode of ventilation that uses two levels of CPAP
9 Mode in which the patient controls the timing and the tidal volume (two words)
11 Abbreviation for inverse ventilation with pressure control
12 Type of control variable
13 Mode of ventilation that uses only time-triggered breaths (two words)
14 Term used when ventilator supplies all the energy necessary to maintain alveolar ventilation (three words)
15 Occurs when the patient and the ventilator are not working together

Down

1 Abbreviation for mode of ventilation in which all breaths are mandatory and can be volume or pressure targeted
2 Type of ventilatory support in which the patient participates in WOB
4 Patient-triggered, volume- or pressure-targeted ventilation (hyphenated word)
6 Mode that supports a spontaneously breathing patient to help reduce WOB (two words)
7 Type of breath in which the timing and/or the tidal volume is controlled by the ventilator
8 Guarantees a specific volume delivery (two words)
9 Ventilator setting used to determine the ventilator's response to the patient's inspiratory effort
10 Cross between mandatory and spontaneous breaths

Review Questions

1. Give seven criteria upon which the choice of a particular type of ventilator is based.

   _____

   _____

   _____

2. Match the type of ventilatory support with the appropriate ventilator connection or interface (there may be more than one answer):

   _____ Negative pressure   (a) Oral endo-
          ventilation   tracheal tube
   _____ Continuous positive   (b) Nasal mask
          airway pressure   (c) Face mask
   _____ Positive pressure   (d) Chest cuirass
          ventilation   (e) Tracheostomy
   _____ Noninvasive positive   tube
          pressure ventilation

3. Continuous positive airway pressure is commonly used

   in the hospital setting for _____

   and in the home setting to treat _____.

4. The most commonly used ventilatory technique in

   the treatment of acute-on-chronic respiratory failure is

   _____.

5. What type of ventilation reduces the requirement for heavy patient sedation? _____

6. Define *full ventilatory support* and *partial ventilatory support*.

   _____

   _____

   _____

   _____

   _____

7. The minimum rate setting that would be considered full

   ventilatory support is _____, and the

   tidal volume range should be _____

   _____.

8. Partial ventilatory support is any amount of mechanical

   ventilation with set machine rates that are less than

   _____.

9. What type of ventilatory support should be used when the patient has acute ventilatory failure caused by ventilatory muscle fatigue or a high WOB? Why?

   _____

   _____

   _____

10. Identify each of the breaths described below as mandatory, spontaneous, or assisted.

    (a) Flow triggered, pressure targeted, time cycled

    _____

    (b) Time triggered, volume targeted, volume cycled

    _____

    (c) Pressure triggered, pressure targeted, time cycled

    _____

    (d) Flow triggered, pressure triggered, flow cycled

    _____

11. What is the main advantage of volume ventilation?

    _____

    _____

12. A patient develops bronchospasm during volume ventilation. What will happen to

    (a) the peak inspiratory pressure? Why?

    _____

    _____

    (b) the amount of volume delivered to the patient? Why?

    _____

    _____

13. A bronchodilator is administered to the patient in

    question 12. The peak inspiratory pressure would be

    expected to _____

    because the patient's lung condition has improved.

14. What are the advantages and disadvantages of using noninvasive positive pressure ventilation in acute respiratory failure?

Advantages	Disadvantages
_____	_____
_____	_____
_____	_____
_____	_____
_____	_____
_____	_____

15. When the patient's lung condition worsens during volume ventilation, the peak inspiratory pressure _____ (increases; decreases), which may lead to alveolar _____ (hyperinflation; hypoventilation). When the patient's lung condition improves, _____ (more; less) pressure is generated during volume delivery.

16. What may result when sensitivity is set too low?

_____

_____

17. When pressure is targeted as the control variable, what varies with changing lung characteristics?

_____

18. When a patient's lung condition worsens during pressure-targeted ventilation, volume delivery _____ (increases; decreases), which may lead to alveolar _____ (hyperventilation; hypoventilation). When a patient's lung condition improves, _____ (more; less) volume is delivered.

19. Complete the following table.

Type of Ventilation	Advantages	Disadvantages
Volume ventilation	_____	_____
	_____	_____
	_____	_____
	_____	_____
	_____	_____
Pressure ventilation	_____	_____
	_____	_____
	_____	_____
	_____	_____
	_____	_____

20. Which type of ventilation is more beneficial for a spontaneously breathing patient when used with a descending flow pattern?

_____

21. Name the three breath delivery techniques.

_____

_____

22. CMV is also known as

(a) _____

(b) _____

(c) _____

23. What trigger is used when a ventilator is in the control mode?

_____

24. Controlled ventilation is appropriate for what types of patients?

_____

_____

_____

_____

25. What patient situations may call for the use of sedation or paralysis induced with medication (or both)?

_____

_____

_____

26. In what two patient situations might deliberate (iatrogenic) hyperventilation be beneficial? Why?

_____

_____

27. What happens when the ventilator is made totally insensitive to patient effort?

_____

_____

28. What three triggers may begin inspiration in the A/C mode?

_____

_____

29. What can happen to a patient's acid-base status if the patient's ventilatory drive increases while the person is ventilated in the A/C (CMV) mode?

_____

_____

30. If inspiration is active with VC-CMV and the set gas flow is inadequate, how much of the work of inspiration is done by the patient?

_____

_____

31. What are the control variables in PC-CMV?

_____

_____

32. A safety mechanism that prevents excessive system pressure is the _____,

which is set about _____

above the PIP setting and causes _____

to end when reached.

33. What ventilator mode should be used when guarding against increasing pressures is more important than guaranteeing a tidal volume?

_____

34. When is the use of PCIRV appropriate?

_____

_____

35. How does IMV differ from CMV?

_____

_____

36. How does SIMV differ from IMV?

_____

_____

_____

_____

37. Spontaneous breathing through a ventilator circuit may be obtained in what two ways?

_____

_____

38. _____

may be used to reduce the WOB for spontaneous

breaths during ventilation in the SIMV mode.

39. What are the advantages and risks/disadvantages of the A/C mode?

_____

_____

_____

_____

_____

_____

_____

_____

_____

40. What are the advantages and risks/disadvantages of the IMV/SIMV mode?

_____

_____

_____

_____

_____

_____

_____

_____

_____

41. The three basic ways to provide support for continuous spontaneous breathing during mechanical ventilation are _____,

_____,

and _____.

42. What are the advantages and disadvantages of having an intubated patient breathe spontaneously through a ventilator circuit?

_____

_____

_____

_____

43. What type of patient would be appropriate for PSV?

_____

_____

44. In PSV the operator sets the _____,

the _____,

and _____.

45. What determines the patient's tidal volume in PSV?

_____

_____

46. What situation causes a mechanical ventilator in the PSV mode to time cycle?

_____

47. What situation causes a mechanical ventilator in the PSV mode to pressure cycle?

_____

_____

_____

48. What are the three basic functions of PSV?

_____

_____

_____

_____

_____

_____

_____

_____

_____

49. The time required for the ventilator to rise to the set pressure at the beginning of inspiration is known as

_____.

50. A very high flow setting in PSV may cause inspiration to _____.

51. PSV ends inspiration by _____ cycling.

52. What are the triggers for bilevel pressure assist?

_____

53. What variables end inspiration in the bilevel pressure assist mode?

_____

54. Varying tidal volume delivery during pressure ventilation can be prevented by using closed loop techniques such as _____, _____,

and _____.

55. How does PAug work?

_____

_____

_____

_____

56. In PAug, if the set volume is achieved before flow cycling occurs, what happens to the breath?

_____

57. In PAug, if the set volume is not reached before flow drops to the set level, how does the ventilator respond?

_____

_____

58. Under what condition can a patient receive more volume than that set in PAug?

_____

_____

_____

59. Describe PRVC in terms of trigger, limit, and cycle.

_____

_____

_____

_____

60. In the PRVC mode, if the upper pressure limit is set at 40 cm H_2O and the volume is set at 600 mL, when will the ventilator's pressure alarm activate?

_____

61. Describe VS in terms of trigger, limit, and cycle.

_____

62. What is the difference between PRVC and VS?

_____

_____

_____

_____

63. The mode of ventilation that provides whatever part of the $\dot{V}_E$ the patient is unable to accomplish is known as _____ .

64. In MVV, what alarms must be set to protect against the problem of rapid shallow breathing?

_____

65. The mode of ventilation that requires two levels of CPAP and allows the patient to breathe spontaneously at both levels is known as _____ .

66. The optimum duration of the release time for the mode mentioned in question 65 is a function of the _____ of the respiratory system.

67. APRV was originally intended to ventilate patients with _____ .

68. With PAV, what variables are proportional to the patient's spontaneous effort?

_____

69. In the PAV mode, what two factors determine the amount of pressure produced by the ventilator?

_____

_____

70. What are the advantages and disadvantages of PAV?

Advantages	Disadvantages
_____	_____
_____	_____
_____	_____
_____	_____

Critical Thinking Questions

1. A patient is waking up after surgery and is receiving mechanical ventilation in the PC-CMV mode. During rounds the respiratory therapist notes the patient's use of accessory muscles, diaphoresis, patient-ventilator dyssynchrony, and the absence of assisted breaths. What is the most probable cause of this patient's clinical appearance? How can this be corrected?

_____

_____

_____

_____

_____

_____

_____

_____

_____

2. If a patient's ventilatory drive increases during VC-CMV, what changes occur in the acid-base balance? What can be done to regulate this?

_____

_____

_____

_____

_____

_____

_____

_____

3. A home care patient with central sleep apnea would benefit from which mode of ventilation? Why?

_____

_____

_____

_____

_____

_____

_____

_____

4. Match the patient condition (column A) with the ventilator mode most likely to benefit the person (column B). Some answers will be used more than once.

Column A

_____ Intubated with quadriplegia from a spinal cord injury

_____ Intubated with acute respiratory distress syndrome

_____ Obstructive sleep apnea at home

_____ Intubated with spontaneous breathing with acute lung injury

_____ Intubated with consistent spontaneous respiratory pattern

_____ Nonintubated, spontaneously breathing with refractory hypoxemia

_____ Intubated with drug overdose

Column B

(a) Nasal mask CPAP

(b) CPAP through ventilator

(c) Pressure support

(d) VC-CMV

(e) PC-CMV with PEEP

Case Studies

Case Study #1

A respiratory therapist approaches a patient receiving mechanical ventilation in the intensive care unit. The ventilator monitor shows the pressure-time scalar in following figure.

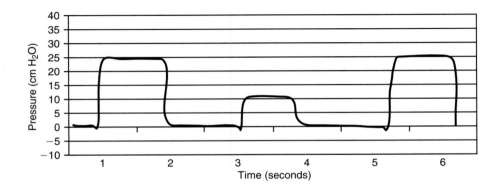

1. What mode of ventilation is the ventilator set to deliver? _____

2. What is the inspiratory time for the mechanical breaths? _____

3. What is the ventilator expiratory time? _____

Case Study #2

A 6′ 3″ man who was involved in a motor vehicle accident is brought to the emergency department with chest and facial injuries. Because of the nature of the facial injuries, he is intubated with a size 7 Fr endotracheal tube. After resuscitative measures are completed, the patient is transferred to the intensive care unit.

1. What type of ventilatory support would this patient require initially? _____

2. What ventilator mode would be appropriate when this patient awakes and has the desire to breathe spontaneously if he has a PaO_2 of 58 mm Hg with an F_IO_2 set at 0.5?

_____

Case Study #3

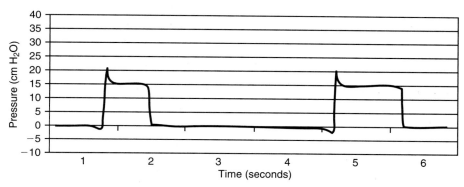

1. What mode of ventilation does the scalar in the preceding figure represent? _____

2. Identify the problem with this pressure tracing. _____

3. What can be done to remedy the identified problem? _____

NBRC–Style Questions

1. When a patient is to be switched from CMV to SIMV to facilitate weaning from mechanical ventilation, which of the following could be used in addition to SIMV to assist this process?
   a. PCV
   b. PSV
   c. PAV
   d. APRV

2. A patient who had thoracic surgery currently is on VC-CMV with 60% oxygen. The person has these ABG values: pH = 7.45, $PaCO_2$ = 36 mm Hg, PaO_2 = 68 mm Hg. The patient's peak inspiratory pressures are averaging 55 cm H_2O. The most appropriate ventilator mode at this time is which of the following?
   a. PSV
   b. VC-SIMV with PEEP
   c. PC-CMV with PEEP
   d. MMV

3. A 38-year-old female has suffered a deceleration injury in a motor vehicle accident. She is alert and oriented but in respiratory distress. A piece of the patient's right anterior chest wall is moving in a paradoxical motion. Breath sounds are decreased on the right, and the trachea is midline. ABG data are as follows: pH = 7.48, $PaCO_2$ = 31 mm Hg, PaO_2 = 63 mm Hg. The respiratory therapist should recommend which of the following for this patient at this time?
   a. Mask CPAP with supplemental oxygen
   b. Intubation and VC-CMV with PEEP
   c. NPPV with supplemental oxygen
   d. Intubation with PCIRV

4. The physician asks the respiratory therapist to recommend a ventilatory therapy for a patient with post-polio syndrome who complains of increasing daytime weakness. The patient's vital capacity is 12 mL/kg, and the MIP is −32 cm H_2O. ABG results on room air are as follows: pH = 7.38, $PaCO_2$ = 46 mm Hg, PaO_2 = 74 mm Hg. The respiratory therapist should suggest which of the following?
   a. Tracheostomy with PSV
   b. Tracheostomy with VC-CMV
   c. Bilevel PAP via nose mask at night
   d. Mask CPAP with supplemental oxygen

5. During a pressure-triggered breath in VC-CMV, the pressure-time curve on the graphic does not rise smoothly, and it looks somewhat concave. This indicates which of the following?
   a. Flow rate is inadequate.
   b. Rise time is set too slow.
   c. A pressure overshoot is occurring.
   d. Inspiratory time is too short.

6. Every breath from the ventilator is time or patient triggered, pressure targeted (limited), and time cycled. This describes which of the following ventilator modes?
   a. PAug
   b. APRV
   c. PC-CMV
   d. VC-SIMV

7. PAug may be beneficial for a mechanically ventilated patient in which of the following situations?
   I. Patient has noncardiogenic pulmonary edema.
   II. Patient has acute respiratory distress syndrome.
   III. Patient has just had upper abdominal surgery.
   IV. Patient is heavily sedated or is receiving paralyzing agents.
   a. I and II
   b. I and III
   c. II and IV
   d. III and IV

8. The ventilator mode that allows the patient to breathe spontaneously at two levels of positive pressure is known as which of the following?
   a. BiPAP
   b. PAug
   c. PRVC
   d. APRV

9. A patient is intubated and on PSV. The respiratory therapist notices that the inspiratory time has increased from 1 second to 2 seconds consistently on every breath since last ventilator rounds. What action should the respiratory therapist take first?
   a. Change to the SIMV mode
   b. Check the ET tube cuff pressure
   c. Increase the inspiratory flow setting
   d. Suction and lavage the patient's airway

10. Which of the following occurs when lung compliance decreases while a patient is receiving mechanical ventilation with PC-CMV?
   a. Peak pressure increases.
   b. Peak pressure decreases.
   c. Tidal volume increases.
   d. Tidal volume decreases.

Helpful Internet Sites

- Lawson W: New ventilator modes. Department of Respiratory Care, University of Texas Health Science Center at San Antonio. Available at www.uthscsa.edu/respiratorycare/vent_modes.htm
- Gregg BL, editor: Ventilator review. School of Allied Health, Kansas University Medical Center. Available at www.kumc.edu/SAH/resp_care/ labfin.html

CHAPTER 7

Initial Ventilator Settings

Learning Objectives

Upon completion of this chapter the reader will be able to do the following:

1. Calculate tubing compliance.
2. Determine volume loss caused by tubing compliance.
3. Calculate minute ventilation from rate and tidal volume.
4. Calculate total cycle time, inspiratory time, expiratory time, flow in L/sec, and inspiratory to expiratory ratios when given the necessary patient data.
5. Select an appropriate flow rate and pattern.
6. Calculate the initial minute ventilation ($\dot{V}_E$), tidal volume (V_T) and rate (f) of volume ventilation based on the patient's sex, height, and ideal body weight.
7. Determine the problem when an inspiratory pause cannot be measured.
8. Establish the initial mode, $\dot{V}_E$, V_T, f, and PEEP settings based on the patient's lung pathology, body temperature, metabolic rate, altitude, and acid-base balance.
9. Evaluate the response in peak inspiratory pressure and plateau pressure when the flow waveform is changed.
10. Recommend the selection of and initial settings for the various modes of pressure ventilation, including bilevel positive airway pressure, pressure support ventilation, pressure control ventilation, and servo-controlled (dual modes) ventilation.
11. Identify a problem in pressure support ventilation from a pressure-time graph.
12. Measure plateau pressure from pressure-time and flow-time waveforms during pressure control mechanical ventilation.
13. Identify the possible causes of a change in pressure during pressure-regulated volume control.
14. Name the mode of ventilation based on the trigger, target, and cycle criteria.

Key Terms Crossword Puzzle

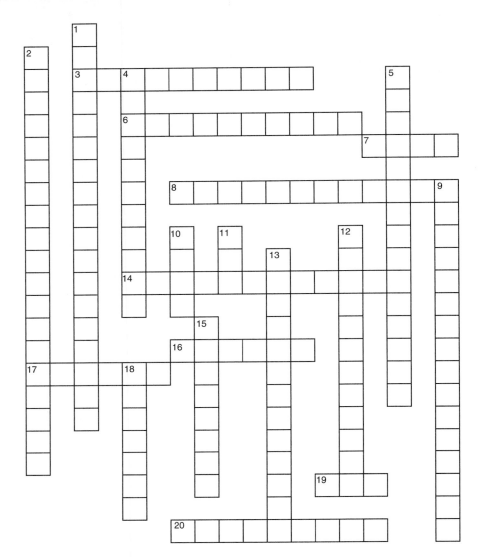

Across

3 This can be directly measured by measuring heat production

6 Flow pattern that occurs naturally with pressure ventilation

7 Name for volume support on the Newport E-500 (abbreviation)

8 Raw × C_L (two words)

14 Control found on ventilators manufactured in Europe (two words)

16 Chart used to determine BSA

17 A constant flow pattern creates this waveform

19 This can be used to estimate metabolism (abbreviation)

20 Type of flow pattern created by a progressive increase in flow

Down

1 Amount lost in the patient circuit (two words)

2 Adding tubing to the patient's endotracheal tube adds this (three words)

4 Ventilators manufactured in the United States have this control (two words)

5 This is difficult to measure accurately if the patient is breathing actively (two words)

9 System compressibility (two words)

10 Peak pressure is high with this flow pattern when airway resistance is high

11 Amount of time for one complete breath cycle (abbreviation)

12 Units of measure for BSA (two words)

13 Excessive pressure in the alveoli can cause this

15 Name for PRVC on the Dräger E-4 (two words)

18 Name of the breathing nomogram

Review Questions

1. To meet oxygen and carbon dioxide transport requirements, mechanical ventilation must support the patient's

   _____.

2. List eight parameters that must be considered in setting up VV.

   _____

   _____

   _____

3. Normal total body oxygen consumption is approximately _____, and carbon dioxide production is

   approximately _____.

For questions 4 through 6, refer to Figure 7-1.

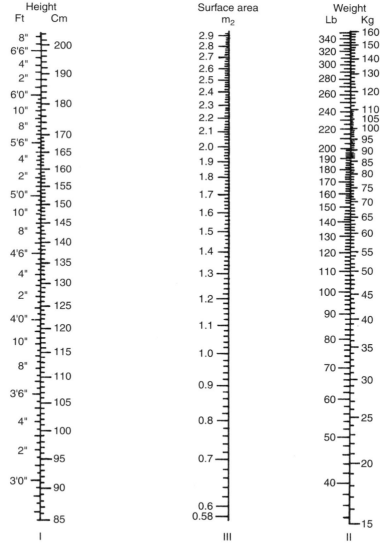

Fig. 7–1. Dubois body surface chart. (From Boothby WM, SandiFord RB: *Boston Med Surg J* 185:337, 1921.)

4. Find the BSA for a person who weighs 200 lb and is 6′ 2″ tall.

   _____

5. Find the BSA for a person who weighs 75 kg and is 155 cm tall.

   _____

6. Find the BSA for a person who weighs 178 lb and is 5′ 7″ tall.

   _____

Calculate the $\dot{V}_E$ for each of the following individuals.

	Gender	BSA	Body Temperature	Other Factors	$\dot{V}_E$
7.	F	1.6 m²	39° C	N/A	_____
8.	M	2.8 m²	37° C	6000 ft above sea level	_____
9.	M	2.3 m²	101° F	N/A	_____
10.	F	1.9 m²	98.6° F	Metabolic acidosis	_____

11. The initial V_T setting for adults should be within what range? _____

12. The initial V_T setting for infants and children should be within what range? _____

13. The estimated V_T range for a 5′ 4″ female is _____.

14. The estimated V_T range for a 6′ 2″ male is _____.

15. What is the normal range for spontaneous V_T in a human being? _____

16. What is the normal range for the spontaneous breathing rate in a human being? _____

17. The normal $\dot{V}_E$ is about _____.

18. Calculate the initial V_T, respiratory rate, and $\dot{V}_E$ for a 5′ 2″ female who has just arrived in the postoperative care unit.

    _____

    _____

19. Calculate the initial V_T, respiratory rate, and $\dot{V}_E$ for a male 71″ tall who has COPD.

    _____

    _____

20. Calculate the initial V_T, respiratory rate, and $\dot{V}_E$ for a male 69″ tall who has pulmonary fibrosis.

    _____

    _____

21. Calculate the tubing compliance when the measured V_T is 300 mL and the static pressure is 110 cm H_2O.

    _____

22. Calculate the tubing compliance when the measured V_T is 210 mL and the static pressure is 115 cm H_2O.

    _____

23. The tubing compliance for a patient circuit is 2.5 mL/cm H_2O. Calculate the volume lost when the estimated V_T is 300 mL and the PIP to deliver each breath is approximately 28 cm H_2O.

    _____

24. Calculate the actual delivered V_T when the tubing compliance is 1.8 mL/cm H_2O, the set V_T is 450 mL, and the PIP is 30 cm H_2O.

   _____

25. What should the respiratory therapist do for ventilators that do not compensate for tubing compliance?

   _____

26. Calculate and fill in the missing information in the following table.

V_T	Respiratory Rate	$\dot{V}_E$
(a) 750 mL	12 breaths/min	_____
(b) 580 mL	10 breaths/min	_____
(c) _____	15 breaths/min	6.9 L/min
(d) _____	20 breaths/min	8.3 L/min
(e) 460 mL	_____	5.2 L/min
(f) 660 mL	_____	9.5 L/min

27. Calculate the TCT for the following respiratory frequencies (i.e., rate setting).

   (a) 30 breaths/min _____

   (b) 15 breaths/min _____

   (c) 12 breaths/min _____

   (d) 10 breaths/min _____

28. Use the corresponding frequencies in question 27 to calculate the T_E for each, given the following T_I:

   (a) T_I = 1 second _____

   (b) T_I = 0.75 second _____

   (c) T_I = 1.25 seconds _____

   (d) T_I = 2 seconds _____

29. Use the corresponding information from question 28 to reduce the I:E ratio to its simplest form.

   (a) _____

   (b) _____

   (c) _____

   (d) _____

30. Calculate T_I, T_E, and TCT for an I:E ratio of 1:3 and a rate of 12 breaths/min.

   _____

   _____

   _____

   _____

   _____

   _____

31. Calculate T_I, T_E, and TCT for an I:E ratio of 1:2 and a rate of 25 breaths/min.

_____

_____

32. Calculate V_T when T_I is 1 second and flow is 50 L/min.

_____

_____

33. Calculate T_I when V_T is 700 mL and flow is 50 L/min.

_____

_____

34. High flow rates during ventilation of an apneic patient with CMV cause the T_I to _____, the PIP to _____, and gas distribution to _____.

35. Explain what happens to T_I, T_E, PIP, and gas distribution when slower flow rates are used.

_____

_____

_____

_____

36. What are the guidelines for setting the T_I, I:E ratio, and flow rates?

_____

_____

37. The type of flow waveform created by pressure ventilation is the _____.

38. The flow waveform that creates the highest PIP during VV when Raw is elevated is the _____.

39. The flow waveform(s) most appropriate for normal lungs is (are) _____.

40. Why is the descending flow pattern beneficial for patients with hypoxemia and low lung compliance?

_____

_____

41. The inspiratory pause is most often used for what?

_____

42. The respiratory therapist attempts to measure $P_{plateau}$ by adding a 1 second inspiratory pause. The set VC-CMV rate is 12 breaths/min, the current rate is 20 breaths/min, and the $P_{plateau}$ is unattainable. What is the cause of this problem?

_____

_____

43. The pressure ventilation modes that have time triggering are

_____

44. The pressure ventilation modes that allow for patient triggering are

_____

45. Flow cycling is used by which pressure ventilation modes?

_____

46. Time cycling is used by which pressure ventilation modes?

_____

47. What are the advantages and disadvantages of using pressure ventilation?

_____

_____

_____

_____

_____

_____

48. Explain the use of low levels of PEEP for ventilator patients with COPD.

_____

_____

_____

_____

49. How is V_T established during pressure ventilation?

_____

_____

50. A patient on PC-CMV has a set PIP of 18 cm H_2O. The measured V_T is 400 mL. The desired V_T is 750 mL. How should the pressure be adjusted to achieve the desired V_T?

_____

_____

_____

_____

51. A patient on PC-CMV has a set PIP of 14 cm H_2O. The measured V_T is 550 mL. The desired V_T is 800 mL. How should the pressure be adjusted to achieve the desired V_T?

_____

_____

52. What formula can be used to estimate the level of pressure support a patient needs?

_____

53. During VC-CMV a patient's respiratory rate is 12 breaths/min and the V_T is 600 mL. The measured PIP is 28 cm H_2O, and the $P_{plateau}$ is 20 cm H_2O. The patient is now ready for VC-SIMV with pressure support. The most appropriate initial pressure support level for this patient is

_____

54. The following figure presents a pressure-time curve for a patient with COPD who is receiving CPAP at 5 cm H_2O with PSV. What problem does the graphic indicate?

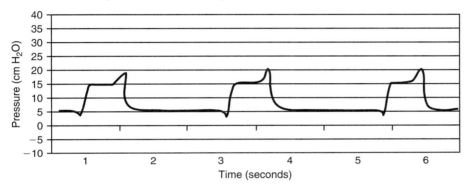

_____

55. What can be done to correct the problem identified in question 54?

_____

56. The flow cycle percent is set at 20%, and the peak inspiratory flow is 50 L/min. At what flow rate does the ventilator cycle?

_____

57. The flow cycle percent is set at 40%, and the peak inspiratory flow is 50 L/min. At what flow rate does the ventilator cycle?

_____

58. Compare your answers for questions 56 and 57. Which PS setup provides the shortest T_I? Why?

_____

_____

59. List the three methods of establishing the initial PIP during PCV.

_____

_____

_____

60. What are the initial setting ranges for bilevel PAP?

_____

_____

_____

61. The ventilator mode in which the breath is pressure limited and time cycled and uses V_T as a feedback control is _____.

62. During ventilation of a patient with PRVC, an audible alarm activates and the ventilator displays a digital message, "Pressure limit, please evaluate." List four possible causes of this problem.

_____

_____

_____

_____

Critical Thinking Questions

1. What factors does the respiratory therapist need to consider before initiating mechanical ventilation?

_____

_____

_____

_____

2. Explain the clinical importance of the tubing compression factor.

_____

_____

_____

_____

3. Volume lost to tubing compression is most critical in which type of patient?

_____

_____

4. How do changes in compliance affect the airway pressure and exhaled V_T in the volume control mode compared with the pressure control mode?

_____

_____

_____

_____

5. Name the two safety systems on ventilators for ending inspiration during PSV.

_____

_____

_____

_____

Case Studies

Case Study #1

A 28-year-old woman comes to the emergency department complaining of general muscle weakness, dysphagia, and difficulty breathing. The history of present illness reveals that she was diagnosed with infectious mononucleosis 10 days ago, and she has recently experienced ptosis and also weakness in her legs and arms. She weighs 150 lb and is 5' 8" tall. ABG results on room air are as follows: pH = 7.3, $PaCO_2$ = 50 mm Hg, PaO_2 = 78 mm Hg, SaO_2 = 83%, HCO_3^- = 23 mEq/L. MIP is 15 cm H_2O, and VC is 13 mL/kg.

1. What is the most appropriate action at this time?

_____

_____

_____

2. Calculate the patient's $\dot{V}_E$ using the Dubois body surface chart in Figure 7-1.

_____

3. What ranges for V_T and respiratory rate would be appropriate for this patient?

_____

_____

_____

Fifteen minutes after her arrival in the emergency department, the patient's breathing is very shallow and she is unresponsive. The patient is intubated immediately.

4. Which type of ventilation is most appropriate for this patient?

_____

5. What ventilator settings are appropriate?

_____

_____

_____

Case Study #2

An 8-year-old boy requires mechanical ventilation after surgical repair of a broken femur and humerus. His IBW is 80 lb. The respiratory therapist sets the ventilator to deliver 250 mL at 12 breaths/min with 3 cm H_2O PEEP in VC-SIMV, occludes the patient Y-connector, and manually triggers a breath. The PIP reading is 68 cm H_2O.

1. Calculate the compliance factor for this circuit.

_____

_____

The patient is connected to the ventilator; PIP is now 27 cm H_2O.

2. Calculate the volume lost.

_____

_____

3. Calculate the delivered V_T.

_____

_____

_____

_____

4. How can the respiratory therapist compensate for the lost V_T?

_____

_____

_____

NBRC–Style Questions

1. A male patient who is 6′ tall and has pulmonary fibrosis is ventilated with VC-CMV. The rate is 10 breaths/min, the V_T is 600 mL, the F_IO_2 is 0.5, and PEEP is 10 cm H_2O. PIP is 53 cm H_2O, and $P_{plateau}$ is 47 cm H_2O. The decision is made to switch the patient to PC-CMV. What set PIP will deliver 6 mL/kg IBW?
   a. 30 cm H_2O
   b. 35 cm H_2O
   c. 38 cm H_2O
   d. 43 cm H_2O

2. Which of the following are the most appropriate initial settings for a 5′ 4″ female postoperative patient with no lung disease?
   a. PC-CMV, PIP = 35 cm H_2O, f = 20 breaths/min, PEEP = 10 cm H_2O
   b. PC-SIMV, PIP = 20 cm H_2O, f = 6 breaths/min, PEEP = 8 cm H_2O
   c. VC-CMV, V_T = 570 mL, f = 10 breaths/min, PEEP = 5 cm H_2O
   d. VC-CMV, V_T = 700 mL, f = 14 breaths/min, no PEEP

3. A patient is ready to be changed from VC-SIMV to PSV. The VC-SIMV settings are as follows: V_T = 450 mL, f = 4 breaths/min, PEEP = 5 cm H_2O. PIP is 31cm H_2O, and $P_{plateau}$ is 23 cm H_2O. The initial PSV setting for this patient should be which of the following?
   a. 5 cm H_2O
   b. 8 cm H_2O
   c. 10 cm H_2O
   d. 12 cm H_2O

4. The most appropriate flow waveform for a patient with high Raw is which of the following?
   a. Rectangular
   b. Descending
   c. Ascending
   d. Exponential

5. What is the I:E ratio when the set rate is 35 breaths/min and the T_I is 1 second?
   a. 1:1
   b. 1.4:1
   c. 1.7:1
   d. 2:1

6. What flow rate is necessary to deliver a V_T of 500 mL at a rate of 15 breaths/min with an I:E ratio of 1:3?
   a. 30 L/min
   b. 35 L/min
   c. 40 L/min
   d. 45 L/min

7. Which of the following is the appropriate $\dot{V}_E$ for a male with a BSA of 2.3 m² and a body temperature of 40° C?
   a. 8.2 L/min
   b. 9.6 L/min
   c. 10.6 L/min
   d. 11.7 L/min

8. A 5′ 1″ female patient receiving PSV at 6 cm H_2O is showing signs of accessory muscle use and exhales a V_T of 220 mL at a rate of 28 breaths/min. Which of the following is the most appropriate action at this time?
   a. Adjust the F_IO_2
   b. Increase the set flow rate
   c. Increase PSV to 10 cm H_2O
   d. Adjust the flow cycle percent

9. Calculate the delivered V_T when tubing compliance is 3.3 cm H_2O, the set V_T is 375 mL, and PIP is 18 cm H_2O.
   a. 300 mL
   b. 316 mL
   c. 357 mL
   d. 365 mL

10. A 5′ 7″ female multiple trauma patient has been managed on VC-CMV for the past 24 hours; the settings are as follows: f = 12 breaths/min, V_T = 640 mL, PEEP = 5 cm H_2O, F_IO_2 = 0.60 with a constant waveform. Currently PIP is 45 cm H_2O and $P_{plateau}$ is 38 cm H_2O. The patient has been diagnosed with ARDS, and the respiratory therapist wants to switch her to PC-CMV. Which of the following is the initial pressure setting for targeting the appropriate V_T for this patient?
    a. 10 cm H_2O
    b. 20 cm H_2O
    c. 38 cm H_2O
    d. 45 cm H_2O

Helpful Internet Sites

- Budinger ERS: Mechanical ventilation. Loyola University Medical Center, Chicago. PowerPoint presentation available on LUMEN summarizing many aspects of mechanical ventilation. Available at www.lumen.luc.edu/lumen/MedEd/medicine/pulmonar/lecture/ vent/case_f.htm
- Brown MK: Lung-protective strategies for acute, severe asthma. *RT J Respir Care Pract* Feb/Mar 2002. Available at www.rtmagazine.com/Articles.ASP?articleid=r0202A03

CHAPTER 8

Final Considerations in Ventilator Setup

Learning Objectives

Upon completion of this chapter the reader will be able to do the following:

1. Recommend F_IO_2 settings when beginning mechanical ventilation.
2. Discuss the pros and cons of using the sigh mode during mechanical ventilation.
3. Compare the use of sigh with the concept of a recruitment maneuver in adult respiratory distress syndrome.
4. List the necessary considerations for preparation of final ventilator setup.
5. Explain the concept of using extrinsic PEEP in patients with airflow obstruction and air trapping who have trouble triggering a breath during mechanical ventilation.
6. Using the equation for the desired F_IO_2 setting and given a known PaO_2 value, calculate the F_IO_2 to be used with a patient.
7. List the essential capabilities of an adult ventilator.
8. Provide initial ventilator settings from the guidelines for patient management for any of the following patient problems: chronic obstructive pulmonary disease, neuromuscular disorders, acute asthma attacks, closed head injuries, adult respiratory distress syndrome, and acute pulmonary edema.

Key Terms Crossword Puzzle

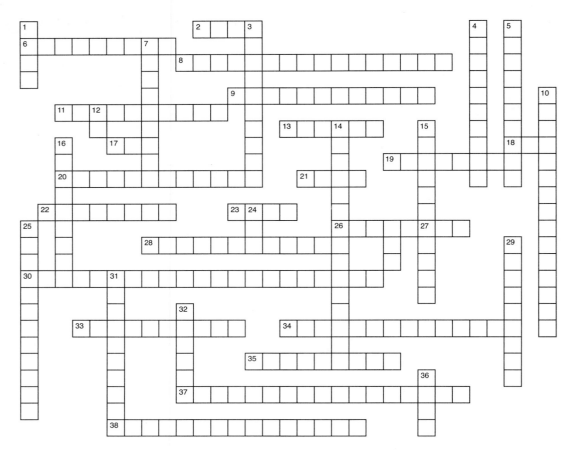

Across

2 Preferred method of triggering with a slightly faster response
6 Pharmacological agent given to improve cardiac contractility
8 Neuromuscular disease that has a rapid onset (two words)
9 Look-and-see type of pulmonary diagnostic procedure
11 Trauma caused by excessive pressure in the lungs
13 Color of sputum in the presence of respiratory infection
17 Type of pressures measured with a closed head injury (abbreviation)
18 Neuromuscular disease made famous by a baseball player (abbreviation)
19 Type of humidifier
20 Not in sync
21 Deep breath that occurs regularly
22 Interface for noninvasive ventilation (two words)
23 Chemical administered to maintain an acceptable pH range (abbreviation)
26 Sound made by alveoli popping open during inspiration
28 A humidifier is filled with this (two words)

Down

1 Type of humidifier that uses capillary action
3 These are placed at gravity-dependent parts of the circuit to catch excess rain-out (two words)
4 Knowingly allowing carbon dioxide levels to rise during mechanical ventilation is known as _____ hypercapnia
5 Warns that the patient has stopped breathing (two words)
7 Pharmacological agent that improves cardiac contractility
10 Dramatic intrapleural pressure changes that alter blood flow through the thorax and heart
12 Percentage of absolute humidity compared with capacity (abbreviation)
14 Ventilator strategy for opening collapsed lung tissue (two words)
15 Pharmacological agent that can improve myocardial oxygenation and reduce preload and afterload
16 Process of adding fluids
24 An artificial nose
25 Enlarged heart
27 Maintaining cerebral blood flow requires this pressure (abbreviation)

Across—Cont'd

30 Another name for auto-PEEP (two words)
33 Warns that T_I is exceeding T_E (two words)
34 Type of percussion note heard over area with increased air
35 Type of drugs that reduce vascular fluid load
37 Asthmatic episode that does not respond to normal therapy (two words)
38 Normal response to acute increases in ICP (two words)

Down—Cont'd

29 Low oxygen level in the blood
31 The point at which inhaled air reaches 100% RH is called the _____ saturation boundary
32 Warns of possible dangers
36 A chest physician group (abbreviation)

Review Questions

1. The clinically acceptable arterial oxygen tension range is

   _____.

2. Before elective intubation a patient's PaO_2 was 90 mm Hg with a nasal cannula running at 2 L/min. What F_IO_2 should be set on the ventilator?

   _____

3. Calculate the estimated F_IO_2 using the following information: known F_IO_2 = 0.5, known PaO_2 = 60 mm Hg, desired PaO_2 = 90 mm Hg.

   _____

   _____

   _____

4. What F_IO_2 should be set on the ventilator for a patient who has had cardiac arrest? _____

5. What is the acceptable goal for SpO_2?

   _____

6. How long after the start of mechanical ventilation should the patient's ABG values be analyzed?

   _____

7. Use of high concentrations of oxygen can cause what three problems?

   _____

   _____

8. Why does flow triggering have a faster response time than pressure triggering?

   _____

   _____

   _____

   _____

9. How does auto-PEEP interfere with pressure triggering?

   _____

   _____

   _____

   _____

   _____

10. In the tracheobronchial tree, the point at which inhaled gas contains 44 mg/L of water, has reached 100% relative humidity, and is 37° C, is called the ————— _____; this point is located at the level of the _____ _____.

11. The absolute humidity of a ventilator's humidification system must be _____ at temperatures between _____ and _____.

12. Give two advantages of a closed humidification system.

    _____

    _____

13. What causes excessive rain-out (condensation) in a ventilator circuit?

    _____

    _____

    _____

    _____

    _____

14. How much water can an HME provide with V_Ts of 500 to 1000 mL? _____

15. How much water can a hygroscopic HME provide with V_Ts of 500 to 1000 mL? _____

16. What happens to an HME when moisture and secretions accumulate in it?

_____

_____

17. What two actions can be taken with the HME during aerosol treatment with a small-volume nebulizer? Why?

_____

_____

18. An MDI with a spacer should be placed where in the ventilator circuit? What should be done with the HME?

_____

_____

19. List at least four contraindications to the use of a HME.

_____

_____

_____

_____

_____

_____

20. Name and describe the three levels of alarms.

_____

_____

_____

For questions 21 through 35, identify the alarm situations with the appropriate alarm level.

21. _____ Heater/humidifier malfunction

22. _____ Timing failure

23. _____ Autocycling

24. _____ Auto-PEEP

25. _____ Excessive gas delivery to the patient

26. _____ Inappropriate PEEP/CPAP

27. _____ Exhalation valve failure

28. _____ Inappropriate I:E ratio

29. _____ Electrical power failure

30. _____ Changes in lung characteristics

31. _____ Circuit leak

32. _____ No gas delivery to the patient

33. _____ Partly obstructed circuit

34. _____ Inappropriate oxygen level

35. _____ Changes in ventilatory drive

36. After a patient is placed on VC-CMV with a PEEP of 8 cm H_2O, the respiratory therapist notices that the average PIP is 30 cm H_2O. The low pressure, high pressure, and low PEEP/CPAP alarms should be set up at what values?

_____

37. The maximum value for the apnea alarm in any ventilator is how many seconds? _____

38. In what way are lung recruitment strategies and sigh maneuvers similar?

_____

_____

_____

_____

_____

39. List at least four circumstances in which sighs or deep breaths are appropriate.

_____

_____

_____

_____

40. List the ten factors that must be considered in the preparation for final ventilator setup.

_____

_____

_____

_____

41. List the essential capabilities of an adult ventilator.

(a) Modes: _____

(b) Tidal volume range: _____

(c) Respiratory rate range: _____

(d) Pressure range: _____

(e) PEEP/CPAP range: _____

(f) Flow rate range: _____

(g) Flow waveforms: _____

(h) F_IO_2: _____

(i) Diagnostic measurements: _____

(j) Alarms: _____

42. What lung characteristics do patients with COPD exhibit?

_____

43. What is the primary reason for providing mechanical ventilatory support for patients with COPD?

_____

44. List at least five causes of increased morbidity in patients with COPD who receive ventilatory support.

_____

_____

45. The mode of choice for a patient with COPD, if possible, is _____.

46. The intubation route of choice for a patient with COPD is _____.

47. Complete the following chart, which summarizes the ventilator guidelines for patients with COPD.

Parameter	Preferred Setting or Range
Tidal volume	_____
Rate	_____
Inspiratory time	_____
Flow rate	_____
Flow waveform	_____
PEEP	_____
F_IO_2	_____

48. List at least five neuromuscular disorders that may require ventilatory support.

_____

_____

_____

_____

49. What are the main reasons patients with these neuromuscular disorders require ventilatory support?

_____

_____

_____

50. Complete the following chart, which summarizes the ventilator guidelines for patients with neuromuscular disorders.

Parameter	Preferred Setting or Range
Tidal volume	_____
Rate	_____
Inspiratory time	_____
Flow rate	_____
Flow waveform	_____
PEEP	_____
F_IO_2	_____

51. Define _pulsus paradoxus_.

_____

_____

_____

_____

52. During mechanical ventilation of a patient with acute asthma, the respiratory therapist must be aware of what two main concerns?

_____

53. During ventilation of a patient with asthma, $P_{plateau}$ should be kept _____.

54. The pharmacological agents that may be used to keep pH above 7.2 during permissive hypercapnia are _____ and _____.

55. Complete the following chart, which summarizes the ventilator guidelines for patients with acute severe asthma.

Parameter	Preferred Setting or Range
Tidal volume	_____
Rate	_____
Inspiratory time	_____
Flow rate	_____
Flow waveform	_____
PEEP	_____
F_IO_2	_____

56. Diagnostic percussion during an asthmatic episode will reveal _____.

57. List the common causes of increased ICP.

_____

_____

_____

58. The equation for the cerebral perfusion pressure is

_____ .

59. What are the normal values for the components of this formula?

_____

60. What CPP indicates poor cerebral perfusion?

_____

61. When and how should iatrogenic hyperventilation be used?

_____

_____

_____

62. Complete the following chart, which summarizes the ventilator guidelines for patients with a closed head injury.

Parameter	Preferred Setting or Range
Tidal volume	_____
Rate	_____
Inspiratory time	_____
Flow rate	_____
Flow waveform	_____
PEEP	_____
F_IO_2	_____

63. Explain the open lung approach to ventilating patients with ARDS.

_____

_____

_____

64. Complete the following chart, which summarizes the ventilator guidelines for patients with ARDS.

Parameter	Preferred Setting or Range
Tidal volume	_____
Rate	_____
Inspiratory time	_____
Flow rate	_____
Flow waveform	_____
PEEP	_____
F_IO_2	_____

65. What are the acceptable end points for ABGs in the management of ARDS?

_____

_____

66. Give at least seven examples of precipitating conditions associated with the development of ARDS.

_____

_____

_____

_____

_____

_____

_____

67. Refractory hypoxemia is identified with what diagnostic criteria? _____

68. Describe the appearance of ARDS on a chest radiograph.

_____

69. What values for shunt, total lung compliance, and pulmonary capillary wedge pressure are diagnostic for ARDS?

_____

_____

70. List five common causes of acute pulmonary edema.

_____

_____

_____

71. Complete the following chart, which summarizes the ventilator guidelines for patients with CHF.

Parameter	Preferred Setting or Range
Tidal volume	_____
Rate	_____
Inspiratory time	_____
Flow rate	_____
Flow waveform	_____
PEEP	_____
F_IO_2	_____

Critical Thinking Questions

1. Discuss the pros and cons of using sighs with mechanical ventilation.

_____

_____

_____

_____

_____

_____

_____

_____

_____

2. Explain the progression of an asthmatic episode from arrival at the emergency department to intubation and mechanical ventilation.

_____

_____

_____

_____

_____

_____

_____

_____

_____

_____

_____

3. Discuss why the use of PSV may not be appropriate for patients with COPD.

_____

_____

_____

_____

_____

_____

_____

_____

_____

4. Why does the exhalation valve not need to close at the beginning of a flow-triggered breath?

_____

_____

_____

_____

_____

_____

_____

_____

5. Why is it important to maximize the expiratory time when ventilating a patient with increased airway resistance, such as with asthma or COPD?

_____

_____

_____

Case Studies

Case Study #1

The patient, a 62-year-old male who weighs 256 lb and is 73″ tall, has a history of congestive heart failure and is placed on a nonrebreathing mask. Physical assessment reveals that the patient is alert and oriented but anxious and diaphoretic. Other findings are as follows: pulse = 142 and thready, BP = 105/68 mm Hg, T = 37° C, respiratory rate = 26 breaths/min, shallow and labored. Breath sounds reveal bilateral inspiratory coarse crackles. ABG values on the nonrebreathing mask are these: pH = 7.24, $PaCO_2$ = 51 mm Hg, PaO_2 = 42 mm Hg, and HCO_3^- = 23 mEq/L. The patient's cardiogram shows a widened QRS complex with occasional premature ventricular contractions

1. What respiratory care intervention is indicated at this time?

   _____

   _____

   _____

   _____

2. If this patient were to be intubated and placed on mechanical ventilation, what mode, tidal volume, and rate would be appropriate?

   _____

   _____

   _____

   _____

   _____

Case Study #2

A 37-year-old female victim of a motor vehicle accident arrives at the hospital by ambulance. The patient has sustained a closed head injury. Physical assessment reveals the following: pulse = 145, respiratory rate = 32 breaths/min, BP = 155/97 mm Hg. The patient's neck veins are distended, and she is diaphoretic and anxious. She is 68″ tall and weighs 175 lb. The patient has no history of cardiac or respiratory disease. An oral airway is in place, and the patient has a weak gag reflex. ABG values on 60% oxygen are these: pH = 7.22, $PaCO_2$ = 64 mm Hg, PaO_2 = 78 mm Hg, SaO_2 = 92%, HCO_3^- = 25 mEq/L.

1. This patient appears to have what type of respiratory

   failure? _____

   _____

2. What acid-base imbalance is present?

   _____

3. What type of mechanical ventilatory support would benefit this patient?

   _____

4. What are the appropriate parameters for this patient? Include minute ventilation, tidal volume, inspiratory time, flow rate, and PEEP.

   _____

   _____

   _____

   _____

   _____

   _____

Case Study #3

A 40-year-old female who is 66″ tall and weighs 156 lb is admitted to the emergency department. She is alert, very anxious, and unable to complete a sentence without stopping to take a breath; she is sitting in a tripod position. Physical examination findings are as follows: HR = 136 beats/min and regular, respiratory rate = 30 breaths/min and very labored with use of accessory muscles, BP = 168/84 mm Hg, T = 37.2° C. Breath sounds are decreased bilaterally with expiratory wheezes, and the patient has a weak, nonproductive cough. The patient has been receiving continuous albuterol aerosol therapy and is being given Solu-Medrol intravenously. The patient's best peak flow after bronchodilator therapy is 65 L/min. ABG results on nasal cannula at 6 L/min are these: pH = 7.34, $PaCO_2$ = 42 mm Hg, PaO_2 = 48 mm Hg, SaO_2 = 79%, and HCO_3^- = 22 mEq/L.

1. How should these ABG values be interpreted?

   _____

   _____

   _____

   _____

   _____

   _____

   _____

   _____

2. Does the situation warrant intubation and mechanical ventilation? Why or why not?

_____

_____

_____

_____

3. What type of mechanical ventilatory support would benefit this patient?

_____

_____

4. If PC-CMV is used for this patient, what are the appropriate settings? Include PIP, resulting tidal volume, respiratory rate, inspiratory time, waveform, and PEEP.

_____

_____

_____

_____

NBRC–Style Questions

1. Which of the following is (are) true concerning the use of permissive hypercapnia in the management of ARDS?
   I. Bicarbonate may be administered to keep the pH above 7.2.
   II. $PaCO_2$ should not exceed 60 mm Hg.
   III. The pH may be allowed to drop as low as 7.1.
   IV. The $PaCO_2$ is permitted to rise rapidly to the acceptable level.
   a. I and III
   b. II and IV
   c. I and IV
   d. II and III

2. A mechanically ventilated patient has been using an HME for humidification for the past 72 hours. On rounds the respiratory therapist notices a steady increase in PIP over the past 2 days. The respiratory therapist suctions the patient to assess the secretions and finds that they are very thick and tenacious. The most appropriate action at this time is which of the following?
   a. Suction the patient more often
   b. Add a passover humidifier to the system
   c. Switch to a heated wick–type humidifier
   d. Use normal saline to lavage before suctioning

3. A 75-year-old female, admitted through the emergency department earlier today, is increasingly distressed and unable to breathe comfortably except in the upright position. She has a history of coronary artery disease and on admission was complaining of chest pain. She is becoming increasingly short of breath and appears cyanotic. Vital signs are as follows: pulse = 142, BP = 150/92 mm Hg, respiratory rate = 30 breaths/min and labored. ABG values on nasal cannula at 3 L/min are these: pH = 7.18, $PaCO_2$ = 81 mm Hg, PaO_2 = 35 mm Hg, SaO_2 = 79%, and HCO_3^- = 29 mEq/L. The respiratory therapist should recommendation which of the following?
   a. Nasal mask CPAP at 10 cm H_2O
   b. Nonrebreathing mask with oxygen at 15 L/min
   c. Bilevel PAP (IPAP = 15 cm H_2O and EPAP = 5 cm H_2O)
   d. Intubation and mechanical ventilation with PC-CMV

4. For an otherwise healthy, 26-year-old male patient who is 6′ 1″ and weighs 185 lb and who was brought to the emergency department because of a drug overdose, appropriate ventilatory parameters include which of the following?
   a. VC-CMV, tidal volume = 1 L, set rate = 8 breaths/min
   b. VC-SIMV, tidal volume = 600 mL, set rate = 6 breaths/min
   c. PC-CMV, set pressure = 25 cm H_2O, inspiratory time = 1.5 second
   d. Pressure support ventilation (15 cm H_2O) with CPAP (5 cm H_2O)

5. Before intubation a patient's PaO_2 was 78 mm Hg with an F_IO_2 of 0.6. What F_IO_2 setting on the ventilator will bring the PaO_2 up to 90 mm Hg? (Assume that this patient's cardiopulmonary status and respiratory quotient are constant.)
   a. 0.7
   b. 0.75
   c. 0.8
   d. 0.85

6. A patient has just been intubated in the emergency department. The patient is a 64-year-old obese male; drug overdose is suspected. The patient is 6′ tall and weighs 435 lb. The most appropriate tidal volume for ventilating this patient is which of the following?
   a. 350 mL
   b. 850 mL
   c. 1000 mL
   d. 1200 mL

7. Which of the following ventilatory parameters is appropriate for mechanically ventilating a patient with COPD?
   a. Rectangular flow waveform
   b. Tidal volume of 10 to 15 mL/kg
   c. Peak inspiratory flow rates above 60 L/min
   d. PEEP of 5 to 10 cm H_2O

8. A patient with acute respiratory distress syndrome has been switched from VC-CMV to PC-CMV. When this change was made, the mean airway pressure increased. Which of the following statements about elevated mean airway pressures is true?
   a. The mean airway pressure increases with longer expiratory times.
   b. An increased mean airway pressure may improve oxygenation.
   c. Elevated mean airway pressures reduce the risk of barotrauma.
   d. High mean airway pressures increase the risk of cardiovascular side effects.

9. A female patient who is 5′ 4″ tall and weighs 125 lb has just been intubated because of a severe asthmatic episode. Which of the following ventilator parameters would be most appropriate for her?
   a. PSV = 20 cm H_2O with CPAP = 10 cm H_2O
   b. PC-CMV, rate = 8 breaths/min, PIP = 25 cm H_2O, T_I = 0.75 second, descending waveform
   c. VC-SIMV, rate = 12 breaths/min, V_T = 800 mL, flow = 50 L/min, rectangular waveform
   d. VC-CMV, rate = 10 breaths/min, V_T = 570 mL, flow = 35 L/min, descending waveform

10. HMEs may not be appropriate for use with infants, children, and small adults because of which of the following?
    a. Presence of mechanical dead space in the HME
    b. Increased rate of ET occlusion with these patients
    c. Patients' inability to overcome resistance across the HME
    d. HME's inability to provide adequate humidity for these patients

Helpful Internet Sites

- Brown MK: Lung-protective strategies for acute, severe asthma, *RT J Respir Care Pract* Feb/Mar 2002. Available at www.rtmagazine.com/Articles.ASP?articleid=r0202A03
- American Thoracic Society: Standards for the diagnosis and care of patients with chronic pulmonary disease: inpatient management of COPD. Available at www.epocnet.com/area_m/normas/b_4_03e.html
- Brown EA, Kirk JD: Role of noninvasive ventilation in the management of acutely decompensated heart failure, *Rev Cardiovasc Med* vol 3(suppl 4), 2002. Available at www.medreviews.com/pdfs/articles/RICM_3suppl4_s35.pdf
- ARDSNet Web site: www.ardsnet.org/studies.php
- Trauma.Org: Control of intracranial hypertension. Available at www.trauma.org/neuro/icpcontrol.html#hyperventilation

Initial Assessment of the Mechanically Ventilated Patient

Learning Objectives

Upon completion of this chapter the reader will be able to do the following:

1. Recognize appropriate times for performing an operational verification check.
2. State the recommended times when an oxygen analyzer is used to measure F_IO_2 during mechanical ventilation.
3. Identify causes of an increase in transairway pressure, peak pressure, and plateau pressure.
4. Calculate alveolar volume from tidal volume and dead space values.
5. Use pressure-time and flow curves obtained during pressure-controlled continuous mandatory ventilation to determine the plateau pressure.
6. Identify a system leak from a volume-time curve.
7. Use physical examination and radiographical data to determine whether pneumonia, pneumothorax, asthma, pleural effusion, or emphysema is present.
8. Determine whether a lung compliance problem or an airway resistance problem is present using the ventilator flow sheet and time, volume, peak inspiratory pressure, and plateau pressure data.
9. Evaluate a static pressure-volume curve for static compliance and dynamic compliance to determine changes in compliance or resistance.
10. Estimate a patient's alveolar ventilation based on ideal body weight, tidal volume, and respiratory rate.
11. Detect a cuff leak by listening to breath sounds.
12. Recognize inappropriate endotracheal tube cuff pressures and an inappropriate tube size and recommend measures to correct these problems.
13. Evaluate flow sheet information for a patient on pressure control ventilation and recommend methods for determining whether compliance and airway resistance have changed.
14. Explain the technique for measuring endotracheal tube cuff pressure using a manometer, syringe, and three-way stopcock.
15. Describe two methods of dealing with a cut pilot tube (pilot balloon line) without changing the endotracheal tube.

Key Terms Crossword Puzzle

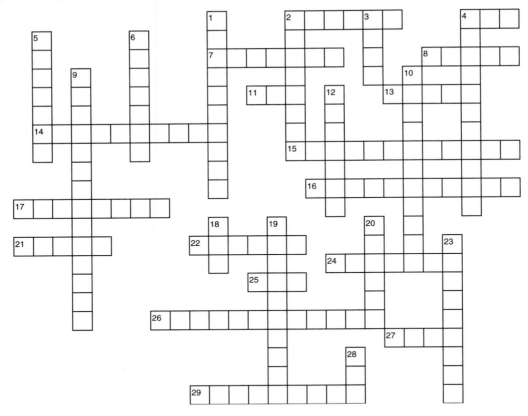

Across

2 Place to measure temperature
4 Something in the ventilator circuit that adds dead space (abbreviation)
7 Cause of abdominal distention due to fluid
8 The _____ inflection point indicates a time at which a large number of alveoli are becoming overinflated.
11 Test to check that a ventilator is working properly (abbreviation)
13 An ET has a _____ balloon
14 Common place for leaks
15 It puts air in the pleural space and reduces lung compliance.
16 Setting that allows patient triggering
17 Cell death
21 The _____ inflection point indicates the pressure at which a large number of alveoli are being recruited
22 Type of compliance measured at no flow
24 Type of compliance measured during gas movement
25 Pressure that can be measured continuously by a flow-directed catheter (abbreviation)
26 What's left in the tubing is called _____ volume
27 Another name for base flow is _____ flow
29 Form on which the patient-ventilator check is recorded (two words)

Down

1 Type of pressure that is important to tissue oxygenation and affects both lung volume and cardiac output (two words)
2 Dynamic hyperinflation (two words)
3 When the exhaled tidal volume is less than the set tidal volume, there is a _____
4 Condition of low body temperature
5 Breath sound that indicates suctioning may be needed
6 Type of recoil
9 It puts fluid in the alveoli and reduces lung compliance (two words)
10 Location of the central venous pressure catheter (two words)
12 Breath sound that indicates bronchodilator therapy may be needed
18 Amount of pressure required to overcome airway resistance (abbreviation)
19 Heart rate, respiratory rate, and blood pressure are all part of this (two words)
20 Tidal volume times frequency equals _____ ventilation
23 Secondary respiratory muscles
28 Method of ensuring that no leaks occur around an ET (abbreviation)

Review Questions

1. List the information that may be obtained from direct observation of a patient.

   _____

   _____

   _____

   _____

2. Documentation of patient information and ventilator settings should be performed _____ and recorded on the _____.

3. Before a ventilator can be used for a patient, the therapist must perform _____.

4. List six instances when ventilator checks should be performed in addition to regularly timed checks.

   _____

   _____

   _____

   _____

   _____

   _____

5. The F_IO_2 must be measured at least every _____ in adults and _____ in infants.

6. Give the appropriate pressure range (sensitivity setting) for a patient to trigger a breath.

   _____

7. An inappropriate sensitivity setting may result in

   _____

   or _____.

8. Define *auto-PEEP*.

   _____

9. List the steps that may be taken to eliminate or reduce auto-PEEP.

   _____

   _____

   _____

10. Calculate how much volume is lost to the patient's ventilator circuit when C_T is 3.27 mL/cm H_2O and PIP is 48 cm H_2O.

    _____

    _____

11. Alveolar minute ventilation is defined as _____ _____ and is written in formula form as _____.

12. How does attaching an HME to the ET affect alveolar ventilation?

    _____

    _____

13. Calculate the alveolar minute ventilation if the set V_T is 775 mL, the IBW is 160 lb, and the added V_D is 85 mL.

    _____

    _____

14. List three factors that determine alveolar ventilation.

    _____

    _____

15. An increase in PIP may be due to _____ in compliance or _____ in airway resistance.

16. What control must be used to measure $P_{plateau}$?

    _____

17. List the circumstances that may result in an inaccurate $P_{plateau}$ measurement.

    _____

    _____

    _____

18. PIP is used to measure _____ compliance, and $P_{plateau}$ is used to measure _____ _____ compliance.

19. Transairway pressure is defined as _____ _____ and is written in formula form as _____.

20. An increase between PIP and $P_{plateau}$ usually indicates

    _____.

21. List the most common causes for an increase in Raw.

    _____

    _____

    _____

22. Why should the mean airway pressure be monitored?

    _____

    _____

23. The PIP alarm usually is set approximately _____ cm H_2O above the measured PIP and when activated will _____.

24. List the most common causes of activation of the maximum safety pressure alarm.

    _____

    _____

    _____

    _____

    _____

25. The low PIP alarm usually is set approximately _____ cm H_2O below the measured PIP and when activated usually indicates _____ _____.

26. List the most common causes of activation of the low pressure alarm.

    _____

    _____

    _____

27. If the leak is not obvious, the patient must be _____ while the leak is checked.

28. List several ways to determine whether a leak is present.

    _____

    _____

    _____

29. If a leak is detected, what steps should be taken to find the source?

    _____

    _____

    _____

    _____

    _____

    _____

    _____

    _____

    _____

    _____

    _____

    _____

    _____

30. What effect would a leak have during pressure support ventilation?

    _____

    _____

31. List the factors that can affect a patient's heart rate.

    _____

    _____

    _____

32. List the factors that can cause hyperthermia.

    _____

    _____

33. List the factors that can cause hypothermia.

    _____

    _____

    _____

34. CVP directly reflects _____

    _____.

35. Monitoring of pulmonary artery pressures is useful for what type of patient?

    _____

    _____

36. Calculate airway resistance for a ventilated patient with the following data: PIP = 48 cm H_2O, $P_{plateau}$ = 30 cm H_2O, set flow rate = 40 L/min.

    _____

    _____

37. ET cuff pressures below _____ are believed to reduce the risk of _____ and _____.

38. In what type of patient may a cuff pressure of 25 mm Hg cause tracheal damage?

_____

39. List the five-step protocol designed to minimize the risk of tracheal necrosis associated with cuff overinflation.

_____

_____

_____

_____

_____

_____

40. Give two situations in which a higher than acceptable cuff pressure may be required to maintain a minimal occlusion.

_____

_____

_____

_____

41. If the source of a leak is determined to be either the pilot balloon or valve, the cuff can be inflated and a _____ attached to the pilot balloon and turned to the _____ position. If the pilot balloon is still leaking, the problem can be temporarily solved by placing a _____ on the pilot line.

42. Describe the procedure for maintaining cuff pressure if the pilot balloon is cut accidentally.

_____

_____

_____

43. What is the rationale for repositioning an ET in the patient's mouth every 8 to 12 hours?

_____

_____

44. List the possible causes of a decrease in C_S.

_____

_____

_____

45. The normal value for C_S is _____.

46. During pressure ventilation, if the set inspiratory pressure remains constant, how would a decrease in C_S affect the tidal volume?

_____

47. C_S is written in formula form as

_____.

48. C_D decreases whenever C_S _____ or Raw _____.

49. C_D is written in formula form as

_____.

50. During volume ventilation, how would a decrease in C_D affect PIP and the delivered tidal volume?

_____

_____

51. Calculate the C_S when the V_T is 740 mL, the $P_{plateau}$ is 44 cm H_2O, and the end-expiratory pressure is 8 cm H_2O.

_____

_____

52. Calculate the Raw when the PIP is 58 cm H_2O, the $P_{plateau}$ is 51 cm H_2O, and the flow rate is 0.5 L/sec.

_____

_____

Critical Thinking Questions

1. During a ventilator check the respiratory therapist notices the patient making inspiratory efforts (the patient is using accessory muscles), but the ventilator is not triggering. What could be causing the problem? What steps could be taken to correct it?

_____

_____

_____

_____

2. A mechanically ventilated 250-lb adult male has a 6.5-mm (inner diameter) ET in place. A cuff pressure of 40 cm H_2O is required to maintain an adequate seal. What is the problem in this situation, and what recommendations should be made to correct it?

_____

_____

_____

3. A patient with ARDS is maintained on PCV with a set inspiratory pressure of 30 cm H_2O. According to the ventilator flow sheet, measured tidal volumes for the past 3 days have ranged from 400 to 450 mL. During the first ventilator-patient check of the day, the respiratory therapist notes that the measured tidal volume now is 550 mL without any change in set parameters. What would cause the tidal volume to increase?

_____

_____

_____

_____

_____

4. When the PIP is 43 cm H_2O and the $P_{plateau}$ is 18 cm H_2O, how much pressure is required to overcome the resistance of the airways?

_____

Case Studies

Case Study #1

A respiratory therapist is called to a code in the ICU. After the patient's condition has stabilized, the physician writes the following order for mechanical ventilation: Volume control, V_T = 700 mL, f = 12 breaths/min, F_IO_2 = 1.0, PEEP = 5 cm H_2O. The therapist notes that the PIP is 42 cm H_2O.

1. At what levels should the high and low pressure alarms be set?

_____

_____

2. At what level should the low V_T alarm be set?

_____

3. What would the therapist need to do to obtain a $P_{plateau}$?

_____

4. What might the therapist conclude if the $P_{plateau}$ is 38 cm H_2O?

_____

Case Study #2

An obtunded patient in the ICU has been receiving VC-CMV for the past 3 days. Today the patient appears to be awakening. The high pressure, low minute volume, and low tidal volume alarms are activating frequently, and the patient appears to be agitated and confused.

1. Give possible causes of activation of the high pressure alarm.

_____

2. Give possible causes of activation of the low minute volume and low tidal volume alarms.

_____

_____

_____

3. What are the possible underlying causes, and what would you recommend to resolve those problems?

_____

_____

_____

_____

_____

_____

NBRC–Style Questions

1. An increase in the peak inspiratory flow rate would increase which of the following?
   a. Tidal volume
   b. Total cycle time
   c. Expiratory time
   d. Inspiratory time

2. C_S declines in a patient receiving volume-cycled mechanical ventilation. Which of the following will most likely occur?
   a. Increase in V_T
   b. Decrease in minute ventilation
   c. Increase in PIP
   d. Increased I:E ratio

3. While monitoring endotracheal cuff pressures during a ventilator check, the therapist obtains a reading of 44 cm H_2O. What should the therapist do next?
   a. Use a syringe to add air to the cuff
   b. Insert a smaller diameter ET
   c. Release air from the cuff until minimal occluding volume is achieved
   d. Make no changes; the cuff pressure is within the acceptable range

4. Which of the following can cause a mechanically ventilated patient's PIP to increase from 20 to 40 cm H_2O while C_S remains relatively unchanged?
   a. Removal of mucous plugs
   b. Increased airway resistance
   c. Tension pneumothorax
   d. Decreased elastance

5. An increase in PIP and $P_{plateau}$ with a stable transairway pressure may be caused by which of the following?
   a. Acute respiratory distress syndrome
   b. Acute asthma exacerbation
   c. Retained secretions in the airways
   d. ET that is too small

6. While responding to a ventilator alarm, the respiratory therapist notes that the low pressure alarm has activated. There is an audible leak, and the exhaled volume is 200 mL less than the set tidal volume. The measured cuff pressure is 15 mm Hg. What action should the therapist take?
   a. Replace the ET with a larger size
   b. Increase the patient's V_T to compensate for the leak
   c. Instill enough volume into the cuff to maintain a pressure of 30 cm H_2O
   d. While auscultating the larynx, instill air into the cuff until a slight leak is heard on inspiration

7. Why is end-expiratory pressure subtracted from $P_{plateau}$ in the calculation of C_S?
   a. To compensate for a loss in volume caused by a leak
   b. To determine auto-PEEP
   c. To determine the actual pressure change
   d. To calculate the actual PEEP level

8. Which of the following may cause an increase in heart rate?
   I. Hypoxemia
   II. Hypothermia
   III. Anxiety
   IV. Pain
   a. I
   b. I and III
   c. I, II, and III
   d. I, III, and IV

9. Which of the following physical findings would you expect when assessing an asthmatic patient?
   I. Late inspiratory crackles
   II. Hyperresonant percussion note
   III. Accessory muscle use
   IV. Tracheal shift
   a. I
   b. I and III
   c. II and III
   d. II, III, and IV

10. Evaluate the following data from a patient's flow sheet:

Time	Set V_T	PIP (cm H_2O)	$P_{plateau}$ (cm H_2O)
1600	700 mL	38	32
1700	700 mL	41	34
1800	700 mL	47	32

Which of the following statements is true?
   a. C_L is improving.
   b. C_L is unchanged.
   c. Raw is improving.
   d. Raw has increased.

Helpful Internet Sites

- Massachusetts General Hospital, Department of Respiratory Care: *Electronic reference manual: measuring lung compliance and airway resistance.* Available at www.mgh.harvard.edu/ rcpolicies/Internal/Procedures/Diagnostics/c&r.htm
- University of California, Berkeley, Department of Molecular and Cell Biology: Work of breathing. Available at http:// mcb.berkeley.edu/courses/mcb136/topic/Respiration/ SlideSet2/Resp2.pdf
- Orme F: Welcome to human physiology. Available at http://members.aol.com/Bio50/LecNotes/lecnot19.html

CHAPTER 10

Ventilator Graphics

Learning Objectives

Upon completion of this chapter the reader will be able to do the following:

1. Identify ventilator variables (e.g., the target variable and trigger variable) and ventilator parameters and their values (e.g., peak inspiratory pressure and plateau pressure) from pressure, flow, and volume scalars in the following modes: volume-controlled continuous mandatory ventilation, volume-controlled synchronized intermittent mandatory ventilation plus pressure support ventilation and continuous positive airway pressure, pressure-controlled continuous mandatory ventilation, pressure-controlled synchronized intermittent mandatory ventilation, and pressure support ventilation.

2. Identify ventilator variables and ventilator parameters and their values from flow-volume and pressure-volume loops.

3. Recognize problems from ventilator scalars and loops, including changes in compliance and airway resistance, inappropriate sensitivity setting, inadequate inspiratory flow, auto-PEEP, leaks, active exhalation during pressure support ventilation, and an inspiratory pressure spike during pressure support ventilation.

4. Calculate airway resistance and compliance from information obtained from scalars and loops during ventilation.

5. Explain the changes that occur in scalars and loops during volume-targeted and pressure-targeted ventilation when airway resistance increases and when lung compliances decreases.

6. Given a compliance value obtained during pressure control ventilation, determine whether compliance is normal, determine tidal volume delivery, and recommend ways to adjust the set pressure to gain a desired tidal volume.

Key Terms Crossword Puzzle

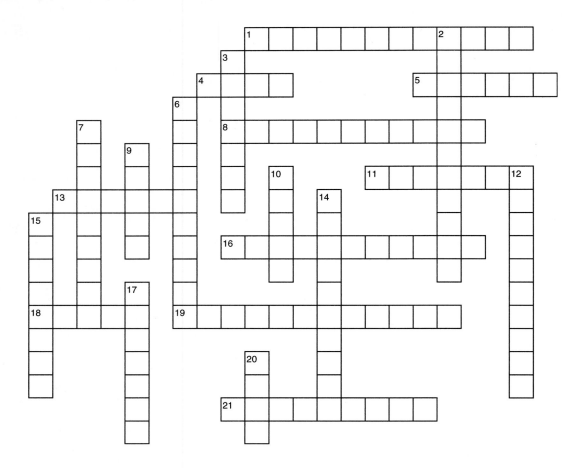

Across

1 When patient and ventilator are not working together
4 Volume per unit of time
5 One variable plotted against time
8 Flow multiplied by airway resistance equals _____ pressure.
11 Begins inspiration
13 Flow multiplied by inspiratory time
16 Rapid rise or decay on a graph
18 A line that is not exactly straight has a slight _____
19 The assisted breath in the SIMV mode is _____
21 Easy to inflate

Down

2 Looks like a long box
3 Pressure reading when inspiration is held
6 Lagging of two associated phenomena
7 Another name for air trapping
9 When flow drops to zero at the end of inspiration, an inspiratory _____ is present
10 Control that adjusts the rate at which the flow valve opens
12 Nonelastic work
14 Type of volume curve
15 The flow-time curve is a straight line parallel to the x axis with a _____ flow
17 Another name for a graph
20 Two variables plotted against each other

Review Questions

1. Identify the scalar shapes in the following figure.

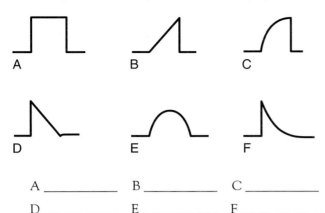

A _____ B _____ C _____

D _____ E _____ F _____

2. Monitored data used for calculations and graphic displays is obtained from what two places on a mechanical ventilator?

_____

_____

_____

_____

3. If the ventilator measures time and gas speed, how does it display volume?

_____

4. What two factors are determined by the pressure gradient between the ventilator and the lungs?

_____

5. As lung compliance increases, the pressure required to deliver the volume to the patient _____.
When lung compliance decreases, the pressure required to deliver the volume to the patient _____.

6. Complete the formula: P_{awo} = _____ + _____.

7. When does the flow-time curve run parallel to the x axis?

_____

8. Calculate the T_I in seconds when the volume is 600 mL and the flow rate is 60 L/min.

_____

_____

9. Calculate P_A when the delivered volume is 800 mL and static compliance is 25 mL/cm H_2O.

_____

10. Identify the labeled parts of the flow-time scalar in the following figure.

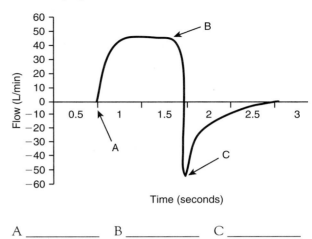

A _____ B _____ C _____

For questions 11 through 14, refer to the flow waveform in the following figure.

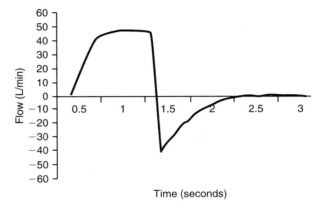

11. What type of flow waveform is represented in the preceding graph? _____

12. What is the peak inspiratory flow rate? _____

13. What is the peak expiratory flow rate? _____

14. What is the approximate inspiratory time? _____

15. _____ prevents the flow curve from returning to zero at the end of exhalation.

16. What would invalidate an auto-PEEP measurement?

_____

_____

17. At what point in the breath cycle does the auto-PEEP measurement occur?

_____

18. In the following figure, what is the reason for the increase in flow (point A) at the end of inspiration?

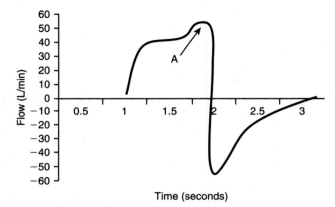

_____

19. What is the appropriate pressure trigger setting for an adult patient? _____

20. Dyssynchrony between the patient and the ventilator may be caused by inappropriate setting of which two parameters? _____

21. How does changing the flow pattern affect PIP during volume ventilation?

_____

For questions 22 through 28, refer to the pressure, volume, and flow curves for VC-CMV in the following graphs.

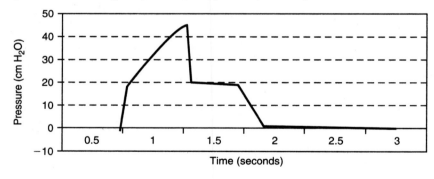

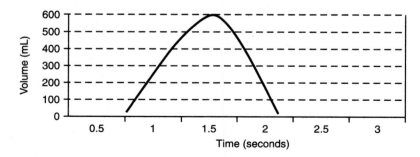

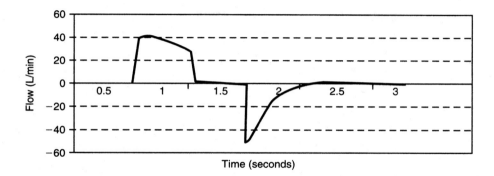

22. What is the PIP? _____

23. What is the set flow pattern and rate? _____

24. What is the tidal volume? _____

25. Calculate the static compliance. _____

26. Calculate the airway resistance.

_____

27. Is auto-PEEP present? _____

28. Why does the flow rate drop to zero before the end of inspiration?

_____

_____

29. During PCV the patient's lung compliance drops. How will this affect the delivered volume?

_____

30. During PC-CMV, why does flow return to zero before the end of inspiration?

_____

31. What type of flow waveform is used during PCV?

_____

32. When does the highest pressure gradient between the ventilator and the lungs occur?

_____

33. What parameters need to be set to deliver PSV?

_____

34. Identify the ventilator mode from the following figure.

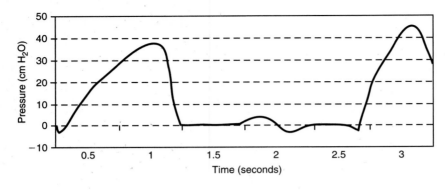

For questions 35 and 36, refer to the following figure.

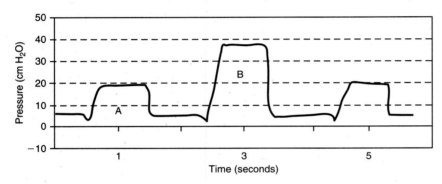

35. Identify the mode of ventilation. _____

36. Identify waves A and B. _____

37. Explain how automatic tube compensation works on inspiration and expiration.

    _____

    _____

38. If the peak flow rate for a PS breath is 45 L/min and the flow cycle percent is set at 25%, at what flow rate will inspiration end?

    _____

For questions 39 through 42, refer to the flow curve for a PSV breath in the following figure.

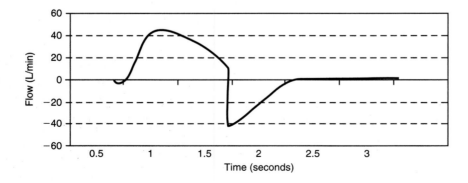

39. What is the T$_I$ for this breath? _____

40. What is the peak inspiratory flow rate for this breath? _____

41. At what flow rate did inspiration end? _____

42. What is the flow cycle percent setting? _____

_____

43. What is the peak expiratory flow rate? _____

44. Explain why a patient with COPD requires a higher flow cycle percent for PS breaths.

_____

_____

_____

45. Explain why a patient with stiff lungs gains the most benefit during PSV with a low flow cycle percent setting.

_____

_____

For questions 46 through 51, refer to the flow, pressure, and volume scalars represented below. The scalars labeled A are the flow, pressure, and volume scalars for a single ventilator breath. The scalars labeled B refer to a second ventilator breath.

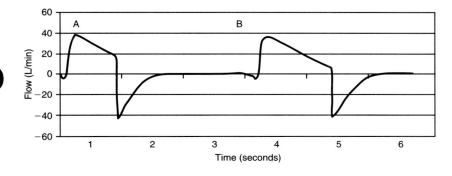

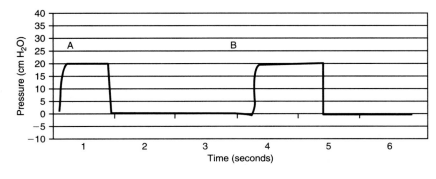

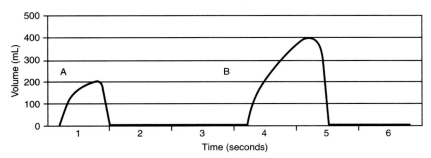

46. What is the approximate flow cycle percent in A? _____

47. What is the patient tidal volume in A? _____

48. What is the approximate flow cycle percent in B? _____

49. What is the patient tidal volume in B? _____

50. What are the approximate inspiratory times in breaths A and B? _____

51. Why is the T_I longer for B than for A?

_____

For questions 52 through 55, refer to the pressure-volume loop in the following figure.

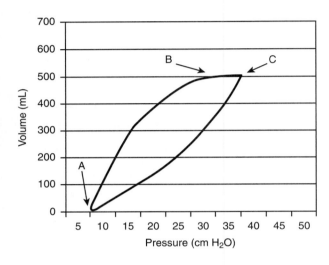

52. Identify points A, B, and C.

_____

53. What is the PIP? _____

54. What is the tidal volume? _____

55. Why does the loop begin and end at 5 cm H_2O? _____

56. What happens to a pressure-volume loop when lung compliance decreases during VC-CMV?

_____

_____

57. What happens to a pressure-volume loop when lung compliance decreases during PC-CMV?

_____

_____

58. What causes the pressure-volume loop to widen or bulge?

_____

For questions 59 through 64, refer to the pressure-volume loops in the following figure.

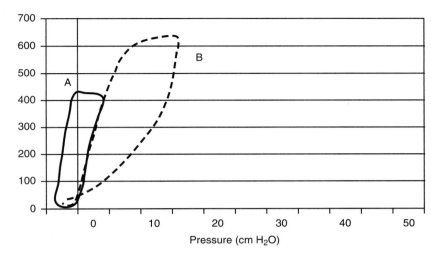

59. What type of breath does loop A represent? _____

60. In which direction does loop A move? Why?

    _____

61. What type of breath does loop B represent? _____

62. In which direction does loop B move? Why?

    _____

63. The set flow is 45 L/min; calculate the Raw.

    _____

64. The difference between the inspiratory and expiratory curves on a volume-pressure loop is called

    _____.

For questions 65 through 68, refer to the flow-volume loop in the following figure.

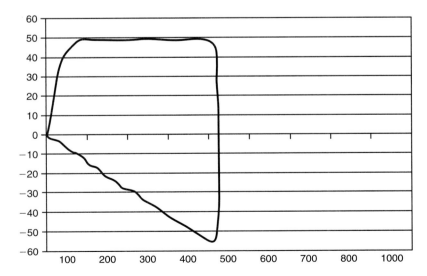

65. In which direction does this loop move? _____

66. What type of flow waveform is represented? _____

67. The set inspiratory flow rate is _____, and the peak expiratory flow rate is _____?

68. What is the tidal volume? _____

69. What can cause the expiratory side of a flow-volume loop to end at a volume above zero?

_____

70. What can cause a gap between the inspiratory side and expiratory side on the zero intercept of the y axis (flow) of a flow-volume loop?

_____

Critical Thinking Questions

For questions 1 through 8, refer to the following graphs:

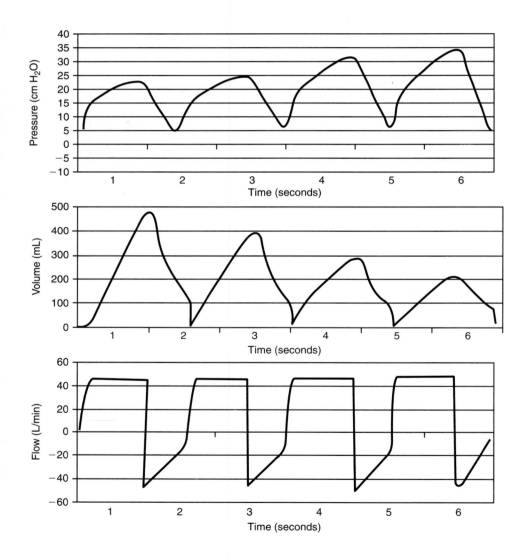

1. What mode of ventilation is being delivered?

   _____

2. Is this patient assisting?

   _____

3. What are the total cycle time, T_I, expiratory time, and set rate?

   _____

   _____

4. Describe the problem that is noticeable on the pressure-time curve.

   _____

5. Describe the two problems that are noticeable on the volume-time curve.

   _____

   _____

   _____

6. Describe the problem that is noticeable on the flow-time curve.

   _____

   _____

   _____

7. Taking into consideration the three scalars, what is causing these waveform problems?

   _____

   _____

   _____

   _____

8. What can be done to eliminate the cause of these problems?

   _____

   _____

Case Studies

Case Study #1

A 68-year-old female who is 63″ tall and weighs 120 lb was admitted through the emergency department with crushing chest pain. The patient has a history of COPD. Angiography was performed, and the patient subsequently underwent coronary artery bypass surgery. She now is in the cardiovascular ICU receiving mechanical ventilation. The following figure shows a current pressure-volume loop for this patient.

1. What accounts for the shape of this loop?

   _____

   _____

   _____

   _____

2. Is the patient triggering the ventilator? Explain.

   _____

   _____

   _____

3. What is the set tidal volume?

   _____

4. What is the PIP? _____

Blood is drawn for ABG analysis. The results are as follows: pH = 7.58, $PaCO_2$ = 45 mm Hg, PaO_2 = 65 mm Hg, SaO_2 = 95%, HCO_3^- = 40 mEq/L.

5. How should the ventilator settings be changed at this time?

_____

_____

_____

_____

_____

_____

Case Study #2

You are the respiratory therapist in the ICU of a large municipal hospital. During rounds you note the pressure-volume loop in the following figure for one of your patients.

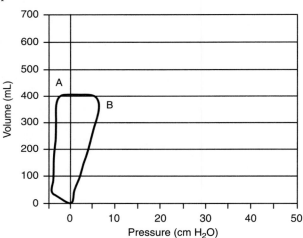

1. What type of breath is represented?

_____

2. The portion of the loop labeled A represents

_____.

3. The portion of the loop labeled B represents

_____.

4. This type of loop moves in what direction?

_____

5. Has PS been set for this patient? Explain.

_____

_____

_____

At the next patient-ventilator system check for this individual, the respiratory therapist notes the pressure-volume loop shown in the following figure.

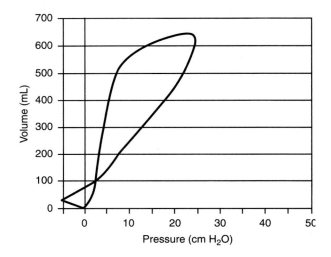

6. What type of ventilatory support is the patient receiving?

_____

7. Is the patient making some inspiratory effort?

_____

8. What ventilator adjustment is most appropriate for this patient at this time? Why?

_____

_____

The respiratory therapist changes the graphic display and now sees the graph shown in the following figure.

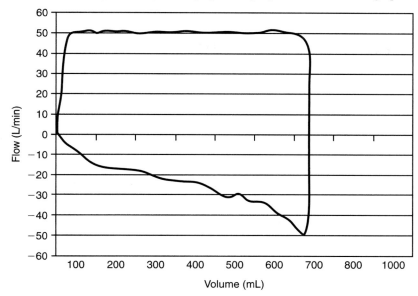

9. What data can be obtained from this loop?

_____

_____

An hour later the respiratory therapist receives an urgent page to come to this patient. The following figure shows the current flow-volume loop.

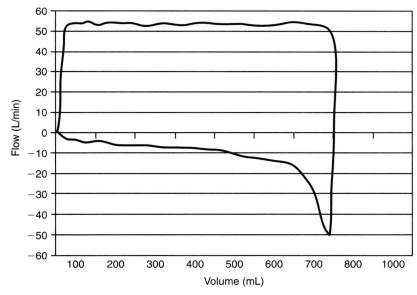

10. Explain the difference between the two flow-volume loops shown on this page.

_____

11. What is the most likely cause of this difference?

_____

12. What therapeutic intervention should the respiratory therapist recommend for this patient?

_____

NBRC–Style Questions

1. In the pressure-time scalar below, line A represents which of the following?

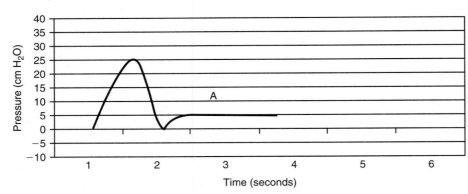

   a. Auto-PEEP
   b. $P_{plateau}$
   c. PS
   d. Transairway pressure

2. In the pressure-time scalar below, the difference between curve A and curve B is due to which of the following?

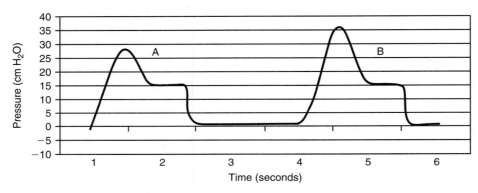

   I.   Atelectasis
   II. Bronchospasm
   III. Increased airway secretions
   IV. Pulmonary edema
   a. I and II
   b. I and III
   c. II and III
   d. II and IV

3. Using curve B in the figure above (question 2), calculate the Raw if the set inspiratory flow rate is 40 L/min.
   a. 0.5 cm H_2O/L/sec
   b. 2 cm H_2O/L/sec
   c. 30 cm H_2O/L/sec
   d. 52 cm H_2O/L/sec

4. The problem with the pressure-time scalar below is which of the following?

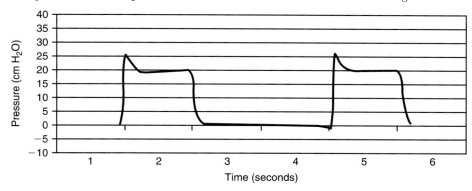

a. Patient is actively exhaling.
b. Pressure rise is too rapid.
c. Sensitivity setting is incorrect.
d. Inspiratory pause is too long.

5. Correction of the problem identified in question 4 includes which of the following?
a. Shorten the T_I
b. Reduce the sensitivity
c. Adjust the inspiratory slope
d. Eliminate the inspiratory pause

6. During PSV for a patient with COPD, the respiratory therapist notices a pressure increase toward the end of inspiration on the pressure-time scalar. This phenomenon can be corrected by which of the following?
a. Shorten the set inspiratory time
b. Increase the flow cycle percent
c. Lower the set PS level
d. Increase the inspiratory flow setting

7. A pressure-volume loop during VC-CMV extends farther to the right and flattens out with which of the following conditions?
a. Pneumonia
b. Bronchitis
c. Asthma
d. Emphysema

8. A flow-volume loop is incomplete because the volume does not return to zero. This can be caused by which of the following conditions?
a. Air trapping
b. Flow starvation
c. Bronchopleural fistula
d. Overdistention of alveoli

9. The pressure-time scalar for VC-CMV shown in the figure below demonstrates which of the following problems?

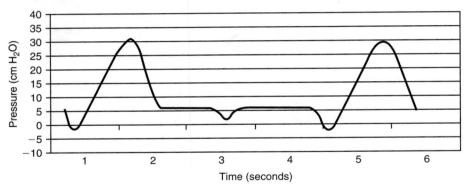

   a. Flow starvation
   b. Active exhalation
   c. Patient-ventilator dyssynchrony
   d. Incorrect sensitivity setting

10. The flow-volume loop for VC-CMV shown in figure below demonstrates which of the following problems?

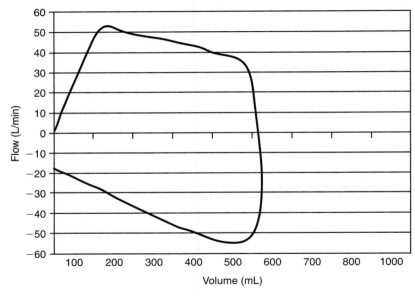

   a. Atelectasis
   b. Auto-PEEP
   c. Flow starvation
   d. Bronchopleural fistula

Helpful Internet Sites

- Kallet RH, Luce JM: Detection of patient-ventilator asynchrony during low tidal volume ventilation using ventilator waveform graphics. *Respir Care* 47, 2002. Available at www.rcjournal.com/contents/02.02/02.02.0183.asp
- Rittner F, Döring M: *Dräger: curves and loops in mechanical ventilation.* PDF format. Available at www.draeger-medical.com/MT/internet/pdf/CareAreas/CriticalCare/cc_loops_book_en.pdf

CHAPTER 11

Noninvasive Assessment of Respiratory Function

Learning Objectives

Upon completion of this chapter the reader will be able to do the following:

1. Describe the operating principle of the pulse oximeter.
2. Identify conditions that can influence the accuracy of pulse oximetry readings.
3. Name the test used to determine disparities between arterial oxygen saturation (SaO_2), oxygen saturation as measured by pulse oximetry (SpO_2), and the patient's clinical condition.
4. Discuss the normal components of a capnogram.
5. Give examples of pathophysiological conditions that can alter the contour of the capnogram.
6. Identify the normal value for the arterial-to-end tidal partial pressure of carbon dioxide ($P[a\text{-}et]CO_2$).
7. Describe the various components of a volumetric carbon dioxide (CO_2) tracing and discuss the ways such tracings can be used to assess gas exchange during mechanical ventilation.
8. Explain the theory of operation of $PtcO_2$ and $PtcCO_2$ monitors.
9. List the clinical data that should be recorded for transcutaneous measurements.
10. Describe the major components of an indirect calorimeter.
11. Provide the respiratory quotient values associated with substrate utilization patterns in healthy subjects.
12. Discuss some clinical applications of metabolic monitoring in critically ill patients.
13. Briefly describe devices used to measure airway pressure, volume, and flow during mechanical ventilation.
14. Calculate static compliance, dynamic compliance, airway resistance, and mean airway pressure.
15. Describe the effects of changes in airway resistance and respiratory system compliance on measurement of the work of breathing.
16. Identify pathological conditions that alter lung compliance and airway resistance.
17. Define the pressure-time product and discuss its application in the management of mechanically ventilated patients.

Key Terms Crossword Puzzle

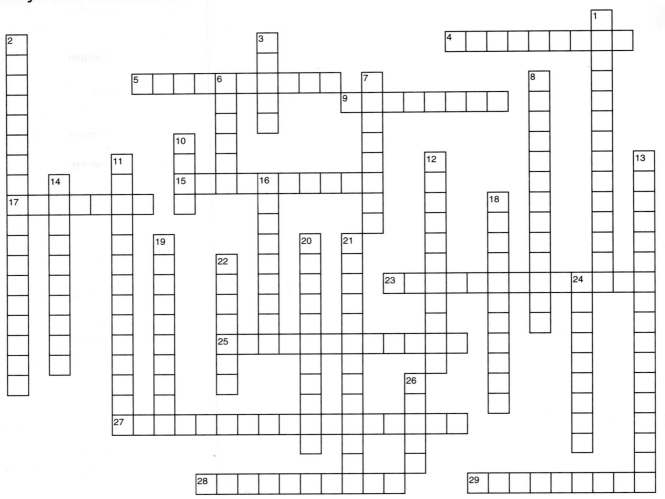

Across

4 Type of pressure measured by occluding the airway during the first 100 msec of spontaneous inspiration
5 Method of sampling respired gases
9 Type of dead space that is free of CO_2
15 Opposition to airflow
17 Type of pressure that reflects alveolar pressure
23 Continuous, noninvasive method of assessing arterial oxygen saturation (two words)
25 Qualitative estimates of exhaled CO_2 are made with a _____ detector.
27 Relies on the Beer-Lambert law

Down

1 Factor that affects pulse oximetry readings because of movement
2 Difference between gastric and esophageal pressures
3 Common problem when monitoring is done at the skin surface
6 Cause of an increase in the volume of CO_2 produced
7 An estimation of energy expenditure from measurements of oxygen consumption and CO_2 production is known as _____ calorimetry
8 States of low perfusion
10 Force times distance
11 Monitoring at the skin surface is known as _____ monitoring
12 Low perfusion state
13 Type of hemoglobin that has attached carbon monoxide
14 Type of device in which the analyzer is directly attached to the endotracheal tube

Across—Cont'd

28 Type of hemoglobin that is calculated by dividing the oxyhemoglobin concentration by the concentration of hemoglobin capable of carrying oxygen

29 Breakdown product of heme metabolism that causes yellow discoloration of the skin

Down—Cont'd

16 Shape of the oxyhemoglobin dissociation curve

18 Measurement of the CO_2 concentration in respired gases

19 Lung volume achieved for a given amount of applied pressure

20 Instrument accuracy depends on this.

21 Absorbs more light at 940 nm

22 Cyclical changes in light transmission allow _____ plethysmography to estimate the pulse rate.

24 Term for CO_2 at the end of the alveolar phase (hyphenated word)

26 Type of hemoglobin that absorbs both red and infrared light (abbreviation)

Review Questions

1. List five ways to monitor the respiratory function of mechanically ventilated patients noninvasively.

    _____

    _____

    _____

2. Name four causes of hypoxemic events in mechanically ventilated patients.

    _____

    _____

    _____

3. List four sites where a pulse oximetry sensor may be placed.

    _____

    _____

    _____

    _____

4. The two principles on which pulse oximetry is based

    are _____ and

    _____.

5. What is the Beer-Lambert law?

    _____

    _____

    _____

6. How are oxyhemoglobin and deoxyhemoglobin differentiated by pulse oximetry?

    _____

    _____

    _____

    _____

    _____

7. How is the pulse rate determined by a pulse oximeter?

    _____

    _____

    _____

    _____

    _____

8. What determines the accuracy of any diagnostic instrument?

    _____

9. What is the minimum oxygen saturation at which a pulse oximeter is accurate?

    _____

10. Identify four conditions that can influence the accuracy of pulse oximetry readings.

    _____

    _____

    _____

11. Give three factors that contribute to low perfusion states in patients.

_____

_____

12. Name the four types of hemoglobin typically found in adult blood.

_____

_____

13. What is the difference between fractional hemoglobin saturation and functional hemoglobin saturation?

_____

_____

_____

_____

_____

14. When COHb is present in the blood, the SpO_2 is

_____ .

15. The presence of MetHb in the blood is a complication of what two medications?

_____

16. What effect does MetHb have on SpO_2?

_____

_____

_____

17. How does nail polish affect SpO_2?

_____

_____

18. What effect does skin pigmentation have on SpO_2?

_____

19. What test is used to determine disparities among SpO_2, SaO_2, and the patient's clinical condition?

_____

20. The continuous display of CO_2 concentrations as a graphic waveform is called a _____ .

21. In what specific clinical situation would a chemical capnometer be particularly useful?

_____

_____

22. What effect does the presence of water vapor and nitrous oxide have on the accuracy of CO_2 measurements?

_____

_____

23. Describe the two methods of gas sampling used by IR analyzers.

_____

_____

_____

_____

_____

24. The normal percentage of CO_2 in expired air is

_____ .

25. Identify and explain the labeled parts of the capnogram in the following figure.

A _____

B _____

C _____

D _____

E _____

26. What determines the amount of CO_2 produced? Explain this process.

_____

_____

_____

_____

27. What pathophysiological conditions increase or decrease a patient's metabolic rate?

_____

_____

_____

28. What is the relationship between $P_{ET}CO_2$ and $PaCO_2$ in a healthy individual?

_____

29. What pathophysiological conditions cause a decrease in ventilation relative to perfusion, resulting in an abnormally high $P_{ET}CO_2$?

_____

_____

30. Where is the lowest $P_{ET}CO_2$ reading in the lungs found?

_____

31. What pathophysiological conditions cause a decrease in perfusion relative to ventilation, resulting in an abnormally low $P_{ET}CO_2$?

_____

_____

32. Name at least four pathophysiological conditions that can alter the contour of a capnogram.

_____

_____

_____

_____

33. What do the labeled capnogram waveforms in the following figure represent?

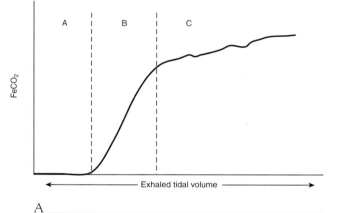

A _____

B _____

C _____

34. What pathological condition mimics esophageal intubation identified by capnography?

_____

_____

35. In what situations might the gastric PCO_2 be at an almost normal $P_{ET}CO_2$ level?

_____

_____

36. Measurement of CO_2 at the end of a forced vital capacity is called the

_____.

37. What should the $P(a\text{-}et)CO_2$ measurement be during normal tidal breathing?

_____

38. What are the x and y axes in a volumetric CO_2 tracing?

_____

_____

39. Identify and explain the phases represented by the letters in the volumetric CO_2 measurement in the following figure.

A _____

_____

B _____

_____

C _____

_____

40. Label all the blanks in the volumetric CO_2 measurement in the following figure.

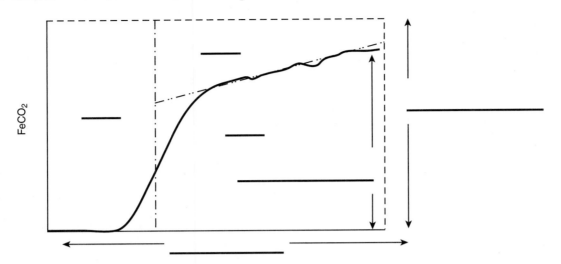

41. Explain the three areas of a volumetric CO_2 tracing.

_____

_____

_____

42. What four major events influence the way CO_2 is exhaled through the lungs?

_____

43. How can trending of VCO_2 be used during the weaning process?

_____

_____

44. What type of electrode is used in a transcutaneous oxygen monitor? _____

45. Why is the transcutaneous oxygen probe heated?

_____

_____

46. Transcutaneous oxygen monitoring is best suited to what type of patient? _____

47. List five causes of erroneous $PtcO_2$ readings.

_____

_____

_____

48. What type of electrode is used for transcutaneous CO_2 measurements? _____

49. What effect does heating of the transcutaneous CO_2 probe have on the measurements?

_____

50. How often should the transcutaneous electrode and sensor membrane be changed? _____

51. What steps need to be taken in placing a transcutaneous electrode on the patient's skin?

_____

52. The high and low values for a two-point calibration of a transcutaneous oxygen monitor are _____ _____ and _____.

53. The high and low values for a two-point calibration of a transcutaneous CO_2 monitor are _____ _____ and _____.

54. List the clinical data that should be documented for transcutaneous measurements.

_____

_____

_____

_____

_____

55. How often should a transcutaneous sensor be repositioned?

_____

56. What device is most commonly used to perform indirect calorimetry?

_____

57. Describe the major components of an indirect calorimeter.

_____

_____

_____

_____

_____

_____

_____

58. What position should the patient be in and for how long before an indirect calorimetric measurement is obtained?

_____

_____

59. The room temperature should be between _____ and _____ when indirect calorimetry readings are obtained.

60. Why is a urinary nitrogen level necessary for calculating energy expenditure?

_____

_____

_____

61. What is the EE of a healthy adult?

_____

62. A hypermetabolic state exists when the EE is _____; a hypometabolic state exists when the EE is _____.

63. List seven conditions that cause hypermetabolic states and five conditions that cause hypometabolic states.

_____

_____

_____

_____

_____

64. What is the RQ range for a healthy adult consuming a typical American diet? _____

65. The RQ for feedings of large amounts of glucose is _____ and for prolonged starvation is _____.

66. When CO_2 production increases, what happens to the RQ? _____

67. How can diet cause a patient to fail to wean from mechanical ventilatory support?

_____

_____

_____

_____

_____

68. The devices used to measure airway pressures in the current generation of adult and neonatal ventilators are _____.

69. What are the most common airway pressure measurements?

_____

70. Explain how a static pressure is obtained on newer ventilators.

_____

_____

71. What factors influence $P_{plateau}$?

_____

_____

72. What devices are used during mechanical ventilation to measure flow?

_____

_____

73. Which flow measuring device can be used to detect bidirectional flow?

_____

74. What potential problems can cause increases in PIP?

_____

_____

75. What is the formula for calculating mean airway pressure?

_____

_____

76. Calculate the $\overline{P}$aw for the following clinical data: PIP = 30 cm H_2O, PEEP = 5 cm H_2O, set respiratory rate = 12 breaths/min, T_I = 1 second.

_____

_____

77. Calculate the dynamic compliance for the following clinical data: PIP = 30 cm H_2O, PEEP = 5 cm H_2O, V_T = 550 mL, C_T = 2.5 mL/cm H_2O.

_____

_____

_____

_____

_____

78. Calculate static compliance for the following clinical data: $P_{plateau}$ = 28 cm H_2O, PEEP = 10 cm H_2O, V_T = 400 mL, C_T = 2 mL/cm H_2O.

_____

_____

_____

_____

79. Calculate airway resistance for the following clinical data: PIP = 35 cm H_2O, $P_{plateau}$ = 25 cm H_2O, flow rate = 50 L/min.

_____

_____

_____

_____

80. Work to overcome the normal elastic and resistive forces plus the work to overcome a disease process affecting normal workloads in the lung and thorax is known as

_____.

81. List five factors that increase extrinsic work of breathing.

_____

_____

82. Give the mathematical formula for the work of breathing.

_____

83. Explain how increased airway resistance affects work of breathing measurements.

_____

_____

_____

_____

84. How does a decrease in static compliance affect the patient's work of breathing?

_____

_____

_____

_____

_____

_____

85. List at least five pathological conditions associated with decreases in lung compliance.

_____

_____

_____

_____

86. What condition is associated with reductions in both C_S and C_D?

_____

87. What pathological conditions are associated with increases in airway resistance?

_____

_____

88. What is transdiaphragmatic pressure and how is it measured?

_____

_____

_____

_____

89. What is the pressure-time product?

_____

_____

90. What is occlusion pressure and how is it measured?

_____

_____

_____

_____

Critical Thinking Questions

1. Why does pulse oximetry become unreliable when dysfunctional hemoglobins (COHb and MetHb) are present in a patient's blood?

_____

_____

_____

_____

_____

_____

_____

_____

2. While trying to use a finger probe for pulse oximetry, the respiratory therapist finds that the pulse rate and the ECG monitor are not consistent and there is no SpO_2 reading. The patient is not wearing nail polish. What are the two most likely causes of this problem and what can be done to resolve them?

_____

_____

_____

_____

_____

_____

3. How do cardiac arrest and decreased cardiac output affect CO_2 detection?

_____

_____

_____

_____

4. A 48-year-old female patient who is 5′ 7″ and weighs 170 lb has a measured CO_2 production of 380 mL/min and oxygen consumption of 420 mL/min. Is this patient in a normal, a hypermetabolic, or a hypometabolic state?

_____

_____

Case Studies

Case Study #1

A respiratory therapist is assessing a patient receiving mechanical ventilatory support in the intensive care unit. The pulse oximeter shows an SpO_2 of 74%. The F_IO_2 is set at 0.4.

1. Is the pulse oximeter reading accurate? Why or why not?

_____

_____

_____

2. The patient's physician asks the respiratory therapist for a recommendation on which laboratory studies to order to clarify or confirm the pulse oximeter reading. What studies are appropriate for this patient at this time?

_____

_____

Case Study #2

A patient is brought to the emergency department after an apartment fire; he is receiving oxygen from a nonrebreathing mask. Because the patient has facial burns, he is intubated and placed on mechanical ventilatory support with 50% oxygen. The pulse oximeter is reading 99%.

1. Is the pulse oximeter reading accurate? Why or why not?

_____

_____

An ABG analysis shows an oxygen saturation of 95% on the 50% oxygen.

2. Is this saturation value accurate? Why or why not?

_____

_____

3. In this situation, what laboratory test should be suggested and why?

_____

_____

_____

Case Study #3

A patient is in the process of being weaned from mechanical ventilatory support; the SIMV mode is used with monitoring of $P_{ET}CO_2$. The respiratory therapist has just reduced the ventilator rate to 4 breaths/min; the set V_T is 500 mL. The following figure shows the tracings resulting from this change.

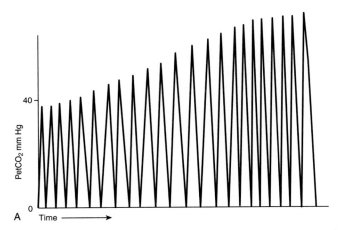

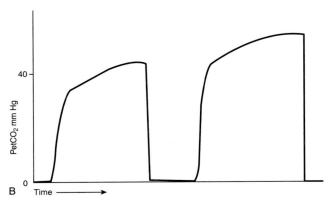

1. Analyze both the CO_2 trend (A) and waveform (B).

_____

_____

_____

2. What are the possible causes of the CO_2 trend (A)?

_____

_____

The respiratory therapist observes the patient using accessory muscles during spontaneous breathing. In addition, the spontaneous V_T is decreasing and the spontaneous respiratory rate is increasing.

3. How do these findings correlate with the $P_{ET}CO_2$ findings?

_____

_____

_____

_____

_____

4. How can the problem be resolved?

_____

_____

_____

Case Study #4

A respiratory therapist is monitoring the $P(a\text{-}et)CO_2$ difference for a patient with COPD receiving mechanical ventilatory support. Over the past 24 hours the $P(a\text{-}et)CO_2$ has risen from 5 to 18 mm Hg.

1. Is this an expected increase for a patient with COPD? Why or why not?

_____

_____

_____

2. What would a single breath CO_2 curve look like in this situation?

_____

_____

_____

NBRC–Style Questions

1. A pulse oximeter generally is considered accurate for oxygen saturations greater than which of the following?
   a. 65%
   b. 70%
   c. 75%
   d. 80%

2. A respiratory therapist encounters a patient whose pulse oximetry reading is 73%. The most appropriate action is which of the following?
   a. Change the sensor and move it to a different location
   b. Contact the patient's physician for further instructions
   c. Confirm the value with arterial blood CO-oximeter analysis
   d. Accept the value and document it in the patient's medical record

3. The response time of a pulse oximeter is most directly affected by which of the following?
   a. The type of pulse oximeter
   b. The location of the sensor or probe
   c. The percentage of oxygen saturation
   d. The position of the patient in the bed

4. The oxyhemoglobin concentration divided by the concentration of hemoglobin capable of carrying oxygen determines which of the following?
   a. Dysfunctional hemoglobin
   b. Fractional hemoglobin
   c. Functional hemoglobin
   d. Methemoglobin

5. On rounds a respiratory therapist encounters a patient receiving supplemental oxygen whose SpO_2 constantly displays 85%. The respiratory therapist notes that the patient is also receiving dapsone. Which of the following is the most appropriate action to take?
   a. Use an ear lobe probe to obtain more accurate readings
   b. Contact the patient's physician for further instructions
   c. Confirm the value with arterial blood CO-oximeter analysis
   d. Accept the value and document it in the patient's medical record

6. The $P_{ET}CO_2$ is read at what point on a capnogram?
   a. During phase 1
   b. End of phase 2
   c. During phase 3
   d. End of phase 4

7. The arterial to _maximum_ expiratory PCO_2 gradient is greatest for a patient with which of the following?
   a. COPD
   b. Asthma
   c. Left-heart failure
   d. Pulmonary embolism

8. The most reliable method of ruling out esophageal intubation is which of the following?
   a. Presence of CO_2 in the patient's exhaled gas
   b. Presence of condensation in the endotracheal tube
   c. Presence of bilateral breath sounds on auscultation
   d. Increased resistance to squeezing of the manual resuscitator bag

9. In cardiac arrest, a calorimetric CO_2 detector is most likely to display which of the following?
   a. <1% CO_2
   b. 1% to 2% CO_2
   c. 2% to 5% CO_2
   d. >5% CO_2

10. A respiratory therapist is called to the bedside of a patient who is being transcutaneously monitored for PO$_2$ and PCO$_2$. The signal is drifting and does not stabilize during calibration. The most appropriate action includes which of the following?
    I. Recalibrate the monitor with 15% and 20% CO$_2$
    II. Clean the electrode and change the sensor membrane
    III. Remove excess electrolyte solution from the electrode
    IV. Add a drop of electrolyte solution to the electrode surface
    a. I and II
    b. I and III
    c. II and IV
    d. III and IV

11. A difficult to wean patient with COPD has an RQ of 0.98. The most likely cause of this patient's inability to wean is which of the following?
    a. Reliance on lipid metabolism is causing hypoxemia.
    b. Lipogenesis is causing the patient to retain CO$_2$.
    c. A highly restricted carbohydrate metabolism is generating hypoxia.
    d. Excessive carbohydrates are overloading the patient's ventilatory reserve.

12. The tracing of a trending capnograph is not returning to zero with every exhalation. The most likely cause of this finding is which of the following?
    a. The F$_1$O$_2$ was decreased.
    b. The patient is hyperventilating.
    c. CO$_2$ is being rebreathed.
    d. The capnograph needs to be recalibrated.

13. A respiratory therapist monitoring a patient receiving mechanical ventilatory support finds that over the past 2 hours the patient's PIP has increased but the static pressure has remained stable. This could be caused by which of the following?
    a. Atelectasis
    b. Pneumothorax
    c. Retained secretions
    d. Right mainstem intubation

14. Intrinsic work of breathing is increased by which of the following?
    a. Bronchospasm
    b. Presence of an endotracheal tube
    c. Machine sensitivity
    d. Use of a heat and moisture exchanger

15. The pressure-volume curve in the following figure is indicative of which of the following?

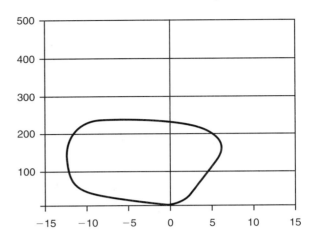

    a. Mechanical breath with little work of breathing
    b. Spontaneous breath under normal circumstances
    c. Spontaneous breath with high impedance to breathing
    d. Patient breathing through a freestanding CPAP system

Helpful Internet Sites

- Kodali B-S: Capnography: A comprehensive educational website. Harvard Medical School. Available at www.capnography.com/Physiology/PhysiologyM.htm
- Global Anesthesiology Server Network: Pulse oximetry (three scientific presentations and links to equipment). Available at www.gasnet.org/pomtp/index.php
- Thompson JE, Jaffe JB: Capnographic waveforms in the mechanically ventilated patient, *Respir Care* 50: Jan 2005. Available at www.rcjournal.com/contents/01.05/01.05.0100.pdf

CHAPTER 12

Hemodynamic Monitoring

Learning Objectives

Upon completion of this chapter the reader will be able to do the following:

1. Discuss the pressure, volume, and flow events that occur in the heart and great vessels during the cardiac cycle.
2. Describe the physiological events that produce heart sounds.
3. Discuss how changes in heart rate, preload, contractility, and afterload can alter cardiac function and cardiac output.
4. Identify indicators of left ventricular contractility.
5. Name the major components of a hemodynamic monitoring system.
6. Explain the proper technique for insertion and maintenance of a systemic arterial line and list the most common complications that can occur with this type of monitoring system.
7. Describe the procedures for insertion and placement of a central venous line and a balloon flotation, flow-directed pulmonary artery catheter and list potential complications associated with these devices.
8. Interpret the waveforms generated during the insertion of a pulmonary artery catheter.
9. Label the waveforms in a ventricular pressure–volume graph.
10. Calculate arterial and venous oxygen content, cardiac output, cardiac index, stroke index, cardiac cycle time, left ventricular stroke work index, right ventricular stroke work index, and pulmonary and systemic vascular resistance.
11. List normal values for measured and derived hemodynamic variables.
12. Describe the most common problems associated with pulmonary artery catheterization and discuss strategies for minimizing these complications.
13. Compare the effects of spontaneous and mechanical ventilation breathing on hemodynamic values.
14. Define the terms *incisura, pulse pressure, stroke index, stroke work, systemic vascular resistance, pulmonary vascular resistance,* and *ejection fraction.*
15. Explain the use of pulmonary capillary wedge pressure measurements for the evaluation of left ventricular function.
16. Differentiate between cardiogenic and noncardiogenic pulmonary edema using hemodynamic parameters.
17. Given a patient case, describe how hemodynamic monitoring can be used in the diagnosis and treatment of certain critically ill patients.

Key Terms Crossword Puzzle

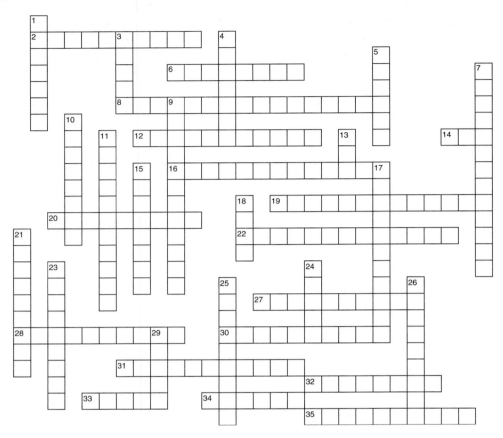

Across

2 The period between closure of the semilunar valves and opening of the AV valves is known as isovolumetric _____

6 Cardiac relaxation and filling

8 Ratio of the stroke volume to the ventricular end-diastolic volume

12 Stroke volume divided by body surface area (two words)

14 Left ventricle must pump against this resistance (abbreviation)

16 Contraction at the beginning of ventricular systole

19 Difference between the systolic and diastolic pressures (two words)

20 One of the atrioventricular valves

22 Pumping strength of the heart

27 The type of electrical circuit used in pressure transducers is known as a _____ bridge

28 Another name for atrial systole (two words)

30 Work done by the ventricle to eject a volume of blood into the aorta (two words)

31 Heart rate less than 60 beats/min

32 Decrease in atrial pressure that occurs as the AV valves open (two words)

33 Gradual ascent resulting from filling of the atria (two words)

34 Valve between the left atrium and left ventricle

35 Moving in the opposite direction

Down

1 Filling pressure of the ventricle at the end of ventricular diastole

3 Atrial systole on an atrial pressure tracing (two words)

4 Contraction that causes ejection of blood from the heart

5 Adult pulmonary artery catheters are available in size 7 or 8 _____

7 Type of catheter line that is inserted into the right atrium (two words)

9 Cardiac output divided by body surface area (two words)

10 Small negative deflection on the aortic and pulmonary artery tracing

11 Heart rate greater than 100 beats/min

13 Right ventricle must pump against this resistance (abbreviation)

15 Atrial contraction pressure drops, creating the _____ on the atrial pressure tracing (two words)

17 Quantification of the amount of pressure generated by the heart during systole (two words)

18 Principle used to calculate cardiac output

21 Flow-directed, multiple lumen catheter with a balloon tip (hyphenated word)

23 Impedance the left and right ventricles must overcome to eject blood into the great vessels

24 Wave that corresponds with atrial depolarization on an ECG (two words)

25 Long period of reduced filling of the heart

26 Both the aortic and pulmonary valves are this type of valve

29 Atrial pressure wave that coincides with the period of ventricular systole (two words)

Review Questions

1. List six common invasive hemodynamic measurements.

   _____

   _____

   _____

2. When the heart rate is 90 beats/min, how many seconds long is one cardiac cycle?

   _____

3. Which wave on the ECG corresponds with atrial depolarization?

   _____

4. Atrial depolarization is also called

   _____ .

5. What percentage of ventricular filling is due to atrial contraction?

   _____

6. In sequence, beginning with the atria, what is the order of events in a cardiac cycle?

   _____

   _____

   _____

7. During atrial systole, which heart valves are open and which are closed?

   _____

   _____

8. Ventricular systole begins with what event?

   _____

9. What produces S_1?

   _____

10. What produces S_2?

    _____

11. Identify and explain the different atrial waveforms in the following figure.

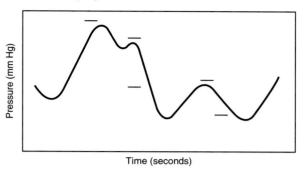

   _____

   _____

   _____

   _____

   _____

12. What four main factors influence the outputs of the right and left ventricle?

    _____

    _____

13. Define the term *preload*.

    _____

    _____

14. Describe how ventricular systole occurs.

    _____

    _____

    _____

    _____

15. What measurements are used to estimate RVEDP and LVEDP?

    _____

    _____

16. What do the systemic vascular resistance and the pulmonary vascular resistance reflect?

    _____

    _____

17. List the major components of a hemodynamic monitoring system.

_____

_____

_____

18. The mid-thoracic line of the patient is called the

_____ and is used to perform a

_____ on the transducer.

19. Why is positioning of the transducer important for accurate measurements?

_____

_____

_____

20. Explain the proper technique for insertion and the maintenance of a systemic arterial line.

_____

_____

_____

_____

21. What problems might occur with an arterial catheter line?

_____

_____

22. What type of fluid is used to flush an arterial line? What should the flow setting be?

_____

_____

23. What factors increase the risk of infection with an arterial line?

_____

_____

24. Why is prolonged or frequent flushing a problem for neonates and pediatric patients who weigh less than 20 kg?

_____

25. List the uses for a central venous line.

_____

_____

26. What pressure is estimated by a CVP measurement obtained at the end of ventricular diastole?

_____

_____

27. The veins most often used for insertion of a CVP line are _____

_____.

28. CVP measurements usually are obtained during which phase of breathing and with the patient in what position?

_____

_____

29. Common problems and potential complications of CVP insertion include

_____

_____.

30. The normal range for CVP is _____.

31. What are the pediatric and adult pulmonary artery catheter lengths and available sizes? How are they marked off for insertion purposes?

_____

_____

_____

32. How are clots prevented in a pulmonary artery catheter?

_____

_____

_____

33. Identify the structures lettered A through G on the four-channel pulmonary artery catheter in the following figure.

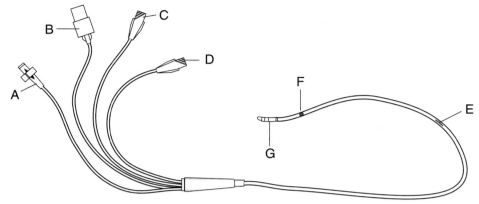

(From Hess DR, MacIntyre NR, Mishoe SC, et al: *Respiratory care: principles and practice*, Philadelphia, 2002, WB Saunders.)

A _____

B _____

C _____

D _____

E _____

F _____

G _____

34. List the insertion sites, both percutaneous and surgical cutdown, for a pulmonary artery catheter.

_____

_____

35. List at least eight complications associated with pulmonary artery catheterization and the cause of each.

_____

_____

_____

_____

_____

_____

_____

_____

_____

36. What are the two ways the catheter's position can be determined during insertion?

_____

37. Trace the insertion of a pulmonary artery catheter from an internal jugular vein to a pulmonary vein. When is the balloon inflated? Into which lung zone should the catheter be inserted?

_____

_____

_____

38. Explain why the pulmonary artery catheter needs to be placed in the lung zone you chose in question 37.

_____

_____

_____

39. What are the pressure relationships in each lung zone?

    Zone   **Pressure Relationship**

      1   _____

      2   _____

      3   _____

40. The volume of an adult PAC balloon is _____; the balloon should be inflated for only _____ seconds when PAWP is measured.

41. Identify the position of the catheter represented by the letters A through D in the PAC waveforms in the following figure.

    A _____

    B _____

    C _____

    D _____

42. How are the following common problems with pulmonary artery catheterization minimized?

    (a) Ventricular arrhythmias _____

    (b) Pulmonary artery infarction _____

    (c) Pulmonary artery rupture _____

    (d) Balloon rupture _____

43. Explain the relationship between heart rates above 200 to 220 beats/min and a decrease in cardiac output.

_____

44. What happens to the systemic arterial diastolic pressure when vasoconstriction occurs?

_____

45. Arterial systolic and diastolic pressures are affected by _____ and _____.

46. When in the breathing cycle is pulmonary artery pressure measured?

_____

47. How does PEEP or auto-PEEP above 15 cm H_2O affect PAWP?

_____

_____

48. Name three pathological conditions that can increase pulmonary vascular resistance and subsequently the pulmonary artery pressure.

_____

49. What does inhaled nitric oxide alter in the pulmonary vasculature?

_____

50. Compare the effects of spontaneous breathing and mechanical ventilation on the pulmonary artery pressure.

_____

_____

51. Complete the table below with the appropriate hemodynamic values.

Parameter	Normal Value
Arterial blood pressure	_____
Mean arterial pressure	_____
Pulse pressure	_____
Central venous pressure	_____
Pulmonary artery pressure	_____
Pulmonary artery wedge pressure	_____

52. Complete the following chart with the formulas used to calculate each parameter.

Parameter	Formula	Normal Value
Cardiac output	_____	_____
Cardiac index	_____	_____
Stroke index	_____	_____
Arterial oxygen content	_____	_____
Mixed venous oxygen content	_____	_____
Systemic vascular resistance	_____	_____
Pulmonary vascular resistance	_____	_____

53. What are the effects of the following factors on cardiac output?

Factor	Effect on Cardiac Output
Tachycardia	_____
Beta-adrenergic blockade	_____
Increased parasympathetic tone	_____
Increased preload and contractility	_____
Bradyrhythmias	_____
Decreased parasympathetic tone	_____

In questions 54 through 57, calculate the oxygen content for the information provided.

54. PaO_2 = 43 mm Hg, SaO_2 = 75%, Hb = 10 gm%

_____

55. PaO_2 = 64 mm Hg, SaO_2 = 94%, Hb = 13 gm%

_____

56. $P\bar{v}O_2 = 40$ mm Hg, $S\bar{v}O_2 = 75\%$, Hb = 15 gm%

_____

_____

57. $P_vO_2 = 70$ mm Hg, $S_vO_2 = 85\%$, Hb = 16 gm%

_____

_____

58. Explain why mixed venous oxygen values decrease when cardiac output is reduced.

_____

_____

_____

59. What are the two most important factors that influence vascular resistance? Give examples of each.

_____

_____

_____

60. How do alveolar hypoxia and high intraalveolar pressures affect pulmonary vascular resistance?

_____

_____

61. List at least three mathematically derived indicators of left ventricular contractility.

_____

_____

Critical Thinking Questions

1. Explain how measurements of pulmonary capillary wedge pressure can be used to evaluate left ventricular function.

_____

_____

_____

_____

_____

_____

_____

_____

_____

2. Differentiate between cardiogenic and noncardiogenic pulmonary edema using hemodynamic parameters.

_____

_____

_____

_____

_____

_____

_____

_____

_____

_____

_____

3. Match the following terms with the appropriate letter or line number on the ventricular pressure-volume loop shown in the figure below.

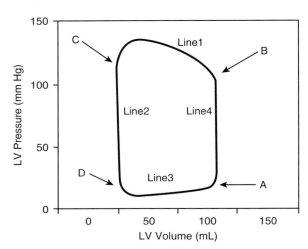

_____ Aortic valve closing   _____ Aortic valve opening

_____ Mitral valve closing   _____ Mitral valve opening

_____ Ventricular ejection   _____ Ventricular filling

_____ Isovolumetric contraction _____ Isovolumetric relaxation

4. What conditions can lead to an increased pulse pressure and a decreased pulse pressure?

_____

_____

_____

_____

_____

_____

Case Studies

Case Study #1

A 53-year-old male who is 6' tall and weighs 195 lb was admitted for head trauma caused by a motor vehicle accident. A craniotomy was performed to relieve pressure. He currently is in the surgical intensive care unit receiving mechanical ventilation with VC-SIMV; the rate is 8 breaths/min, the V_T is 800 mL, and the F_IO_2 is 0.6. The patient is receiving dobutamine and nitroprusside. A PAC is inserted, and the following information is collected:

PAP 38/20 mm Hg	PAWP 10 mm Hg	Cardiac output 5.1 L/min
CVP 12 mm Hg	SBP 145/68 mm Hg	HR 92 beats/min
Hb 12.6 gm%		

	Arterial Blood Gas Values	Mixed Venous Blood Gas Values
pH	7.46	7.38
PCO_2	32 mm Hg	43 mm Hg
PaO_2	100 mm Hg	40 mm Hg
SaO_2	99%	75%

Calculate the following values and indicate whether each is normal, high, or low.

1. Pulse pressure _____

2. Stroke volume _____

3. Stroke index _____

4. Cardiac index _____

5. Mean arterial pressure _____

6. Mean pulmonary artery pressure _____

7. SVR _____

8. PVR _____

9. CaO_2 _____

10. $C\bar{v}O_2$ _____

11. $Ca\text{-}\bar{v}O_2$ _____

12. DO_2 _____

13. VO_2 _____

14. RVSW _____

15. RVSWI _____

16. LVSW _____

17. LVSWI _____

18. Comment on the patient data.

_____

_____

_____

_____

_____

_____

_____

Case Study #2

The respiratory therapist is monitoring a patient who is receiving mechanical ventilatory support in one of the intensive care units. Hemodynamic monitoring is being considered because of the concern that the patient's condition is very unstable.

1. What aspect of hemodynamic monitoring should the respiratory therapist suggest for this patient?

_____

_____

The hemodynamic monitoring system is now in place. The catheter was placed via the subclavian route about 1 hour ago. The patient is showing signs of respiratory distress, and breath sounds are absent on the right side.

2. What complication is most likely causing this clinical situation?

_____

_____

3. What is the most likely cause of this complication?

_____

_____

After correction of the problem, the PAWP is 12 mm Hg. However, as the day progresses, the pressure rises to 20 mm Hg and then over the next few hours to 28 mm Hg, where it stabilizes.

4. What is the significance of this finding?

_____

_____

NBRC–Style Questions

1. The respiratory therapist is assisting a physician who is inserting a PAC. The respiratory therapist notes that a damped waveform is displayed on the oscilloscope. This indicates which of the following?
   a. The catheter is not wedged.
   b. The balloon is deflated, and the catheter is not wedged.
   c. The balloon may still be inflated, or the catheter may be wedged.
   d. The balloon is deflated, and the catheter has perforated the right ventricle.

2. The PAWP value most indicative of cardiogenic pulmonary edema is which of the following?
   a. 8 mm Hg
   b. 12 mm Hg
   c. 18 mm Hg
   d. 25 mm Hg

3. The pressure measured from the proximal lumen of a PAC is which of the following?
   a. PAP
   b. RAP
   c. RVP
   d. PAWP

4. The position of a pulmonary catheter is verified by which of the following?
   a. Checking the pressure waveform
   b. Checking the number of centimeters inserted
   c. Obtaining a blood sample through the catheter tip
   d. Obtaining a chest radiograph for catheter tip placement

5. The third lumen of a PAC is used to measure which of the following?
   a. Cardiac output
   b. CVP
   c. PAP
   d. PCWP

6. A low CVP value is indicative of which of the following?
   a. Shock, dehydration, or hemorrhage
   b. Shock, overhydration, or hemorrhage
   c. Hypertension, dehydration, or hypervolemia
   d. Hypertension, overhydration, and hypovolemia

7. The most common long-term complications of systemic arterial catheterization include which of the following?
   a. Hemorrhage and spasm of the artery
   b. Cardiac valve stenosis and prolapse
   c. Arterial laceration and subsequent hemorrhage
   d. Infection and tissue ischemia distal to the catheter

8. The proper location for the distal tip of a central venous catheter is in which of the following?
   a. Left ventricle or aorta
   b. Vena cava or right atrium
   c. Right ventricle or pulmonary artery
   d. Pulmonary artery or pulmonary capillary

9. Preload of the left ventricle may be estimated by which of the following measurements?
   a. RAP
   b. CVP
   c. PAP
   d. PAWP

10. The cardiac index is increased by which of the following?
    a. Shock
    b. Exercise
    c. Hypovolemia
    d. Cardiac failure

11. Calculate the cardiac output when the stroke volume is 65 mL and the heart rate is 76 beats/min.
    a. 4.9 L/min
    b. 4.6 L/min
    c. 4.5 L/min
    d. 4.3 L/min

12. Left ventricular end-diastolic volume is represented by what amount of blood?
    a. The amount ejected by the ventricle during systole
    b. The amount ejected by the ventricle during diastole
    c. The amount in the ventricle at the beginning of diastole
    d. The amount remaining in the ventricle at the end of diastole

13. The c wave on an arterial pressure tracing represents which of the following?
    a. Closing of the bicuspid valves
    b. Opening of the bicuspid valves
    c. Closing of the semilunar valves
    d. Opening of the semilunar valves

14. An increase in pulmonary vascular resistance causes which of the following?
    a. Increased right-heart afterload
    b. Increased right-heart preload
    c. Increased left-heart afterload
    d. Increased left-heart preload

15. Which of the following values indicates a patient problem?
    a. PVR = 225 dynes/sec/cm^{-5}
    b. CI = 3.8 L/min/m^2
    c. SVR = 550 dynes/sec/cm^{-5}
    d. DO$_2$ = 950 mL/min

Helpful Internet Sites

- American Association of Critical Care Nurses, American Association of Nurse Anesthetists, American College of Chest Physicians, American Society of Anesthesiologists, American Thoracic Society, National Heart Lung Blood Institute, Society of Cardiovascular Anesthesiologists, Society of Critical Care Medicine: Pulmonary artery catheter education project (see First Time Visitors). Available at www.pacep.org/pages/start/ref.html?xin=accp

Methods to Improve Ventilation and Other Techniques in Patient-Ventilator Management

Learning Objectives

Upon completion of this chapter the reader will be able to do the following:

1. Recommend ventilator adjustments to reduce work of breathing and improve ventilation based on the patient's diagnosis, arterial blood gas results, and ventilator parameters.
2. Calculate the appropriate suction catheter size and the length and amount of suction pressure needed for a specific size endotracheal tube and patient.
3. Compare the benefits of closed-suction catheters to the open-suction technique.
4. Discuss the pros and cons of instilling normal saline to loosen secretions before suctioning.
5. Explain how silent aspiration and ventilator-associated pneumonia can occur even with a cuffed endotracheal tube.
6. Describe the endotracheal tube that can provide continuous aspiration of subglottic secretions.
7. Based on sputum description and physical findings in a patient, provide a possible cause for findings.
8. List the parameters that are useful in establishing the presence of a respiratory infection.
9. Describe the procedure for prone positioning in ventilated patients with adult respiratory distress syndrome.
10. List potential problems associated with placing the patient in a prone position.
11. Discuss some of the theories about how ventilation-perfusion is improved with prone positioning in adult respiratory distress syndrome.
12. Compare the protocols for the use of metered dose inhalers and small volume nebulizers during mechanical ventilation.
13. Recognize the complications associated with the use of small volume nebulizers powered by external flowmeters during mechanical ventilation.
14. Recommend a change in medication based on the patient's response to a beta-agonist during mechanical ventilation.
15. Explain the equipment needed for in-house transport of a mechanically ventilated patient.
16. Identify complications associated with in-house transport of a mechanically ventilated patient.
17. Describe patient-centered mechanical ventilation and how it might be assessed by the respiratory therapist.

Key Terms Crossword Puzzle

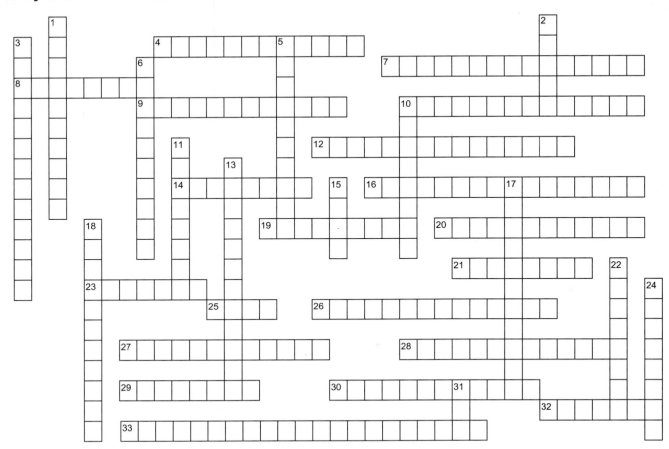

Across

4 "Out of step" with the ventilator
7 In PCV, increasing _____ can increase volume delivery without an increase in pressure (two words)
8 Reduced urine output
9 Enteral feeding route that reduces the risks of vomiting and aspiration
10 Instillation of this solution is probably more effective than saline lavage.
12 Overactive thyroid
14 Respiratory acidosis indicates that this type of ventilation is not adequate.
16 In mechanically ventilated patients, _____ is often the cause of respiratory alkalosis.
19 Ventilation without perfusion (two words)
20 Procedure for visualizing the bronchi
21 Excessive urine output
23 Type of bag historically used to collect a patient's expired air

Down

1 An overdose of this causes a metabolic acidosis.
2 _____ can increase metabolism and carbon dioxide production.
3 Preventative
5 Complication of suctioning
6 Intentionally or purposefully brought about
10 Another name for air trapping (two words)
11 _____ can cause loss of bicarbonate and lead to metabolic acidosis.
13 Blood condition caused by fluid retention (overhydration)
15 Reduces the risk of VAP by removing secretions above the cuff of the ET (abbreviation)
17 Type of cardiac arrhythmia generally attributed to hypoxemia
18 Carinal stimulation with a suction catheter causes this
22 Deficient blood flow to cells
24 Rigid tonsil suction tip
31 Using this aerosol administration device may require dose doubling for ventilator patients (abbreviation)

Across—Cont'd

25 Type of ventilatory support used for an apneic patient

26 Procedure that must be done before and after ET suctioning

27 Metabolic acidosis brought on by alcoholism, starvation, or diabetes

28 Powerful cerebral vessel vasodilator

29 Preprocedural medication used to reduce secretion production and dry the airways

30 Type of therapy used to draw cerebral edema fluid from the brain tissue

32 Fluid filled with cellular debris and protein that accumulates as a result of inflammation

33 Deliberate limitation of ventilatory support to prevent lung injury (two words)

Review Questions

1. Calculate the desired V_T when the known $PaCO_2$ is 55 mm Hg, the known V_T is 500 mL, the known frequency is 14 breaths/min, and the desired $PaCO_2$ is 40 mm Hg.

     _____
     _____
     _____
     _____

2. Calculate the desired frequency when the known $PaCO_2$ is 65 mm Hg, the known V_T is 600 mL, the known frequency is 12 breaths/min, and the desired $PaCO_2$ is 50 mm Hg.

     _____
     _____
     _____
     _____

3. What three factors can affect $PaCO_2$ in patients receiving mechanical ventilation?

     _____
     _____
     _____

4. Identify three ABG components that reflect a patient's ventilatory status.

     _____

5. When the $PaCO_2$ is elevated, the pH is _____ (increased; decreased) because of a (an) _____ (increase; decrease) in alveolar ventilation.

6. Match the pathological process with the appropriate disease.

     ____ Parenchymal lung problem   (a) Asthma
     ____ Airway disease   (b) Drug overdose
     ____ Pleural abnormalities   (c) Myasthenia gravis
     ____ Central nervous system problems   (d) Effusions
     ____ Neuromuscular disorders   (e) Pneumonia

7. Whether in volume or pressure ventilation, an increase in V_T results in a (an) _____ (increase; decrease) in $PaCO_2$ and a (an) _____ (increase; decrease) in pH.

8. The average range for V_T is _____ of ideal body weight.

9. When increasing the V_T, it is important to maintain $P_{plateau}$ below _____.

10. List two methods of increasing V_T in pressure control ventilation.

     _____
     _____

11. Respiratory alkalosis can be defined as a $PaCO_2$ _____ (less than; greater than) 35 mm Hg with a pH _____ (less than; greater than) 7.45; respiratory alkalosis is the result of a (an) _____ (increase; decrease) in alveolar ventilation.

12. List seven common causes of respiratory alkalosis.

_____

_____

_____

_____

_____

13. A patient with a $PaCO_2$ of 25 mm Hg and a pH of 7.55 is sedated and ventilated in a volume-controlled mode. The IBW is 60 kg. The frequency is set at 16 breaths/min, and the delivered V_T is set at 10 mL/kg. What frequency would result in a $PaCO_2$ of 40 mm Hg?

_____

_____

_____

14. Is it more appropriate to change the frequency or the V_T to correct a respiratory alkalosis when the delivered volume is set at less than 10 mL/kg? Explain your answer.

_____

_____

_____

15. For a patient on VC-CVM, the frequency is set at 10 breaths/min, and the total respiratory rate is 20 breaths/min. The $PaCO_2$ is 25 mm Hg with a pH of 7.52. Will decreasing the set rate correct the respiratory alkalosis? Explain your answer.

_____

_____

16. Referring to question 15, what modes of ventilation will not deliver the set V_T with every inspiratory effort?

_____

17. List six common causes of hyperventilation in patients receiving mechanical ventilation.

_____

_____

_____

18. What is the body's physiological response to a metabolic acidosis?

_____

_____

19. Identify six causes of metabolic acidosis and give an example of each.

_____

_____

_____

_____

_____

_____

20. A metabolic alkalosis can be defined as a pH between _____ and _____ and a bicarbonate level of _____.

21. List five common causes of metabolic alkalosis.

_____

_____

_____

_____

22. By what mechanism would an increase in physiological dead space affect pH?

_____

_____

23. Give two examples of pathological processes that would result in an increase in physiological dead space.

_____

_____

24. (a) Give the normal range for the V_D/V_T ratio.

    _____

    (b) Calculate the V_D/V_T ratio based on the following information:

    V_T = 800 mL, $PaCO_2$ = 45 mm Hg, $P_{\bar{E}}CO_2$ = 36 mm Hg

    _____

    _____

    _____

    _____

25. List eight clinical disorders which may result in a hypermetabolic state.

    _____

    _____

    _____

    _____

26. Hyperventilation _____
    (reduces; increases) CO_2 in the blood, resulting in
    _____ (expansion; constriction)
    of cerebral blood vessels and _____
    (increased; decreased) blood flow to the brain.

27. Define the term *permissive hypercapnia*.

    _____

    _____

    _____

28. Permissive hypercapnia in the presence of cerebral edema or increased intracranial pressure is _____
    _____ (contraindicated;
    absolutely contraindicated), and _____
    _____ (contraindicated; absolutely
    contraindicated) in the presence of an intracranial lesion.

29. Match the range of suction pressure with the appropriate patient.

Patient	Suction Pressure
___ Adult	(a) −60 to −100 mm Hg
___ Child	(b) −100 to −120 mm Hg
___ Infant	(c) −80 to −100 mm Hg

30. Suction time must not exceed _____ seconds, and suction should be applied _____ (intermittently; continually).

31. Estimate the correct suction catheter size for a size 9.5 Fr ET.

    _____

32. List seven indications for tracheal suctioning of mechanically ventilated patients, as stated in the AARC Clinical Practice Guidelines.

    _____

    _____

    _____

    _____

    _____

    _____

    _____

33. List the contraindication(s) to suctioning.

    _____

34. Match the complication with its most likely cause.

Complication	Cause
___ Hypoxemia/hypoxia	(a) Suction pressures
___ Tracheal/mucosal trauma	(b) Reduction in lung volume
___ Cardiac/respiratory arrest	(c) Airway trauma
___ Cardiac arrhythmias	(d) Patient or caregiver
___ Atelectasis	(e) Hypoxemia/vagal stimulation
___ Bronchospasm	(f) Extreme response to suctioning and disconnection from the ventilator
___ Infection	(g) Ventilator disconnection and loss of PEEP
___ Bleeding	(h) Reaction to tracheal stimulation

35. (a) Hyperoxygenation *before* suctioning should be achieved with what F_IO_2, and how long should it be performed?

_____

(b) Hyperoxygenation *after* suctioning should be achieved with what F_IO_2, and how long should it be performed?

_____

36. List the advantages and disadvantages of in-line suction catheters.

Advantages	Disadvantages
_____	_____
_____	_____
_____	_____
_____	_____
_____	_____
_____	_____
_____	_____
_____	_____
_____	_____

37. List the indications for use of an in-line suction catheter.

_____
_____
_____
_____
_____
_____
_____
_____
_____
_____
_____
_____
_____
_____
_____

38. List four conditions that may lead to silent aspiration and ventilator-associated pneumonia (VAP).

_____
_____
_____
_____

39. Explain how silent aspiration and VAP occur.

_____
_____
_____
_____

40. Name and describe the type of ET that can provide continuous aspiration of subglottic secretions (CASS).

_____
_____
_____
_____

41. Referring to question 40, what is the major advantage of using this type of tube?

_____
_____

42. List the advantages and disadvantages of instillation of normal saline before suctioning.

Advantages	Disadvantages
_____	_____
_____	_____
_____	_____
_____	_____
_____	_____

43. Name the two alternatives to instillation of saline that can help facilitate suctioning.

_____
_____

44. Which factors may serve as indicators of the effectiveness of a suctioning procedure?

_____
_____

45. What parameters should be monitored before, during, and after suctioning?

_____

_____

_____

_____

_____

46. (a) List five aerosolized medications that can be administered to mechanically ventilated patients.

_____

_____

(b) List the two most common methods of administering an aerosol for ventilated patients.

_____

47. Under what circumstance should a small-volume nebulizer be used instead of an MDI to deliver aerosolized medication to a patient receiving mechanical ventilation?

_____

_____

_____

48. Give nine factors that affect aerosol deposition when an SVN is used during mechanical ventilation.

_____

_____

_____

_____

_____

49. List five possible complications with use of an SVN powered by a continuous gas source.

_____

_____

_____

_____

_____

50. What steps can be taken to reduce the risk of infection when an in-line SVN is used?

_____

_____

_____

51. What three factors would optimize aerosol deposition of bronchodilators during noninvasive positive pressure ventilation?

_____

_____

_____

52. List four methods of monitoring the effectiveness of bronchodilator therapy.

_____

_____

_____

_____

53. If a mechanically ventilated patient's condition improves after bronchodilator therapy, what should happen with the following factors?

PIP _____

P_{TA} _____

PEFR _____

54. What is the goal of chest physiotherapy?

_____

55. Chest physiotherapy includes what two procedures?

_____

_____

56. List the sequence of four recommended positions that aids the clearance of secretions.

_____

_____

_____

_____

57. List the possible hazards of performing chest physiotherapy on patients requiring mechanical ventilation.

_____

_____

58. List the four channels found in a flexible fiberoptic bronchoscope and the purpose of each.

_____

_____

_____

_____

59. List the indications and contraindications for flexible fiberoptic bronchoscopy.

Indications	Contraindications
_____	_____
_____	_____
_____	_____
_____	_____
_____	_____
_____	_____
_____	_____
_____	_____
_____	_____
_____	_____
_____	_____
_____	_____
_____	_____
_____	_____
_____	_____

60. Give the three indications for frequent body position changes in mechanically ventilated patients.

_____

_____

_____

61. Why is an ARDS patient placed in the prone position?

_____

_____

62. List six mechanisms believed to improve oxygenation with prone positioning.

_____

_____

_____

_____

_____

_____

_____

63. Match the type of contraindication to placing a patient in the prone position with the pathological process.

Pathological Process	Type of Contraindication
___ Hemodynamic instability	(a) Absolute contraindication
___ Arrhythmias	(b) Strong relative contraindication
___ Thoracic or abdominal surgery	(c) Relative contraindication
___ Spinal cord instability	

64. (a) Describe the five steps for placing a patient in the prone position.

_____

_____

_____

_____

(b) Once the patient is in the prone position, what steps should be taken?

_____

_____

_____

65. List six potential problems associated with placing a patient in a prone position.

_____

_____

_____

_____

66. Identify two methods of improving the ventilatory status of patients with unilateral lung disease.

_____

_____

_____

67. List four indications for changing a ventilator circuit.

_____

_____

_____

_____

68. Match the sputum characteristic with the possible cause.

Characteristic	Possible Cause
___ Yellow	(a) Old blood
___ Green, thick	(b) *Klebsiella* infection
___ Green, foul smelling	(c) Pulmonary edema
___ Pink tinged	(d) Sputum has been in airway for long time.
___ Fresh blood	(e) *Pseudomonas* infection
___ Brown	(f) May indicate new bleeding or may occur after treatment with aerosolized epinephrine or racemic epinephrine
___ Rust colored	
___ Pink, copious, and frothy or emboli	(g) Presence of pus (WBCs) and possible infection
	(h) Airway trauma, pneumonia, pulmonary infarction

69. (a) Define the term *oliguria*.

_____

(b) Define the term *polyuria*.

_____

70. List six factors that may result in a decrease in urine output.

_____

_____

_____

_____

_____

_____

_____

_____

71. For a patient receiving PPV, the effects of $\bar{P}aw$ can be a (an) _____ (increase; decrease) in cardiac output and a (an) _____ (increase; decrease) in plasma ADH.

72. Describe the objective of patient-centered mechanical ventilation.

_____

_____

_____

_____

73. (a) List the equipment needed for in-house transport of a mechanically ventilated patient.

_____

_____

_____

(b) List the capabilities a transport ventilator should have to ensure patient safety.

_____

_____

_____

74. List four contraindications to in-house transport of a mechanically ventilated patient.

_____

_____

_____

_____

75. Identify 10 hazards and complications associated with in-house transport of a mechanically ventilated patient.

_____

_____

_____

_____

_____

_____

_____

_____

_____

_____

Critical Thinking Questions

1. A patient is being ventilated in a volume-controlled mode. The set V_T is 700 mL and the frequency is 10 breaths/min. The $P_{plateau}$ is 45 cm H_2O, and the $PaCO_2$ is 60 mm Hg. The physician would like to reduce the $PaCO_2$ to 40 mm Hg, but does not want to increase the V_T because of the high $P_{plateau}$. What can the therapist do to reduce the $PaCO_2$ to 40 mm Hg?

_____

_____

_____

_____

_____

_____

_____

2. A postsurgical patient who had multiple traumatic injuries is septic and has a temperature of 40° C. The patient is being ventilated in a volume-controlled mode. The V_T is 800 mL; the set frequency is 15 breaths/min and the patient is triggering to 25 breaths/min. ABG analysis reveals a $PaCO_2$ of 38 mm Hg and a PaO_2 of 42 mm Hg. Why does the patient have a normal $PaCO_2$ with a minute ventilation of 20 L/min?

_____

_____

_____

_____

_____

_____

3. A patient in respiratory distress is intubated and placed on pressure control ventilation with a PEEP of 5 cm H_2O. Soon after, the patient's cardiac output declines from 6 L/min to 4.5 L/min. What can the therapist do to help determine what caused the reduction in cardiac output?

_____

_____

_____

_____

Case Studies

Case Study #1

A patient is ventilated in a volume-controlled mode with a set rate of 12 breaths/min and a V_T of 700 mL. The total rate is 25 breaths/min, the $PaCO_2$ is 30 mm Hg, the pH is 7.52, and the PaO_2 is 45 mm Hg. When the set frequency is reduced to 10 breaths/min in an attempt to correct the respiratory alkalosis, the total rate remains at 25 breaths/min. An attempt at reducing the V_T results in an increase in the total rate.

1. What can the therapist do to correct the respiratory alkalosis?

_____

_____

_____

_____

Case Study #2

A 100 kg (IBW) patient is receiving PCV at a set pressure of 20 cm H_2O at a frequency of 12 breaths/min. The exhaled volume is 550 mL, the $PaCO_2$ is 65 mm Hg, and the pH is 7.29. The physician asks that the patient's $PaCO_2$ be reduced to 45 mm Hg.

1. What would be the most effective means of reducing the $PaCO_2$?

_____

_____

_____

2. What parameter change would result in the desired $PaCO_2$ of 45 mm Hg?

_____

_____

_____

_____

_____

_____

_____

Case Study #3

A patient with ARDS is ventilated in a pressure-controlled mode. PEEP is set at 10 cm H_2O with an F_IO_2 of 0.6. The patient is manually ventilated with 100% O_2 before suctioning. When the ventilator is disconnected from the ET and the therapist begins the procedure, O_2 saturation drops rapidly and the HR increases markedly.

1. What is the possible cause of the problem?

_____

_____

_____

_____

2. What can the therapist do to resolve the situation?

_____

_____

_____

_____

NBRC–Style Questions

1. A patient with severe pneumonia is being mechanically ventilated. The most effective method for delivering aerosolized antibiotics is which of the following?
   a. MDI
   b. MDI with spacer
   c. SVN
   d. Dry powdered capsule

2. Permissive hypercapnia may be beneficial for a patient with which of the following?
   a. High $P_{plateau}$
   b. Intracranial lesion
   c. Pulmonary hypertension
   d. Head trauma

3. A patient requiring mechanical ventilation has an 8 mm ET tube in place. The patient requires frequent suctioning with a 10 Fr catheter. The therapist should recommend which of the following?
   a. Instilling saline with every suctioning procedure
   b. Using a suction frequency of every 2 hours
   c. Increasing the suction pressure to −180 mm Hg
   d. Changing to a size 12 Fr catheter

4. Which of the following statements regarding the Hi-Lo Evac ET is (are) true?
   I. The tube has a suction port above the ET cuff.
   II. The continuous suction pressure should be set at 20 cm H_2O.
   III. The device can reduce the incidence of nosocomial pneumonias.
   IV. This tube is not indicated for all patients.
   a. I
   b. I and II
   c. I, III, and IV
   d. I, II, III, and IV

5. The most effective method of thinning secretions and facilitating suctioning is to lavage with which of the following?
   a. Acetylcysteine
   b. Normal saline
   c. Sterile water
   d. Bronchodilator

6. A patient with a WBC count of 12,000/cm^3 is coughing up moderate amounts of yellow secretions. Physical examination reveals decreased breath sounds and dullness to percussion. These findings are consistent with which of the following?
   a. Airway trauma
   b. Pulmonary embolism
   c. Pneumonia
   d. Pulmonary edema

7. An increase in physiological dead space can be caused by which of the following?
   I. Pulmonary embolism
   II. Increase in V_T
   III. Low cardiac output
   IV. High alveolar pressures
   a. I
   b. I and II
   c. I, III, and IV
   d. I, II, III, and IV

8. A patient receiving mechanical ventilation should not be transported under which of the following conditions?
   I. Patient is hemodynamically unstable.
   II. Cardiac function cannot be monitored.
   III. Patient is nasally intubated.
   IV. Patient has multiple intravenous lines.
   a. I
   b. I and II
   c. I, III, and IV
   d. I, II, III, and IV

9. Methods for managing the ventilatory status of a patient with unilateral lung disease include which of the following?
   - I. Use of a double lumen ET tube
   - II. Instillation of normal saline before suctioning
   - III. Bronchodilator therapy via small-volume nebulizer
   - IV. Positioning of the patient laterally so that the good lung is dependent
   a. I
   b. I, II and II
   c. I, II, III, and IV
   d. I and IV

10. The concept of patient-centered mechanical ventilation includes which of the following?
    a. Determining the patient's comfort level
    b. Maintaining the PaO_2 over 60 mm Hg
    c. Maintaining the $P_{plateau}$ under 40 cm H_2O
    d. Determining the patient's nutritional needs

Helpful Internet Sites

- Brandis K: *Acid-base physiology.* Available at www.anaesthesiamcq.com/AcidBaseBook/
- Collard HR: *Prevention of ventilator-associated pneumonia.* Available at www.ahrq.gov/clinic/ptsafety/chap17a.htm
- Martin GS: *Fluid balance and colloid osmotic pressure in acute respiratory failure: emerging clinical evidence.* Available at http://ccforum.com/content/4/S2/S21
- Op't Holt T: Aerosol therapy during mechanical ventilation. Available at www.aarc.org/ marketplace/ reference_articles/ 07.00.018.pdf

CHAPTER 14

Improving Oxygenation and Management of ARDS

Learning Objectives

Upon completion of this chapter the reader will be able to do the following:

1. Calculate the F_IO_2 needed to achieve a desired PaO_2 based on current ventilator settings and blood gases.
2. Calculate the percent shunt.
3. Identify indications and contraindications for continuous positive airway pressure (CPAP) and PEEP.
4. Name the primary goal of PEEP and the conditions in which high levels of PEEP are most often used.
5. From a PEEP study providing arterial blood gases (ABGs) and hemodynamic data, determine the optimum PEEP level.
6. Explain the increase in peak inspiratory pressure that occurs when PEEP is increased.
7. Describe the most appropriate way to establish an optimum PEEP level in a patient with acute respiratory distress syndrome (ARDS) using recruitment-derecruitment maneuver and the deflection point (lower inflection point during deflation or derecruitment).
8. Explain what happens when a patient with a unilateral lung disease receives PEEP/CPAP therapy.
9. Describe the effects of PEEP in a patient with an untreated pneumothorax.
10. Recommend adjustments in PEEP and ventilator settings based on assessment of the patient, ventilator parameters, and ABGs.
11. Compare static compliance, hemodynamic data, and ABGs as indicators of an optimum PEEP level.
12. Name the first parameter to measure following the administration of PEEP.
13. Identify from patient assessment and ABGs when it is appropriate to change from CPAP to mechanical ventilation with PEEP.
14. Define acute lung injury and ARDS using the PaO_2/F_IO_2 ratio.
15. Explain why it is important to set the PEEP level high enough in ARDS, but not too high.
16. Recommend a tidal volume setting in a patient with ARDS.
17. Provide the maximum plateau pressure value in patients with ARDS.
18. Identify weaning criteria from PEEP or CPAP.
19. Describe ventilator adjustments that can be performed to provide inverse ratio ventilation on a conventional volume ventilator.
20. Recommend a PEEP setting based on the inflection point on the deflation curve using the pressure-volume loop for a patient with ARDS.

Key Terms Crossword Puzzle

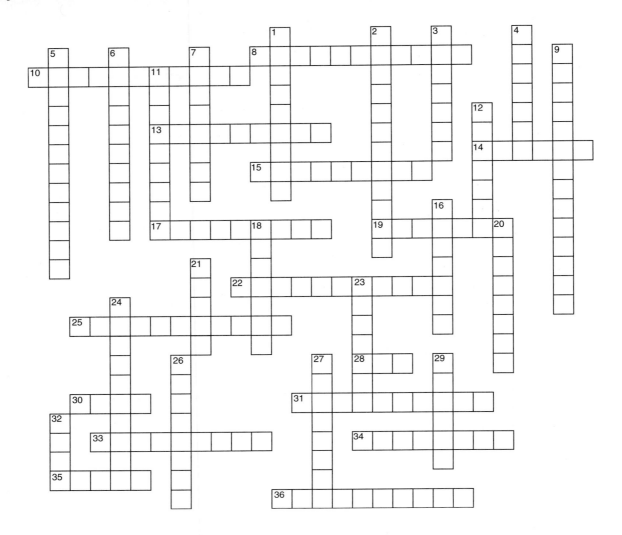

Across

8 Hemorrhaging or dehydration causes this
10 Maneuver for opening collapsed alveoli
13 Phase of ARDS characterized by inflammation and alveolar filling
14 Lung units
15 Point that occurs when a large number of lung units collapse quickly
17 Zone 3 of the lungs is _____
19 PEEP level that has maximum benefit
22 Type of pulmonary edema caused by CHF
25 Collapse of previously expanded areas of the lung
28 Point on a static pressure volume curve where the slope of the line changes significantly (abbreviation)
30 _____-billed appearance of pressure-volume curve indicates overdistention
31 Overinflation of the lungs may lead to this

Down

1 A type of inflammatory mediator
2 Creates resistance to gas flow through an orifice (two words)
3 Alters F_IO_2, depending on oxygen saturation
4 Pressure that pulls fluid out of tissues
5 High thoracic pressures can reduce this (two words)
6 Material produced by type II pneumocytes
7 Has blood flowing through its capillaries
9 F_IO_2 is kept low to prevent this (two words)
11 Resistor that maintains pressure independent of flow
12 Pressure used to calculate static compliance
16 Some CPAP masks are composed of this material
18 Type of pressure-volume loop obtained during gas flow
20 Chemical that causes inflammation
21 A Dräger ventilator
23 A Hamilton ventilator

Across—Cont'd

33. _____ alveolitis is the second phase of ARDS.
34. Direction that is toward the head
35. Perfusion without ventilation
36. A type of hypoxia

Review Questions

1. List at least three factors that affect oxygen delivery.

   _____

2. What is the importance of measuring oxygen delivery?

   _____

   _____

3. Write the formula for calculating oxygen consumption.

   _____

   _____

4. How often should the F_IO_2 be monitored for a patient receiving mechanical ventilation?

   _____

5. How soon after the F_IO_2 is changed can a sample be drawn for ABG analysis?

   _____

6. At what level should the F_IO_2 be maintained to help prevent the complications of oxygen toxicity?

   _____

7. By what mechanism can breathing 100% oxygen contribute to hypoxemia?

   _____

   _____

8. When trying to keep the F_IO_2 low enough to prevent oxygen toxicity, it is important to maintain a PaO_2 in the range of _____ to _____; the CaO_2 should be kept at approximately _____.

9. What conditions are required for a linear relationship between the PaO_2 and F_IO_2?

   _____

   _____

   _____

   _____

Down—Cont'd

24. Point that occurs where a large number of lung units collapse quickly
26. Cellular death
27. Breath sound indicative of pulmonary edema
29. Direction that is toward the base of the spine
32. Specific clinical disorder that benefits from PEEP (abbreviation)

10. Write the equation for selecting the F_IO_2 necessary to obtain a desired PaO_2.

    _____

    _____

11. Thirty minutes after initiation of pressure-targeted ventilation, an ABG sample is drawn and analyzed, with the following results: pH = 7.43, $PaCO_2$ = 43 mm Hg, PaO_2 = 50 mm Hg. The F_IO_2 is set at 0.75, and PEEP is 5 cm H_2O. What F_IO_2 is required to achieve a PaO_2 of 60 mm Hg?

    _____

12. What does the shunt equation measure?

    _____

13. Write the shunt equation.

    _____

    _____

    _____

    _____

14. Use the following information to calculate the ratio of physiological shunt to total perfusion in percent form: $Cc'O_2$ = 20.4 vol%, CaO_2 = 19.8 vol%, $C\overline{v}O_2$ = 13.4 vol%.

    _____

    _____

    _____

    _____

    _____

    _____

15. Define $\overline{P}aw$.

    _____

    _____

16. List the factors that affect P_{aw} during PPV.

_____

_____

17. How does increasing P_{aw} increase PaO_2 in the presence of ventilation/perfusion abnormalities and/or diffusion defects?

_____

_____

_____

18. List three methods of increasing P_{aw}.

_____

19. What is the intended effect of PEEP/CPAP therapy on alveoli and small airways?

_____

_____

20. Explain the difference between PEEP and CPAP therapy.

_____

_____

_____

21. How is PEEP applied to the airway during mechanical ventilation and what is the desired physiological result?

_____

_____

_____

22. List four devices capable of applying PEEP/CPAP to the airway.

_____

23. List three methods of applying noninvasive CPAP.

_____

24. List the patient criteria for placing a patient on mask CPAP.

_____

_____

_____

_____

25. List the hazards associated with the use of mask CPAP.

_____

_____

26. List five hazards associated with the use of nasal CPAP in infants.

_____

_____

_____

_____

_____

27. When CPAP is used, what determines the patient's WOB through the device?

_____

_____

_____

_____

28. On what principle is PEP mask therapy based?

_____

_____

29. How can CPAP therapy reduce WOB in a patient with ARDS?

_____

_____

_____

_____

30. Name an indication for the use of CPAP therapy in a patient's home.

_____

31. What is the goal of PEEP therapy?

_____

_____

_____

_____

32. What is *optimal PEEP?*

_____

_____

_____

33. One method of determining optimal PEEP is to calculate the _____ compliance.

34. To prevent a decrease in distribution of V_T breath to independent (ventral) levels while PEEP is administered, the $P_{plateau}$ should be maintained at _____.

35. (a) List four beneficial effects of PEEP.

_____

_____

_____

_____

(b) List five side effects of PEEP.

_____

_____

_____

_____

_____

36. List seven indications for PEEP therapy.

_____

_____

_____

_____

_____

_____

_____

37. Referring to question 36, if PEEP is indicated, how soon should it be initiated and why?

_____

_____

38. List three specific clinical disorders that may benefit from the use of PEEP/CPAP.

_____

_____

39. List the two levels of PEEP and the corresponding range of pressure for each.

_____

_____

40. Referring to question 39, give an indication for the use of each level of PEEP.

_____

_____

41. In adults, PEEP usually is increased in increments of _____ ; in infants this range generally is _____.

42. What pulmonary condition may require the use of high PEEP levels (15 to 20 cm H_2O) to provide adequate tissue oxygenation?

_____

_____

43. A patient's response to PEEP is evaluated based on which eight goals of therapy?

_____

_____

_____

_____

_____

_____

_____

_____

44. What is the first parameter measured after administration of PEEP?

_____

45. Referring to Figure 14-3 in the text, parameters measured and monitored during a PEEP study.

Ventilatory Data	Hemodynamic Data
_____	_____
_____	_____
_____	_____
_____	_____
_____	_____

46. Why is it important to measure PIP and $P_{plateau}$ during a PEEP study?

_____

_____

47. At what PEEP level is compliance no longer a valid indicator for determining optimum PEEP?

_____

48. Based on the data in the following table, what is the optimum PEEP level? Explain your answer.

PEEP (cm H_2O)	PaO$_2$ (mm Hg)	Cardiac Output (L/min)	P$\bar{v}$O$_2$ (mm Hg)	CS (mL/cm H_2O)
3	50	3.5	27	25
7	75	4	30	30
11	90	4.5	35	37
17	95	4.3	32	35
22	105	4	30	33

_____

_____

49. Why don't patients with emphysema benefit from PEEP therapy?

_____

_____

50. Give an example of a nontherapeutic indication for therapy with a low level PEEP.

_____

51. Why is hypovolemia a relative contraindication to PEEP therapy?

_____

52. Why is untreated pneumothorax an absolute contraindication to PEEP?

_____

53. During volume-controlled ventilation, PEEP is set at 5 cm H_2O, and the PIP is 42 cm H_2O. After PEEP is increased to 10 cm H_2O, the PIP measures 48 cm H_2O. Has the patient's condition worsened? What caused the increase in PIP?

_____

54. Referring to table 14-4 in the text, why didn't the PaO$_2$ improve significantly until PEEP was increased to 15 cm H_2O?

_____

55. List five uses for PEEP other than ALI.

_____

_____

_____

56. List five criteria that may indicate a patient is ready for a trial reduction of PEEP.

_____

_____

57. What is _ARDS_? _____

_____

58. How is ALI distinguished from the ARDS?

_____

59. In ALI/ARDS, inflammation of the pulmonary capillary endothelium and the alveolar epithelium results in

_____ permeability and leads to leakage of _____ from the capil-

lary into the _____ and then the _____.

60. Why is ARDS considered a systemic syndrome and not just a problem confined to the lung?

_____

_____

_____

61. How does cardiogenic pulmonary edema differ from the pulmonary edema associated with ARDS?

_____

_____

62. What effect does ALI/ARDS have on compliance and lung volumes?

_____

_____

63. Identify the two phases of ARDS and the characteristics of each.

_____

_____

64. Explain how the alveoli are affected in primary (direct) ARDS and secondary (indirect) ARDS.

_____

_____

_____

65. Why is the use of a normal V_T (10 to 15 mL/kg) no longer recommended for ventilation of patients with ARDS?

_____

_____

66. What is the goal of lung-protective strategies in the ventilation of a patient with ARDS?

_____

_____

67. List seven guidelines for managing patients with ARDS using the open lung or a lung-protective strategy.

_____

_____

_____

_____

_____

_____

68. List the three components of a recruitment maneuver and the purpose of each.

_____

_____

_____

_____

69. List three possible hazards of recruitment maneuvers.

_____

_____

_____

70. List three contraindications to performing a recruitment maneuver.

_____

_____

_____

71. List four types of recruitment maneuvers.

_____

_____

_____

72. A patient with ARDS is ventilated with PC-CMV. The rate is 10 breaths/min, the I:E ratio is 1:1, the PC is set at 20 cm H_2O above PEEP, and PEEP is 10 cm H_2O. Explain how manipulation of the PEEP level may be used to establish an optimum PEEP for this patient.

_____

_____

_____

_____

_____

_____

_____

_____

Use the following table to answer questions 73 and 74.

Time	PEEP (cm H_2O)	C_S (mL/cm H_2O)	Time	PEEP (cm H_2O)	C_S (mL/cm H_2O)
0800	0	27	0850	32.5	40
0805	5	27	0855	30	38
0810	10	27	0900	27.5	38
0815	15	29	0905	25	38
0820	20	32	0910	22.5	38
0825	25	36	0915	20	37
0830	30	38	0920	17.5	37
0835	35	41	0925	15	28
0840	40	40	0930	12.5	28
0845	35	40	0935	10	27

73. At what time, PEEP level, and C_S did the deflation point occur (inflection point on the deflation curve)?

_____

74. What is the appropriate PEEP setting for this patient? _____

Critical Thinking Questions

1. Use the pressure-volume curve in the figure below to answer the following questions.

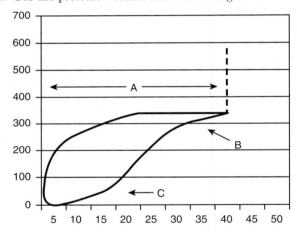

(a) Identify the following points in the graphic:

A _____

B _____

C _____

(b) Identify the point where the lung is most compliant.

_____

(c) Identify the point that may correlate with an increase in $PaCO_2$.

_____

2. Use the pressure-volume curve in the figure below to answer the following questions. The graphic was obtained from a patient receiving volume-controlled ventilation.

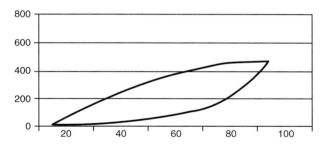

(a) What is the approximate PIP?

_____

(b) What is the approximate exhaled V_T?

_____

(c) Can the respiratory therapist determine from this pressure-volume curve whether the high airway pressure is a result of a decrease in compliance or an increase in airway resistance?

_____

_____

_____

_____

_____

_____

3. A patient with ARDS and refractory hypoxemia is ventilated in a volume-controlled mode. The physician would like to institute an inverse I:E ratio. What ventilatory parameters could the therapist recommend to achieve the inverse ratio in a volume ventilation mode?

_____

_____

_____

Case Studies

Case Study # 1

A 38-year-old patient is admitted to the emergency department and placed on volume-controlled mechanical ventilation for aspiration pneumonia. A postintubation radiograph reveals that the ET is in the proper position ; it also shows complete opacification of the right lung. The left lung appears normal. The PIP is 62 cm H_2O, and the $P_{plateau}$ is 55 cm H_2O. Ventilator settings and ABG results are as follows :

Ventilator Settings		ABG Results	
Mode	A/C	pH	7.43
F_IO_2	1	$PaCO_2$	38 mm Hg
Frequency	20 breaths/min	PaO_2	40 mm Hg
V_T	800 mL	HCO_3^-	23 mEq/L
PEEP	15 cm H_2O	BE	0

1. What is the cause of the severe hypoxemia?

_____

_____

_____

_____

_____

_____

2. What should the therapist recommend?

_____

_____

_____

Case Study #2

A 26-year-old male patient who is 5′ 6″ tall and weighs 125 lb is admitted to the hospital for treatment of a heroin overdose. The patient is intubated and placed on volume-controlled ventilation. A chest radiograph reveals bilateral fluffy infiltrates. Ventilatory data and ABG results are as follows:

Ventilator Data		ABG Results	
Mode	SIMV	pH	7.37
F_IO_2	1	$PaCO_2$	43 mm Hg
Frequency	12 breaths/min	PaO_2	44 mm Hg
V_T	600 mL	SaO_2	85%
PEEP	5 cm H_2O	HCO_3^-	23 mEq/L
PIP	55 cm H_2O	BE	0
$P_{plateau}$	48 cm H_2O		

1. Interpret the ABG results.

_____

2. What is the significance of the $P_{plateau}$?

_____

_____

_____

_____

3. What should the therapist recommend to treat the hypoxemia and high ventilating pressures?

_____

_____

_____

NBRC–Style Questions

1. By what mechanism does PEEP cause an increase in intracranial pressure?
   a. Cardiac output and venous return are increased.
   b. Stroke volume is decreased.
   c. Central venous pressure is increased.
   d. Venous return is decreased, which results in intracranial hemorrhage

2. Which of the following is an absolute contraindication to the use of PEEP or CPAP therapy?
   a. Increased intracranial pressure
   b. Severe hyperventilation
   c. Decreased lung compliance
   d. Untreated pneumothorax or tension pneumothorax

3. A 35-year-old patient diagnosed with ARDS is receiving pressure-controlled mechanical ventilation. Based on ABG results, the respiratory therapist increases the PEEP from 14 to 18 cm H_2O. Which of the following should the therapist monitor immediately after making the change?
   a. Cardiac output
   b. Creatinine
   c. Hemoglobin
   d. Serum potassium

4. How much oxygen is delivered if the total CaO_2 is 16.94 vol% and cardiac output is 12.54 L/min?
   a. 1 L/min
   b. 2.124 L/min
   c. 3.45 L/min
   d. 3.926 L/min

5. Which of the following is the primary mechanism by which PEEP increases PaO_2 and improves compliance?
   a. Reduced mean airway pressure
   b. Increased minute ventilation
   c. Recruitment and distention of collapsed alveoli
   d. Reduced cardiac output

6. What effect does PEEP have on both PaO_2 and $PaCO_2$?
   a. Both should increase.
   b. PaO_2 should increase, and $PaCO_2$ should decrease.
   c. Both PaO_2 and $PaCO_2$ and should decrease.
   d. $PaCO_2$ should remain unaffected, and PaO_2 should increase.

7. Which of the following is (are) considered a direct lung insult that can cause ARDS?
      I. Pneumonia
      II. Aspiration
      III. Sepsis
      IV. Smoke inhalation
   a. I
   b. I and II
   c. I, II, and IV
   d. I, II, III, and IV

8. Which of the following conditions is (are) potential complications when instituting PEEP therapy?
      I. Decrease in cardiac output
      II. Barotrauma
      III. Altered cardiac function
      IV. Decrease in urine output
   a. I
   b. III and IV
   c. I, III, and IV
   d. I, II, III, and IV

9. What is the most likely cause of an increased $PaCO_2$ after an increase in PEEP?
   a. Tension pneumothorax
   b. Lung overdistention
   c. Increased in compliance
   d. Reduced airway resistance

10. When managing a patient with ARDS who is receiving mechanical ventilation + PEEP, what can the respiratory therapist do to help alleviate the problem of excessive lung water?
    a. Ventilate with large V_T.
    b. Increase the amount of IV fluids.
    c. Administer diuretic therapy.
    d. Keep the PIP below 50 cm H_2O.

Helpful Internet Sites

- AARC Clinical Practice Guideline: Patient-ventilator system checks. Available at www.rcjournal.com/online_resources/cpgs/mvsccpg.html
- Cornell University: *Medical calculators, oxygen index.* Available at www-users.med.cornell.edu/~spon/picu/calc/oxyindex.htm
- ARDSNet: *Mechanical ventilation protocol summary card.* Available at www.ardsnet.org/lowvtrefcard.pdf
- ARDS Support Center: Understanding ARDS. Available at www.ards.org/ learnaboutards/whatisards/brochure/

Frequently Used Pharmacological Agents in Ventilated Patients: Sedatives, Analgesics, and Paralytics

Learning Objectives

Upon completion of this chapter the reader will be able to do the following:

1. List the most common sedatives and analgesics used in the treatment of critically ill patients.
2. Discuss the indications, contraindications, and potential side effects of each of the sedatives and analgesic agents reviewed.
3. Describe the most common method of assessing the need for and level of sedation.
4. Describe the Ramsay scale.
5. Compare the advantages and disadvantages of using benzodiazepines, opioids, neuroleptics, and anesthetic agents in the management of mechanically ventilated patients.

6. Discuss the mode of action of depolarizing and nondepolarizing paralytics agent.
7. Explain how the train-of-four method is used to assess the level of paralysis in critically ill patients.
8. Contrast the indications, contraindications, and potential side effects associated with using various types of neuromuscular blocking agents.
9. Recommend a medication for a mechanically ventilated patient with severe anxiety and agitation.
10. From a clinical description, assess drug interaction and recommend a reversing agent.
11. From a clinical situation, recommend an appropriate medication for a ventilated patient with severe muscle contractions.

Key Terms Crossword Puzzle

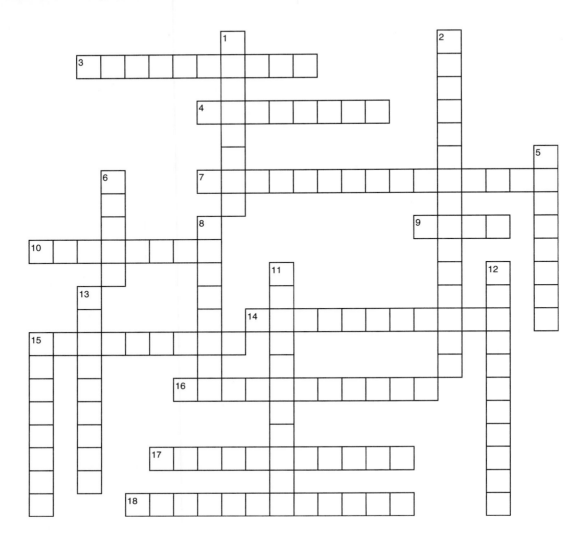

Across

3 Reverses the effects of benzodiazepines
4 Benzodiazepine drug
7 A NMBA
9 Benzodiazepines bind to these receptors on neurons in the brain (abbreviation)
10 Naturally occurring opioid drug
14 Nondepolarizing NMBA
15 Facilitates invasive procedures by preventing movement
16 Haloperidol is included in this category of drugs.
17 Type of amnesia related to the prevention of new memories
18 Agent that resembles acetylcholine in chemical structure

Down

1 Disorganized thought patterns and excessive, nonpurposeful motor activity
2 Agent that inhibits the action of acetylcholine at the neuromuscular junction
5 Opioid narcotic that is stronger than morphine
6 Type of opioid receptor
8 Agent that reduces anxiety and agitation
11 Method of monitoring the depth of paralysis with an electrical current (three words)
12 Method of assessing the level of sedation (two words)
13 Drug of choice for sedating mechanically ventilated patients for longer than 24 hours
15 Anesthetic agent

Review Questions

1. What effects do sedatives have on the body?

   _____

2. Why is paralysis used during mechanical ventilation?

   _____

   _____

3. List the four types of pharmacological agents used for sedation in the ICU. Give at least one example of each.

   _____

   _____

   _____

4. What modes of ventilation often require patients to be sedated?

   _____

5. Name the four JCAHO-defined levels of sedation.

   _____

6. Complete the following table. What type of patient response and ventilatory and cardiovascular function do patients have at each level of sedation?

Sedation Level	Patient Response	Ventilatory Function	Cardiovascular Function

7. What level of sedation is necessary when a patient is "fighting the ventilator"?

   _____

8. What level of sedation is necessary during weaning from mechanical ventilation?

   _____

9. The most popular method of assessing the level of sedation is the _____.

10. Using the sedation assessment method identified in question 9, identify the range of scores that indicates adequate sedation.

    _____

11. What score indicates the need for sedation?_____

12. What scores indicate oversedation of an ICU patient? _____

13. Why are benzodiazepines the drugs of choice for the treatment of anxiety in critical care?

_____

_____

14. What is the mode of action for benzodiazepines?

_____

_____

_____

_____

15. What factors alter the intensity and duration of action of various benzodiazepines?

_____

_____

16. What pathological processes prolong recovery from treatment with benzodiazepines?

_____

17. Why does diazepam have a rapid onset of action?

_____

_____

_____

18. How is diazepam administered?

_____

_____

19. Acutely agitated patients are best treated with which benzodiazepine? Why?

_____

_____

20. How can prolonged sedation occur with midazolam?

_____

_____

_____

21. Which benzodiazepine is best suited for sedating mechanically ventilated patients in the ICU for longer than 24 hours?

_____

22. An overdose of benzodiazepines may be reversed with what drug?

_____

23. Potential side effects of continual use of lorazepam (Ativan) include

_____

24. Two commonly used opioids are _____ and _____.

25. List three effects that opiates have on the body.

_____

26. How do opiates exert their effects on the body?

_____

_____

27. List at least 10 serious side effects of opioids.

_____

_____

_____

_____

_____

_____

28. The severity of the side effects of opioids depends on

_____.

29. Which drug can reverse the respiratory depression caused by opioids?

_____

30. What effects does morphine have on the central nervous system?

_____

_____

31. How does morphine affect the gastrointestinal tract?

_____

_____

_____

32. How does morphine affect the cardiovascular system?

_____

_____

33. Which opioid should be used for a patient whose hemodynamic status is unstable?

_____

34. Complete the following table.

	Morphine	Fentanyl
Is it natural or synthetic?		
Is it lipid soluble?		
Does it cross the blood-brain barrier?		
What is the onset of action?		
What is the duration of action?		
How is it administered?		

35. What class of drugs is routinely used to treat extremely agitated and delirious patients in the ICU?

_____

36. The drug most often used to treat ICU delirium is _____.

37. What are some of the side effects of the drug in question 36?

_____

38. The anesthetic agent that has proved useful for sedation of neurosurgical patients is _____.

39. What are the hemodynamic effects of the drug in question 38?

_____

_____

40. Referring to question 38, what are the advantages and disadvantages of using this drug to sedate neurological patients?

Disadvantages	Advantages

41. Increased intracranial pressure caused by traumatic brain injury may be controlled by a combination of which two drugs?

_____

42. What type of drug is used to reduce oxygen consumption and carbon dioxide production? _____

43. What is the difference between depolarizing and nondepolarizing agents?

_____

_____

44. Give two reasons to use paralyzing agents.

_____

45. What is *TOF?*

_____

46. How is TOF used? _____

_____

47. According to the Society for Critical Care Medicine, what indicates that an adequate amount of NMBA is being administered when TOF is used?

_____

48. What other medication is necessary when a paralytic agent is used?

_____

_____

49. The most widely used depolarizing NMBA is

_____.

50. What are the onset of action and duration of action for the drug in question 49?

_____

51. The drug in question 49 is most often used for what purpose?

_____

52. What are the most common side effects of the drug in question 49?

_____

_____

_____

_____

53. Which nondepolarizing NMBA has the longest duration of action?

_____

54. Which nondepolarizing NMBAs have a medium duration of action?

_____

_____

55. Which of the nondepolarizing NMBAs should not be used with hemodynamically unstable patients? Why?

_____

_____

_____

56. Seizures have been associated with which nondepolarizing NMBA?

_____

57. Mast cell degranulation and histamine release, which may lead to peripheral vasodilation and hypotension, are associated with which nondepolarizing NMBA?

_____

58. Which nondepolarizing NMBAs are ideal for patients with renal and hepatic insufficiency?

_____

59. The nondepolarizing NMBA of choice for patients who are hemodynamically unstable, have cardiac disease, or are at risk of histamine release is

_____.

60. Give two side effects of the long-term use of neuromuscular blocking agents.

_____

_____

Critical Thinking Questions

1. When a neuromuscular blocking agent is administered to a patient receiving ventilatory care, what ventilator alarms should be activated?

_____

_____

_____

2. Which type of opioid is best suited to a patient who has asthma? Why?

_____

_____

_____

Case Study

The respiratory therapist checks on an ICU patient receiving ventilatory support with VC-SIMV. The ventilator settings are as follows: rate = 8 breaths/min, $V_T = 600$ mL, $F_IO_2 = 0.4$, PEEP = 5 cm H_2O. The patient's legs are hanging over the bed railing, and his hands are on the ventilator tubing. The high pressure alarm is activating with every breath at a rate of 35 breaths/min. The patient is anxious and uncooperative.

1. What type of medication is most appropriate for this patient?

_____

The patient does not respond to the initial dose of the medication chosen. Wrist restraints are necessary to prevent him from pulling out the ET. The patient is still extremely agitated and confused and is fighting the ventilator. However, he is hemodynamically stable.

2. The most appropriate type of medication to deliver at this time would be _____.

3. What concerns should the respiratory therapist have about the patient's ventilatory settings?

_____

_____

_____

_____

NBRC–Style Questions

1. The drug that can be used to reverse the effects of benzodiazepines is which of the following?
   a. Pseudocholinesterase
   b. Flumazenil (Romazicon)
   c. Fentanyl citrate (Sublimaze)
   d. Naloxone hydrochloride (Narcan)

2. The respiratory therapist is called to the postanesthesia care unit to assist in the weaning of a postoperative patient who had a cholecystectomy. The patient is 3 hours postop and is still apneic and receiving full ventilatory support. The medication(s) that could be used to facilitate ventilator weaning is (are) which of the following?
   I. Naloxone (Narcan)
   II. Propofol (Diprivan)
   III. Midazolam (Versed)
   IV. Flumazenil (Romazicon)
   a. I and IV
   b. II and IV
   c. I and III
   d. II and III

3. An adult patient is in pain, panicky, and fighting the ventilator. The most appropriate medication to control this patient during mechanical ventilation is which of the following?
   a. Propofol (Diprivan)
   b. Haloperidol (Haldol)
   c. Fentanyl (Sublimaze)
   d. Succinylcholine (Anectine)

4. Which of the following is the fast-acting neuromuscular blocking agent that is often used to facilitate intubation?
   a. Vecuronium (Norcuron)
   b. Pancuronium (Pavulon)
   c. Midazolam (Versed)
   d. Succinylcholine (Anectine)

5. A mechanically ventilated patient who is hemodynamically unstable needs to be placed on PC-IRV and will require paralysis. The most appropriate drug combination for this patient is which of the following?
   a. Succinylcholine (Anectine) and morphine
   b. Propofol (Diprivan) and fentanyl (Sublimaze)
   c. Atracurium (Tracrium) and midazolam (Versed)
   d. Cisatracurium (Nimbex) and flumazenil (Romazicon)

6. A patient with which of the following Ramsay scores is most likely to wean successfully from mechanical ventilation?
   a. 1
   b. 2
   c. 4
   d. 6

7. The depth of paralysis during neuromuscular blockade may be assessed with which of the following?
   a. Ramsay Scale
   b. Serum GABA levels
   c. TOF monitoring
   d. Level of sedation assessment

8. The neuromuscular blocking agent that causes histamine release is which of the following?
   a. Atracurium
   b. Cisatracurium
   c. Vecuronium
   d. Pancuronium

9. The neuromuscular blocking agent most appropriate for facilitating emergency intubation is which of the following?
   a. Pancuronium (Pavulon)
   b. Vecuronium (Norcuron)
   c. Atracurium (Tracrium)
   d. Succinylcholine (Anectine)

10. The neuromuscular blocking agent that can be used in patients with renal or hepatic insufficiency without producing prolonged paralysis is which of the following?
    a. Cisatracurium (Nimbex)
    b. Vecuronium (Norcuron)
    c. Pancuronium (Pavulon)
    d. Succinylcholine (Anectine)

Helpful Internet Sites

- University of Kansas School of Nursing: *Assessment of neuromuscular blockade*. Available at http://classes.kumc.edu/son/nurs420/unit3/neuromusc-bloc.htm

- Cawley MJ: Case report: sedation and analgesia for the mechanically ventilated patient, *RT J Respir Care Pract* September, 2004. Available at www.rtmagazine.com/ Articles.ASP?articleid= R0409F02
- Ramsay MAE: How to use the Ramsay Score to assess the level of ICU sedation. Available at http://5jsnacc.umin.ac.jp/How%20to%20use%20the%20Ramsay%20Score%20to%20assess%20the%20level%20of%20ICU%20Sedation.htm
- Hammerschmidt M: Notes on ICU nursing: sedation and paralysis. Available at www.icufaqs.org/ finalsedationupdate.doc

Effects of Positive Pressure Ventilation on the Cardiovascular, Cerebral, Renal, and Other Organ Systems

Learning Objectives

Upon completion of this chapter the reader will be able to do the following:

1. Explain the effects of positive pressure ventilation on cardiac output and venous return to the heart.
2. Discuss the three factors that can influence cardiac output during positive pressure ventilation.
3. Explain the effects of positive pressure ventilation on gas distribution and pulmonary blood flow in the lungs.
4. Describe how positive pressure ventilation increases intracranial pressure.
5. Summarize the effects of positive pressure ventilation on renal and endocrine function.
6. Describe the effects of abnormal arterial blood gases on renal function.
7. Name five ways of assessing a patient's nutritional status.
8. Describe techniques that can be used to reduce some of the complications associated with mechanical ventilation.

Key Terms Crossword Puzzle

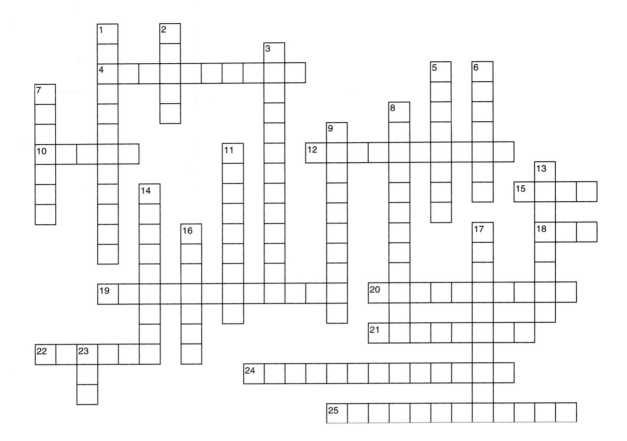

Across

4 Area under the pressure-time curve equals this pressure (two words)
10 Gas always follows the path of _____ resistance
12 Spontaneous inspiration increases blood flow to this (two words)
15 18 across plus ICP equals this (abbreviation)
18 The amount of blood flowing to the brain is determined by this (abbreviation)
19 Unoxygenated blood comes back (two words)
20 Through the wall of an organ
21 ADH release results in this
22 Volume pumped out of a ventricle with one beat.
24 Maneuver that can increase the inspiratory time (two words)
25 Inflammation of many nerves simultaneously

Down

1 Mechanism that maintains BP in healthy individuals receiving PPV
2 Function that can be altered by mechanical ventilation
3 This decreases with the use of PPV (two words)
5 Reduction in perfusion to an organ
6 Structural and functional unit of the kidney
7 Reductions in 19 across decrease this
8 Pressure that falls with spontaneous inspiration
9 Drug used to prevent gastrointestinal bleeding
11 This capillary thins when an alveolus is overfilled
13 Reflex that is blocked by 25 across
14 Compression of the heart
16 Vein that is visible when CVP is elevated
17 Urinary output declines when this capillary pressure drops below 75 mm Hg
23 Measuring this provides information about a patient's daily caloric requirements (abbreviation)

Review Questions

1. List the five bodily functions that PPV can significantly alter.

_____

_____

2. The physiological effects of PPV on the cardiovascular system depend on what two factors?

_____

_____

3. Explain how inspiration facilitates venous return to the right heart.

_____

_____

_____

4. During what part of a spontaneous breath is right ventricular preload increased? Why?

_____

_____

5. During what part of a spontaneous breath is left ventricular preload decreased? Why?

_____

_____

_____

6. How does an increase in CVP affect the pressure gradient between systemic veins and the right heart?

_____

For questions 7 through 9, refer to the following figure.

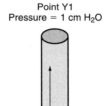
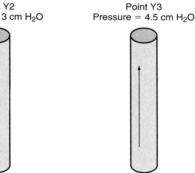

Point Y1
Pressure = 1 cm H_2O

Point Y2
Pressure = 3 cm H_2O

Point Y3
Pressure = 4.5 cm H_2O

Point X1
Pressure = 5 cm H_2O

Point X2
Pressure = 5 cm H_2O

Point X3
Pressure = 5 cm H_2O

A

B

C

7. Which diagram (A, B, or C) represents the largest pressure gradient? _____

8. Which diagram represents the smallest pressure gradient? _____

9. Assume that each tube in the figure represents the inferior vena cava, the X points represent systemic pressure, and the Y points represent CVP; which diagram has the most venous return?

   _____

10. What effect does alveolar overdistention have on the pulmonary capillaries and right ventricular afterload?

    _____

    _____

    _____

    _____

    _____

11. What conditions are required for the interventricular septum to move to the left during PPV?

    _____

    _____

12. How can PPV cause myocardial ischemia?

    _____

    _____

    _____

    _____

    _____

13. List the compensatory mechanisms responsible for maintaining systemic blood pressure during ventilation of healthy individuals.

    _____

    _____

    _____

    _____

14. In patients receiving PPV, what factors can block the body's compensatory mechanisms for maintaining arterial blood pressure?

    _____

    _____

    _____

15. How can a respiratory therapist make sure that normal vascular reflexes are intact when PPV is initiated?

    _____

16. Cardiac output may decline in normovolemic patients when PEEP levels of _____ are used.

17. Give the three factors that can influence cardiac output during PPV.

    _____

    _____

    _____

18. How does PPV benefit the cardiac function of a patient with left ventricular dysfunction?

    _____

    _____

19. What pressure most influences the extent of harmful effects from PPV?

    _____

20. Calculate the mean airway pressure using the following parameters: PIP = 25 cm H_2O, T_I = 1 second, respiratory rate = 12 breaths/min.

    _____

    _____

    _____

21. Calculate the mean airway pressure using the following parameters: PIP = 35 cm H_2O, PEEP = 10 cm H_2O, T_I = 1 second, respiratory rate = 12 breaths/min.

    _____

    _____

    _____

    _____

22. Calculate the mean airway pressure using the same parameters as in question 21 but add a 1 second inspiratory hold.

    _____

    _____

    _____

23. What type of inspiratory flow produces uneven ventilation? _____

24. The I:E ratios least likely to cause air trapping and significant hemodynamic complications are

_____.

25. What type of T_E allows for better alveolar emptying and less chance of the development of intrinsic PEEP?

_____

26. The amount of mean airway pressure required to achieve a certain level of oxygenation may indicate what?

_____

27. List five factors that influence mean airway pressure during mechanical ventilation.

_____

_____

_____

28. Explain why rapid inspiratory flow rates may produce lower mean airway pressures in a patient with healthy conducting airways.

_____

_____

29. What circumstances must exist for PEEP levels to affect cardiac output?

_____

_____

_____

30. Under what circumstance would high levels of PEEP not cause a decrease in cardiac output?

_____

_____

_____

31. Calculate the CPP when the ICP is 18 cm H_2O and the MABP is 85 cm H_2O.

_____

_____

_____

32. How does PPV increase ICP?

_____

_____

_____

33. How can increased ICP be observed clinically?

_____

34. What does hyperventilation do to cerebral vessels?

_____

_____

35. In what three ways is renal function altered by PPV?

_____

_____

_____

_____

36. At what glomerular capillary pressure does urinary output become severely reduced?

_____

37. What happens to kidney function when blood flow to the outer cortex decreases and flow to the inner cortex and outer medullary tissue increases?

_____

_____

38. Name the three hormones involved in fluid and electrolyte balance during PPV.

_____

_____

39. How does PPV affect each of the three hormones?

_____

_____

_____

_____

_____

40. Describe the effects of abnormal arterial blood gas levels on renal function.

_____

_____

_____

_____

_____

41. How does PPV affect the pharmacokinetics of certain drugs?

_____

_____

_____

42. How do PPV and PEEP affect the liver?

_____

_____

_____

_____

_____

_____

_____

43. What causes gastric distention in patients receiving PPV and how can it be reduced?

_____

_____

_____

44. Why are medical and surgical patients subject to malnutrition during serious illness?

_____

_____

_____

45. Name three deleterious effects that nutritional depletion can have on mechanically ventilated patients.

_____

_____

_____

46. How can overfeeding affect a mechanically ventilated patient?

_____

_____

_____

47. Name five ways to assess a patient's nutritional status.

_____

_____

_____

_____

_____

_____

48. How can some of the complications associated with mechanical ventilation be reduced?

_____

_____

_____

Critical Thinking Question

1. Describe the cardiovascular effects (represented by the lettered arrows) of PPV on the heart in the following figure.

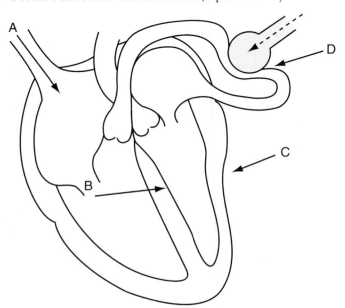

_____

Case Study

A 30-year-old, 5′ 8″ male postoperative patient who has no lung disease is in the surgical intensive care unit. He is receiving full mechanical support with VC-CMV at the following settings: rate = 12 breaths/min, V_T = 560 mL, flow rate = 84 L/min, PEEP = 10 cm H_2O, F_IO_2 = 0.5. His PIP averages about 30 cm H_2O, and $P_{plateau}$ is 23 cm H_2O.

1. Calculate this patient's mean airway pressure.

_____

_____

_____

_____

_____

_____

2. The patient's ABG values with these ventilator settings are as follows: pH = 7.38, $PaCO_2$ = 42 mm Hg, PaO_2 = 78 mm Hg, SaO_2 = 90%, HCO_3^- = 23 mEq/L. Analyze these results.

_____

_____

_____

_____

3. What is the most appropriate ventilator change at this time and why?

_____

_____

_____

_____

_____

_____

NBRC-Style Questions

1. What effect does the normal thoracic pump mechanism have on cardiac output?
   a. Reduces cardiac output in healthy individuals
   b. Improves cardiac output in healthy individuals
   c. Improves cardiac output in individuals with disease
   d. Improves cardiac output in mechanically ventilated patients only

2. Which of the following is true during PPV and PPV with PEEP regarding the thoracic pump mechanism?
   a. Cardiac output and venous return are reduced.
   b. Left ventricular output is reduced, and cardiac output is increased.
   c. Left ventricular stroke volume and cardiac output are reduced.
   d. Right heart venous return and BP are increased.

3. The greatest reductions in venous return and cardiac output are most likely to occur with which of the following ventilator modes and settings?
   a. CPAP = 8 cm H_2O
   b. SIMV = 10 breaths/min, V_T = 450 mL
   c. CMV = 12 breaths/min, V_T = 475 mL
   d. CMV = 10 breaths/min, V_T = 435 mL, PEEP = 6 cm H_2O

4. The patient's inability to compensate for diminished cardiac output during PPV results in which of the following?
   a. Severe hemorrhaging
   b. Increased BP
   c. Compromised perfusion
   d. Maintenance of normal BP

5. Patients with ARDS are less likely to experience hemodynamic changes during PPV even with high ventilatory pressures because of which of the following?
   a. Systemic BP is elevated.
   b. Blood vessel walls have become too thick.
   c. Pressure is not transmitted to the pleural space.
   d. Pressure is lost in the poorly conductive airways.

6. Hazardous cardiovascular side effects in patients with severe bronchospasm are due to which of the following?
   a. Short T_I
   b. Auto-PEEP
   c. Elevated mean airway pressure
   d. Elevated PIP

7. The pressure that most influences the hemodynamic effects of PPV is which of the following?
   a. PEEP
   b. PIP
   c. $P_{plateau}$
   d. Mean airway pressure

8. Methods of increasing the mean airway pressure include which of the following?
   I. Increasing PEEP
   II. Increasing the total cycle time
   III. Shortening the T_I
   IV. Adding an inflation hold
   a. I and II
   b. I and IV
   c. II and III
   d. II and IV

9. The risk of cardiovascular complications is least with which of the following ventilator modes?
   a. PC-CMV
   b. VC-CMV with PEEP
   c. PC-SIMV with PS
   d. CPAP with PS

10. Which of the following is an anticipated effect of PPV on the kidneys?
    I. Diuresis
    II. Sodium retention
    III. Decreased urinary output
    IV. Increased creatinine excretion
    a. I and II
    b. II and III
    c. III and IV
    d. I and IV

Helpful Internet Sites

- Department of Anesthesia and Intensive Care, the Chinese University of Hong Kong: ICU web. Available at www.aic.cuhk.edu.hk/web8/mechanical%20ventilation%20physiology.htm
- Shekerdemian L, Bohn D: The cardiovascular effects of mechanical ventilation. ADC Online. Available at http:// adc.bmjjournals.com/cgi/content/full/archdischild%3b80/5/475
- Anaesthesia UK: Heart-lung interactions. Available at www.frca.co.uk/article.aspx?articleid=100426

Effects of Positive Pressure Ventilation on the Pulmonary System

Learning Objectives

Upon completion of this chapter the reader will be able to do the following:

1. Recognize barotrauma or extraalveolar air based on patient assessment.
2. Recommend appropriate action in patients with barotrauma.
3. Evaluate findings from a patient with adult respiratory distress syndrome to establish an optimum PEEP and ventilation strategy.
4. Identify situations in which chest wall rigidity can alter transpulmonary pressures and acceptable plateau pressures.
5. Name the types of ventilator-induced lung injury caused by opening and closing of alveoli and overdistention of alveoli.
6. Compare the clinical findings in hyperventilation and hypoventilation.
7. Recommend ventilator settings in patients with hyperventilation and hypoventilation.
8. Identify a patient with air trapping.
9. Provide strategies to reduce auto-PEEP.
10. Suggests methods to reduce the work of breathing during mechanical ventilation.
11. Determine the presence of a ventilator-associated pneumonia based on clinical findings.
12. Provide methods to reduce the risk of ventilator-associated pneumonia.
13. List the possible responses to an increase in mean airway pressure in a ventilated patient.
14. Describe the effects of positive pressure ventilation on pulmonary gas distribution and pulmonary perfusion in relation to normal spontaneous breathing.

Key Terms Crossword Puzzle

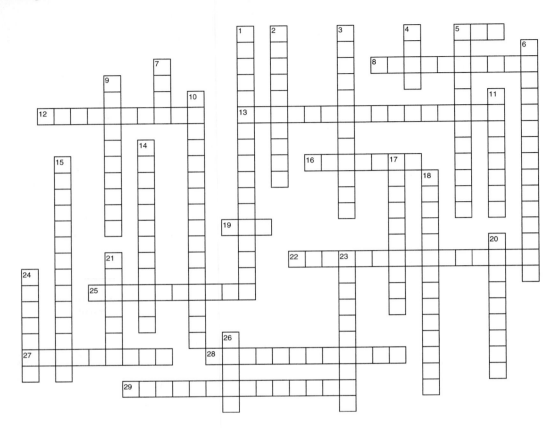

Across

5 Resistance to blood flow in the lungs (abbreviation)

8 Damage from high distending volumes

12 Type of atelectasis caused by high oxygen concentrations

13 Compression of the heart caused by collection of fluid or blood in the pericardium (two words)

16 Type of pressure that is kept under 30 cm H_2O to prevent lung injury

19 Pneumonia acquired 48 hours after intubation in a patient receiving mechanical ventilation (abbreviation)

22 Rising PCO_2

25 An internal source

27 An external source

28 Opposite of synchrony

29 Free air in the area of the diaphragm causes a

_____ on a chest radiograph (three words)

Down

1 Release of these substances causes multiple organ dysfunction syndrome (two words)

2 Trauma associated with pressure

3 Shear stress injury and loss of surfactant

4 Lung injury that occurs at the level of the acinus and resembles ARDS (abbreviation)

5 Around the vessels

6 Type of fungi commonly isolated as a cause of nosocomial pneumonia

7 Lung injury as a consequence of mechanical ventilation (abbreviation)

9 Substance that forms a molecular layer between the air and the liquid alveolar surface

10 Air dissects into the retroperitoneal space, causing a

_____

11 Direction that is toward the head

14 Type of emphysema caused by the collection of air under the skin

15 Too much air in the lungs causes _____

17 Common type of *Pseudomonas* organism that causes pneumonia in mechanically ventilated individuals

18 Lung overinflation

20 Release of mediators from the lungs as a result of overdistention

21 Life-threatening type of pneumothorax

23 Site of organism colonization before VAP develops

24 Type of patient-ventilator problem caused by an insensitive ventilator is called _____ dyssynchrony.

26 Exhalation before the ventilator completes inspiration causes _____ dyssynchrony

Review Questions

1. Define the terms *volutrauma*, *biotrauma*, and *atelectrauma*.

   _____

   _____

   _____

   _____

2. Briefly explain the difference between VILI and VALI.

   _____

   _____

   _____

   _____

3. List five conditions that predispose a mechanically ventilated patient to barotrauma.

   _____

   _____

   _____

   _____

4. During a patient-ventilator system check, the respiratory therapist notes that the patient's neck and face appear puffy. What is the most likely cause of this problem?

   _____

5. Puffiness of the neck, face, and chest with increased peak airway pressures and decreasing lung compliance may be caused by _____.

6. What is the treatment for a tension pneumothorax?

   _____

   _____

   _____

7. A mechanically ventilated patient has developed a tension pneumothorax. How should the patient be ventilated until the appropriate treatment can begin?

   _____

   _____

8. List four signs of a tension pneumothorax.

   _____

   _____

   _____

   _____

9. Describe the appearance of a chest radiograph for a patient with a tension pneumothorax.

   _____

   _____

10. Dissection of air into the retroperitoneal space is known as a _____.

11. What is the minimum transpulmonary pressure that has been associated with lung injury in animals?

   _____

12. Give three examples of situations involving an abnormally high transpulmonary pressure that may cause lung injury.

   _____

   _____

   _____

   _____

13. Explain how volutrauma occurs.

   _____

   _____

   _____

   _____

   _____

   _____

   _____

   _____

14. In the clinical setting, how can chest wall movement be minimized to reduce the risk of lung injury from volutrauma?

   _____

15. What clinical situation puts a ventilated patient at risk of atelectrauma?

   _____

   _____

16. Name the types of VILI caused by opening and closing of alveoli and overdistention of alveoli.

_____

_____

17. Name two chemical mediators that are released when the alveolar epithelial cells are overstretched.

_____

18. Explain how multiple organ dysfunction syndrome develops from overdistention of alveoli.

_____

_____

_____

_____

19. How can multiple organ dysfunction syndrome be prevented during mechanical ventilation?

_____

_____

_____

20. In what areas of the lung are ventilation and perfusion best matched during spontaneous ventilation in the supine position?

_____

21. How are ventilation and perfusion altered during positive pressure ventilation of a sedated, paralyzed patient?

_____

_____

_____

_____

22. What is the cause of increased pulmonary vascular resistance in most patients?

_____

23. List the invasive devices that increase the risk of nosocomial infections.

_____

_____

_____

24. List the factors that predispose a patient to nosocomial infections and pneumonias.

_____

_____

_____

_____

_____

25. Define VAP.

_____

_____

26. What is considered the main cause of VAP?

_____

27. Name three common gram-negative aerobes that cause nosocomial pneumonias.

_____

_____

_____

28. Name two common gram-positive aerobes that cause nosocomial pneumonias.

_____

29. Other than time of onset, what is the difference between early and late onset VAP?

_____

_____

_____

_____

30. What four clinical findings are suggestive of VAP?

_____

_____

_____

_____

31. What laboratory tests may be helpful in diagnosing VAP?

_____

32. How does VAP develop?

_____

_____

_____

_____

_____

_____

33. List the endogenous sources of microorganisms that may cause VAP.

_____

_____

34. List the exogenous sources of microorganisms that may cause VAP.

_____

_____

35. What type of mechanical ventilation has a low incidence of nosocomial pneumonia?

_____

_____

36. What patient position tends to help prevent the development of VAP?

_____

37. What is the relationship between the acidity of gastric contents and gastric colonization by potentially pathogenic organisms?

_____

_____

38. What cuff pressures increase the risk of VAP?

_____

39. What must be done before cuff deflation for whatever reason?

_____

40. How can the respiratory therapist reduce the risk of nosocomial pneumonia when changing a tracheostomy tube or caring for a patient with a tracheostomy?

_____

_____

41. Does continuous aspiration of subglottic secretions increase or reduce the incidence of VAP and why?

_____

_____

_____

42. When should ventilator circuits be changed?

_____

_____

43. A small-volume nebulizer is used in a ventilator circuit to administer a medication; how should it be handled after a treatment?

_____

_____

44. What four factors constitute the important components of a VAP surveillance mechanism?

_____

_____

_____

_____

45. How do acid-base disturbances affect the oxyhemoglobin dissociation curve?

_____

_____

_____

_____

_____

46. What effect does acidosis have at the tissue level?

_____

47. How does hypoventilation lead to cardiac dysrhythmias?

_____

_____

48. Patients may appear to be "fighting the ventilator" while on controlled ventilation when the settings for which two parameters are inadequate?

_____

49. List four clinical signs associated with hyperventilation.

_____

_____

50. How does hyperventilation of a mechanically ventilated patient lead to respiratory muscle atrophy?

_____

_____

_____

51. What happens to the cerebrospinal fluid during prolonged hyperventilation with mechanical ventilation?

_____

_____

_____

52. In what two patient situations is use of intravenous bicarbonate indicated?

_____

_____

_____

53. Write the formula for calculating bicarbonate replacement.

_____

54. List at least five causes of metabolic alkalosis.

_____

_____

_____

55. What are the possible treatments for severe metabolic alkalosis?

_____

_____

_____

56. How can auto-PEEP be detected in a mechanically ventilated patient?

_____

_____

57. How many time constants are required for the lungs to empty 98% of the inspired volume?

_____

58. Define _dynamic hyperinflation_.

_____

_____

59. What ventilator settings put a mechanically ventilated patient at increased risk of developing auto-PEEP?

_____

_____

60. What patient situations increase the risk for the development of auto-PEEP?

_____

_____

_____

61. How does auto-PEEP affect ventilator function?

_____

_____

_____

_____

_____

62. Calculate the static compliance, given the following parameters: V_T = 525 mL, PIP = 43 cm H_2O, $P_{plateau}$ = 30 cm H_2O, set PEEP = 12 cm H_2O, auto-PEEP = 5 cm H_2O.

_____

_____

_____

63. List four strategies that can be used to reduce auto-PEEP in a patient receiving full ventilatory support.

_____

_____

_____

_____

64. List four modes of ventilation that can be used to reduce auto-PEEP in an intubated patient who attempts to breathe spontaneously.

_____

65. When does pulmonary oxygen toxicity become a problem in adults and premature infants?

_____

_____

_____

66. List four ways to assess pulmonary changes associated with oxygen toxicity.

_____

_____

_____

67. What is the normal inspiratory WOB?

_____

68. Inspiratory WOB is considered high when it exceeds

_____.

69. A patient with an increased WOB most likely shows what signs?

_____

70. Calculate the estimated WOB for a mechanically ventilated patient with the following data: PIP = 45 cm H_2O, $P_{plateau}$ = 33 cm H_2O, and V_T = 475 mL.

_____

_____

_____

_____

71. List four strategies for keeping a patient's WOB minimized.

_____

_____

_____

72. List four signs of patient-ventilatory dyssynchrony.

_____

_____

73. Define _trigger dyssynchrony_ and describe a method of preventing it.

_____

_____

_____

74. What should the initial flow setting be when volume ventilation with a constant flow is used?

_____

75. What type of breaths may provide more synchrony for a patient with high flow demands and why?

_____

_____

76. What is _cycle dyssynchrony_ and under what conditions can it occur?

_____

_____

_____

77. What strategies may be used to eliminate cycle dyssynchrony during mechanical ventilation with full support and spontaneous ventilation?

_____

_____

_____

78. What mode of ventilation delivers varying breath types, which may result in mode dyssynchrony?

_____

79. List five points of easy disconnection in a ventilator circuit.

_____

_____

_____

80. List seven hazards and complications associated with the use of heat and moisture exchangers.

_____

_____

_____

_____

_____

_____

Critical Thinking Questions

For questions 1 and 2, refer to the following figure.

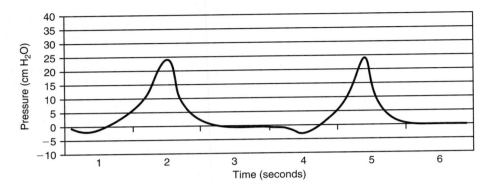

1. What problem is shown in this pressure-time curve for VC-CMV?

_____

_____

2. How can the ventilator settings be changed to solve this problem?

_____

For questions 3 and 4, refer to the following figure.

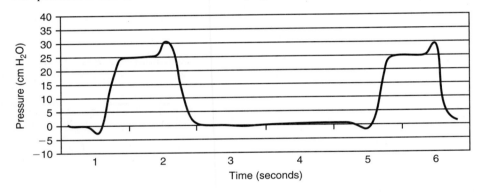

3. What problem is shown in this pressure-time curve for PSV?

_____

_____

4. How can the ventilator settings be changed to solve this problem?

_____

_____

Case Studies

Case Study #1

A patient who received a lung transplant 4 days ago is receiving mechanical ventilation. The remaining lung appears fibrotic on the chest radiograph, and the transplanted lung is hyperinflated. The patient is unresponsive, cyanotic, and hypotensive. Her ideal body weight 135 lb. She is being ventilated with VC-CMV, and the flow sheet for the past few hours shows the following:

Time	Set Rate (breaths/min)	Set V_T (mL)	Flow (L/min)	PIP (cm H_2O)	F_IO_2	PEEP	pH	$PaCO_2$ (mm Hg)	PaO_2 (mm Hg)
0800	20	300	60	52	0.7	0	7.18	86	275
1000	22	300	60	50	1	0	7.15	94	504
1200	24	300	60	55	1	0	7.14	95	95
1400	40	320	60	60	1	0	7.06	110	125

The $P_{plateau}$ at 1400 hours was 38 cm H_2O.

1. What is the most serious problem in this patient's ventilator course?

2. What is the most likely cause of this problem?

3. What complications is this patient at risk of developing?

4. What change in the ventilator parameters should be made first?

Case Study #2

A 26-year-old male patient involved in a motor vehicle accident suffered a closed head injury and multiple facial fractures. He was orally intubated in the emergency department. He currently is comatose and receiving nasogastric tube feedings. The trauma surgeon orders a prophylactic antibiotic. On day 5 the patient has a temperature of 38.8° C, the WBC count is 12,300 mm³, and sputum production is slightly increased.

1. List five factors that put this patient at risk for developing VAP.

2. What two methods can be used to obtain sputum specimens for determination of the causative organism?

NBRC–Style Questions

1. Which of the following is (are) the major hazard(s) of oxygen therapy in association with mechanical ventilation?
   - I. Tachycardia
   - II. Absorption atelectasis
   - III. Oxygen-induced bradypnea
   - IV. Pulmonary oxygen toxicity
   - a. III
   - b. I and II
   - c. II and IV
   - d. I, III and IV

2. Auto-PEEP should be suspected if which of the following is observed?
   - a. There is a prolonged postexpiratory pause.
   - b. The patient coughs severely when suctioned.
   - c. Expiration is continuous up to the next inspiration.
   - d. The SIMV mandatory rate is set at 10 breaths/min.

3. The lung capacity that increases when auto-PEEP is present is which of the following?
   - a. Vital capacity
   - b. Inspiratory capacity
   - c. Total lung capacity
   - d. Functional residual capacity

4. Iatrogenic hyperventilation of a patient diagnosed with COPD may lead to which of the following consequences?
   - I. Tetany
   - II. Air trapping
   - III. Cerebral edema
   - IV. Hypokalemia
   - a. II
   - b. I and III
   - c. II and IV
   - d. I, II and IV

5. A patient who has been mechanically ventilated for 7 days has recently developed subcutaneous emphysema. Further assessment reveals cyanosis, signs of dyspnea, and a markedly elevated PIP. This patient is most likely experiencing which of the following?
   - a. Pneumothorax
   - b. Pneumoperitoneum
   - c. Increased compliance
   - d. Pneumomediastinum

6. The risk of volutrauma is increased for mechanically ventilated patients with which of the following?
   - a. Increased P_{TA}
   - b. Decreased P_A
   - c. Increased P_L
   - d. Decreased P_{awo}

7. The amount of bicarbonate replacement given to a patient with severe metabolic acidosis who weighs 145 lb and has a base deficit of 10 should be which of the following?
   - a. 55 mEq
   - b. 110 mEq
   - c. 220 mEq
   - d. 242 mEq

8. Failure of the ventilator to recognize a patient's trigger efforts is known as which of the following?
   - a. Mode dyssynchrony
   - b. Flow dyssynchrony
   - c. Trigger dyssynchrony
   - d. Closed loop ventilation dyssynchrony

9. An increase in the assist rate followed by a rise in PIP and a decline in $V_T$exh is most often associated with which of the following?
   - a. Auto-PEEP
   - b. Mode dyssynchrony
   - c. PEEP dyssynchrony
   - d. Subcutaneous emphysema

10. Fine, late inspiratory crackles may lead to which of the following lung injuries?
    - I. Biotrauma
    - II. Shear stress
    - III. Surfactant alteration
    - IV. Subcutaneous emphysema
    - a. I and II
    - b. II and III
    - c. I and IV
    - d. III and IV

Helpful Internet Sites

- Kaplan LJ, Bailey H: Barotrauma. eMedicine. Available at www.emedicine.com/med/topic209.htm
- Institute for Healthcare Improvement: Getting started kit: prevent ventilator-associated pneumonia, how to guide. Available at www.ihi.org/NR/rdonlyres/A448DDB1-E2A4-4D13-8F02-16417EC52990/0/VAPGettingHowtoGuideFINAL.pdf
- Wilson J, Peterson M: Auto-PEEP and work of breathing. Virtual Hospital. Available at www.vh.org/adult/provider/internalmedicine/AdultCriticalCare/AutoPeep/AutoPeep.html

Troubleshooting and Problem Solving

Learning Objectives

Upon completion of this chapter the reader will be able to do the following:

1. Identify the various types of technical problems encountered with mechanical ventilation of critically ill patients.
2. Describe the steps for protecting a patient when problems occur.
3. Name at least two possible causes for each of the following alarm situations: low pressure alarm, high pressure alarm, low PEEP/CPAP alarm, apnea alarm, low or high tidal volume alarm, low or high minute volume alarm, low or high respiratory rate alarm, low or high F_IO_2 alarm, low source gas pressure or power input alarm, ventilator inoperative alarm, and technical error message.
4. Determine the cause of a problem using a graphic from a patient-ventilator system.
5. Assess a description of a patient situation and recommend a solution.
6. Describe the signs and symptoms of a patient-ventilator dyssynchrony.
7. Explain the correct procedure for determining whether a problem originates with the patient or the ventilator in patient-ventilator dyssynchrony.
8. List four ways the addition of an externally powered nebulizer can affect ventilator function.
9. Describe the types of problems that can result when a ventilated patient is turned.
10. Recognize a situation of inadequate flow delivery to a patient.
11. Identify potential problems related to electrolyte imbalances and their causes.
12. Recognize the signs and symptoms of a respiratory infection.
13. Identify a problem associated with an artificial airway or a mask used for noninvasive positive pressure ventilation.
14. Recognize the presence of auto-PEEP.
15. Compare findings from a right mainstem intubation and from a pneumothorax.
16. Evaluate problems caused by a heated humidification system during ventilation.
17. Use a ventilator flow-volume loop to assess a patient's response to bronchodilator therapy.
18. Make recommendations about ventilator parameters for a patient with acute respiratory distress syndrome.
19. Recommend adjustment of flow cycle criteria during pressure support ventilation based on ventilator graphics.

Key Terms Crossword Puzzle

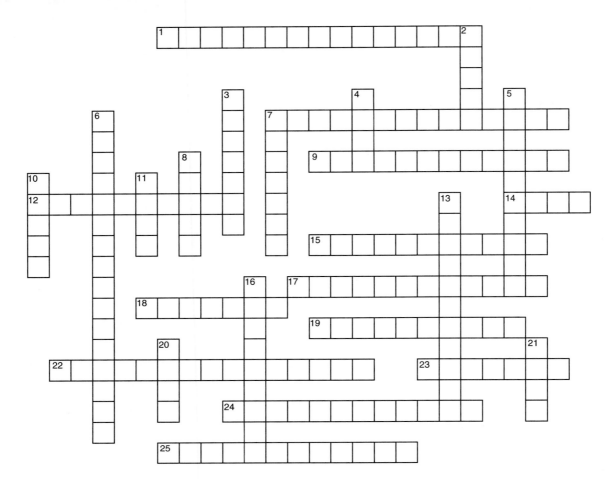

Across

1 Type of interference caused by a cell phone
7 Fluid in the lungs (two words)
9 Life-threatening cause of severe patient distress
12 Artery that may rupture within 3 weeks after a tracheostomy
14 Continuous suction endotracheal tube (abbreviation)
15 Indicator of severe cardiopulmonary distress
17 Out of synchrony with the ventilator
18 Waveform _____ is caused by oscillation of air in the patient-ventilator circuit at the beginning of inspiration.
19 Without synchrony
22 Identification and resolution of technical malfunctions in the patient-ventilator system
23 Abnormal accumulation of edematous fluid in the peritoneal cavity
24 Smooth muscle contraction in the lungs
25 Type of therapy that breaks up blood clots

Down

2 Active exhalation during PSV is a common cause of this type of dyssynchrony.
3 An uncomfortable situation
4 Type of dyssynchrony that occurs when more than one breath type is delivered
5 Inward protrusion of intercostal spaces
6 Blood clot in the lungs (two words)
7 Person attached to the ventilator
8 Alert for a clinician
10 The ET will slip into this bronchus.
11 Unintentional bend in the ET
13 Abnormally profuse perspiration
16 Radiograph of blood vessels
20 Type of dyssynchrony that occurs when gas speed is inadequate
21 Patient disconnection causes this.

Review Questions

1. Define the term *problem*.

   _____

   _____

2. Define the term *troubleshooting* in the context of mechanical ventilation.

   _____

   _____

   _____

3. When the respiratory therapist responds to an activated ventilator alarm, what is the first priority?

   _____

   _____

4. What assessments must be made to establish the first priority?

   _____

   _____

   _____

5. If a serious ventilatory problem is detected, what should the respiratory therapist's next step be?

   _____

   _____

6. What are the advantages and disadvantages of manually ventilating a patient when a problem is detected?

Advantages	Disadvantages
_____	_____
_____	_____
_____	_____
_____	_____
_____	_____
_____	_____
_____	_____
_____	_____

7. List the physical signs of distress that a patient receiving mechanical ventilation might show.

   _____

   _____

   _____

   _____

8. List six patient-related causes of sudden respiratory distress that originate in the lungs.

   _____

   _____

   _____

9. List six nonpulmonary patient-related causes of sudden respiratory distress.

   _____

   _____

   _____

10. List the six types of patient-ventilator dyssynchrony that can cause sudden respiratory distress.

    _____

    _____

    _____

    _____

11. Aside from patient-ventilator asynchrony, what ventilator-related factors can cause sudden respiratory distress in patients?

    _____

    _____

12. How can the respiratory therapist differentiate between severe distress caused by a ventilator-related problem and that caused by a patient-related problem?

    _____

    _____

    _____

    _____

13. Give the seven steps of management of sudden severe distress in a mechanically ventilated patient.

_____

_____

_____

_____

_____

_____

_____

_____

14. What centimeter marking at the teeth for an ET is common for men and women?

_____

15. For what clinical manifestation should a respiratory therapist look when a tension pneumothorax is suspected during positive pressure ventilation?

_____

_____

_____

_____

16. If a tension pneumothorax is strongly suspected and cardiopulmonary arrest is imminent, what action should be taken?

_____

_____

_____

17. When should bronchospasm be suspected during mechanical ventilation?

_____

_____

_____

_____

18. How can problems caused by secretions be minimized during mechanical ventilation?

_____

_____

_____

_____

19. Which type of pulmonary edema can occur suddenly?

_____

_____

20. List the conditions that may stimulate respiratory center output.

_____

_____

_____

21. The rapid onset of hypoxemia, tachycardia, tachypnea, and hypertension, along with a decrease in $P_{ET}CO_2$, is indicative of what type of patient problem? How can this problem be confirmed and treated?

_____

_____

_____

22. What are the common sites of leaks in the patient-ventilator system?

_____

_____

_____

_____

23. List four common causes of a low pressure alarm.

_____

_____

_____

24. List nine common causes of a high pressure alarm.

_____

_____

_____

_____

_____

_____

_____

_____

_____

25. If the PIP is 30 cm H_2O, what should the settings be for the low and high pressure alarms?

_____

_____

26. Give two conditions that would trigger a low PEEP/CPAP alarm.

_____

_____

27. List five possible reasons an apnea alarm might be triggered.

_____

_____

_____

28. List two possible reasons a low source gas pressure alarm might be triggered.

_____

_____

29. Give two possible causes of activation of a power input alarm.

_____

_____

30. What is the most likely cause of a ventilator inoperative alarm?

_____

31. Describe the alarms activated and the ventilator graphics produced by a leak in the patient-ventilator system.

_____

_____

_____

_____

32. What types of graphics allow the respiratory therapist to detect inadequate flow?

_____

_____

_____

_____

33. Auto-PEEP may be detected on which type of ventilator graphic? How would it appear?

_____

_____

_____

_____

_____

34. The phenomenon caused by the oscillation of air in the patient-ventilator circuit and at the upper airway at the beginning of inspiration is known as _____

_____.

35. What can be done to solve the problem caused by the phenomenon in question 34?

_____

_____

_____

36. Name three problems that may cause the expiratory portion of the volume-time curve to drop below baseline.

_____

37. List four ways the addition of an externally powered nebulizer can affect ventilator function.

_____

_____

_____

_____

38. What types of problems can result when a ventilated patient is turned?

_____

_____

_____

_____

_____

39. Which alarms are activated by a leak in the ET cuff?

_____

_____

_____

40. Compare the findings from a right mainstem intubation and from a left and right tension pneumothorax by completing the chart below.

Clinical Findings	Right Mainstem Intubation	Left Tension Pneumothorax	Right Tension Pneumothorax
PIP	_____	_____	_____
P$_{plateau}$	_____	_____	_____
Breath sounds	_____	_____	_____
Chest movement	_____	_____	_____
Percussion	_____	_____	_____
Tracheal shift	_____	_____	_____

41. How can a pulmonary embolism be detected during mechanical ventilation?

_____

_____

42. During mechanical ventilation with PC-CMV, the low V_T alarm is activated on every breath, but there is no leak in the system. What could be the cause of this alarm?

_____

43. How can a respiratory therapist determine the cause of an increasing PIP? _____

_____

44. What type of dyssynchrony most often occurs during PSV? _____

45. How can the dyssynchrony in question 44 be detected on ventilator graphics?

_____

46. What type of problem would cause a high pressure alarm to activate intermittently?

_____

47. What type of problem should the respiratory therapist suspect when a ventilated patient has sudden respiratory distress and a suction catheter cannot be passed through the ET? What action should be taken?

_____

_____

48. What steps can be taken to reduce auto-PEEP?

_____

_____

49. What situations can cause activation of the I:E ratio indicator and alarm?

_____

50. A respiratory therapist responding to a ventilator alarm finds that the high respiratory rate alarm has been activated. The ventilator is set to a VC-CMV rate of 12 breaths/min. What are some possible reasons for activation of this alarm? _____

_____

Critical Thinking Questions

For questions 1 through 4, refer to the following scenario.

You are the respiratory therapist who responds to a ventilator alarm. The patient suffered an exacerbation of congestive heart failure and pneumonia and has been receiving mechanical ventilation for the past 3 days. The patient has been unresponsive to verbal stimuli during this period. Her ventilator settings are as follows: VC-CMV, set rate = 12 breaths/min, V_T = 475 mL, F_IO_2 = 0.5, and PEEP = 5 cm H_2O. PIP has been averaging 28 cm H_2O, and $P_{plateau}$ has been averaging 21 cm H_2O. As you approach the patient, you note that the alarm panel indicates a high pressure condition along with low $V_T$exh and low exhaled $\dot{V}_E$. The patient's high pressure alarm threshold is set at 40 cm H_2O, and the returned volume is 175 mL.

1. What action should the respiratory therapist take at this time?

2. Name three conditions that could have caused this situation.

3. How could each of the three conditions be remedied?

4. Why have the low $V_T$exh and low exhaled $\dot{V}_E$ alarms been activated, along with the high pressure alarm?

For questions 5 and 6, refer to the following scenario.

A patient recently weaned from full ventilatory support has just been placed on CPAP at 10 cm H_2O with PS of 25 cm H_2O. After a few spontaneous breaths, the patient develops respiratory distress. He does not seem to be able to trigger the PS breaths, and the ventilator's apnea alarm has been activated.

5. Give two possible causes of this patient's respiratory distress.

6. What actions could correct these possible causes?

Case Studies

Case Study #1

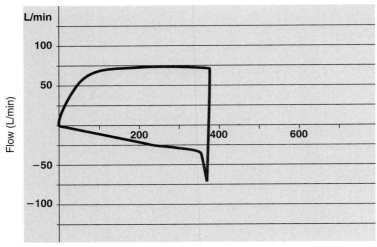

Volume (mL)

1. The preceding figure shows the flow-volume loop for a patient receiving mechanical ventilation. What type of problem is demonstrated in this flow-volume loop?

_____

2. What can be done to solve this problem?

_____

Case Study #2

A 42-year-old male had surgery to repair a crushed hip and femur fractures that occurred in a motor vehicle accident. Five hours after surgery, the patient continues to receive positive pressure ventilation. Up to now the patient's condition has been stable, but he has been unconscious. A sudden change in the patient's vital signs has brought the respiratory therapist to the patient's bedside. The pulse oximeter reading has dropped from 96% to 87%, and BP has risen from 136/82 to 157/98 mm Hg. The table below shows the last patient-ventilator checks.

Date		5/29	5/29	5/29	5/29
Time		1400	1610	1750	1810
Mode		PC-CMV	PC-CMV	PC-CMV	PC-CMV
Set rate	Total rate	12 12	12 12	12 20	12 25
Volume		620 mL	628 mL	625 mL	615 mL
T_I		1 second	1 second	1 second	1 second
Waveform		Square	Square	Square	Square
PIP		30 cm H_2O	28 cm H_2O	32 cm H_2O	33 cm H_2O
$P_{plateau}$		23 cm H_2O	21 cm H_2O	22 cm H_2O	20 cm H_2O
PEEP		5 cm H_2O	5 cm H_2O	5 cm H_2O	8 cm H_2O
F_IO_2		0.4	0.4	0.4	0.6
Breath sounds		Bilateral clear	Bilateral clear	Bilateral clear	Bilateral clear
BP		136/82 mm Hg	132/80 mm Hg	157/98 mm Hg	160/100 mm Hg
HR		96 beats/min	94 beats/min	125 beats/min	128 beats/min
SpO_2		96%	96%	87%	86%
$P_{ET}CO_2$		36 mm Hg	36 mm Hg	26 mm Hg	26 mm Hg
ABGs					
pH		7.43	—	—	7.47
$PaCO_2$		39 mm Hg	—	—	30 mm Hg
PaO_2		98 mm Hg	—	—	78 mm Hg

1. The patient now is in obvious respiratory distress. What action should the respiratory therapist take at this time?

_____

_____

2. Nothing seems to relieve this patient's respiratory distress. What is the most likely cause of this problem?

_____

_____

Case Study #3

A 62-year-old woman is receiving ventilatory support with volume ventilation. She had abdominal surgery 10 hours ago. She has no history of smoking. Over the past few hours, the following patient monitoring values were gathered:

Time	0700	0900	1000
Volume	450 mL	450 mL	450 mL
PIP	18 cm H_2O	24 cm H_2O	27 cm H_2O
$P_{plateau}$	13 cm H_2O	12 cm H_2O	14 cm H_2O

1. What is the most likely cause of the increase in PIP between 7 and 10 AM?

_____

_____

2. List some of the problems that can cause this type of increase in PIP.

_____

_____

3. What actions should the respiratory therapist take to determine the source of this patient's problem?

_____

_____

NBRC–Style Questions

1. During pressure control ventilation, the alarm that identifies worsening lung compliance is which of the following?
   a. Low PEEP/CPAP
   b. High respiratory rate
   c. Low $V_T$exh
   d. High PIP

2. Identify the problem in the following flow-time scalar.

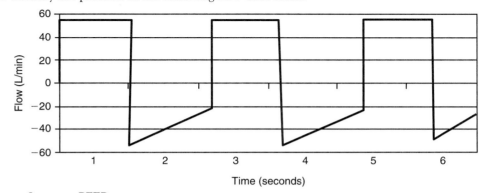

   a. Intrinsic PEEP
   b. Excessively prolonged T_E
   c. Inadequate T_I
   d. Increased airway resistance

3. The problem represented in the pressure-time scalar in below may be solved by which of the following?

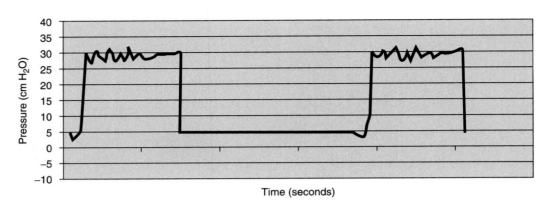

a. Changing the flow waveform
b. Increasing pressure sensitivity
c. Increasing inspiratory rise time
d. PIP

4. The problem indicated in the flow-volume loop below is which of the following?

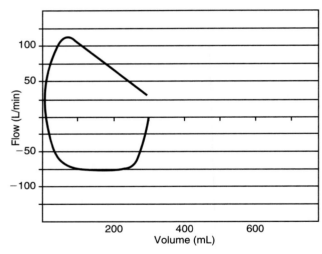

a. Increase in airway resistance
b. Active exhalation against inspiration
c. Leak in the patient-ventilator system
d. Auto-PEEP

5. The problem indicated in the pressure-volume loop below, obtained during VC-CMV, can be solved by which of the following?

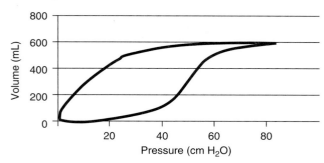

I. Suctioning of the ET tube
II. Switching to PC-CMV
III. Lowering the V_T
IV. Administering a bronchodilator
a. I and II
b. II and III
c. III and IV
d. I and IV

6. The problem that could cause the pressure-time scalar below is which of the following?

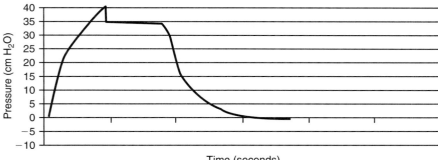

I. Bronchoconstriction
II. High airway resistance
III. Alveolar overdistention
IV. Decreased lung compliance
a. I and II
b. II and III
c. III and IV
d. I and IV

7. The respiratory therapist is assessing a mechanically ventilated patient who has developed sudden respiratory distress. The respiratory therapist notes that the 15-mm ET adapter is at the level of the patient's teeth. The suspected airway problem is which of the following?
a. Cuff rupture or leakage
b. Rupture of the innominate artery
c. Patient biting the ET
d. ET has slipped into the right mainstem bronchus.

8. The respiratory therapist is unable to pass a suction catheter into a patient's ET or to ventilate the patient manually with a resuscitator bag. Deflation of the cuff does not relieve the patient's distress. The most appropriate action is which of the following?
a. Reinflate the cuff and attempt ventilation again
b. Remove the ET and provide bag-mask ventilation
c. Keep the cuff inflated and attempt ventilation again with 100% oxygen
d. Deflate the cuff, suction the upper airway, and provide bag-mask ventilation

9. The respiratory therapist strongly suspects that the patient has a tension pneumothorax. What should the RT do in this life-threatening situation?
   a. Suction the patient's ET vigorously
   b. Insert a chest tube into the sixth intercostal space
   c. Insert a 14- or 16-gauge needle into the second intercostal space
   d. Remove the patient from the ventilator and provide resuscitation

10. While providing mechanical ventilatory support for a conscious patient, the respiratory therapist notes dyspnea, wheezing, and increased use of accessory muscles of breathing. These clinical findings are most closely associated with which of the following?
    a. Cuff leakage
    b. Bronchospasm
    c. Pneumothorax
    d. Increased secretions

11. What should the respiratory therapist check first when a low pressure alarm is activated on a ventilator?
    a. Apnea parameters
    b. Patient connection
    c. 50 psi gas source
    d. Ventilator electronics

12. What problem must be present to cause simultaneous activation of the low pressure, low volume, and low $\dot{V}_E$ alarms?
    a. Inadequate flow setting
    b. Ventilator dyssynchrony
    c. Patient-ventilator system leak
    d. Inappropriate trigger sensitivity

Helpful Internet Sites

- Beamer M: Mechanical ventilator graphics. Available at http://members.aol.com/Grafxsman/
- Gomershall C: Troubleshooting mechanical ventilation. ICU Web, Department of Anaesthesia and Intensive Critical Care, the Chinese University of Hong Kong. Available at www.aic.cuhk.edu.hk/web8/Mech%20vent%20troubleshooting.htm
- Orlando Regional Healthcare Education and Development: Troubleshooting the ventilator: invasive mechanical ventilation. Available at www.orhs.org/classes/nursing/mechvent.pdf
- Kaufman DA, Fuchs B, Lipschik G: Assessment of respiratory distress in mechanically ventilated patients. Up-To-Date Patient Information. Available at http://patients.uptodate.com/topic.asp?file=cc_medi/26665

CHAPTER 19

Basic Concepts of Noninvasive Positive Pressure Ventilation

Learning Objectives

Upon completion of this chapter the reader will be able to do the following:

1. Define noninvasive ventilation and discuss the three basic noninvasive techniques.
2. Discuss the clinical and physiological benefits of noninvasive positive pressure ventilation (NPPV).
3. Identify the selection and exclusion criteria for use of NPPV in the acute and chronic care settings.
4. Compare the types of ventilators used for noninvasive ventilation.
5. Explain the importance of humidification during NPPV.
6. Describe factors that affect the F_IO_2 delivered by a portable pressure-targeted ventilator.
7. Identify possible causes of CO_2 rebreathing during NPPV administration from a portable pressure-targeted ventilator.
8. Compare the advantages and disadvantages of the various types of interfaces used for NPPV.
9. List the steps for initiating NPPV.
10. Identify several indicators of success for patients receiving NPPV.
11. Make recommendations for ventilator changes based on observation of the patient's respiratory, acid-base, and/or oxygenation status.
12. Recognize potential complications of NPPV.
13. Suggest solutions for complications of NPPV.
14. Describe two basic approaches to weaning a patient from NPPV.

Key Terms Crossword Puzzle

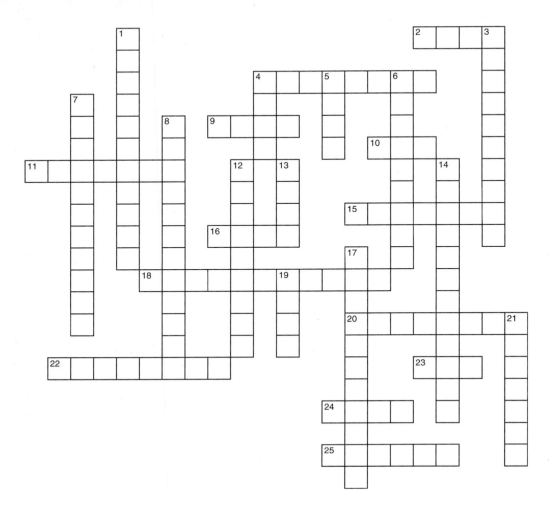

Across

2 First-choice therapy to treat OSA
4 Type of ventilator used during the polio epidemic (two words)
9 Abbreviation for a therapy used to deliver periodic aerosolized medication with positive pressure breaths
10 Another name for bilevel CPAP ventilators (abbreviation)
11 Symptom of chronic hypoventilation
15 Type of apnea that originates in the brain
16 Setting that allows positive pressure levels to increase gradually
18 Antigas agent
20 Type of heated humidifier used to prevent or treat mucosal dehydration with NPPV
22 Type of mask that covers both the nose and mouth
23 Type of pneumonia acquired outside the hospital (abbreviation)
24 Abdominal displacement ventilator (abbreviation)
25 Material that fastens the headgear

Down

1 Type of pulmonary edema caused by a weak heart
3 Type of abdominal displacement ventilator
4 Another name for positive pressure ventilation (abbreviation)
5 Use of positive pressure ventilation with a mask (abbreviation)
6 Type of hypoventilation that occurs at night
7 Type of sleep apnea that occurs from the collapse of the upper airway during sleep
8 Portable negative pressure device (two words)
12 Setting that controls the amount of time required for the positive pressure level to increase gradually (two words)
13 Expiratory setting for bilevel CPAP (abbreviation)
14 Right-heart failure caused by an obstructive pulmonary disease (two words)
17 Secretions that are dried up are _____
19 Inspiratory setting for bilevel CPAP (abbreviation)
21 Type of bed that is motorized and moves continuously in a longitudinal plane

Review Questions

1. Define the term *noninvasive ventilation*.

   _____

   _____

2. How do negative pressure ventilators operate?

   _____

   _____

   _____

   _____

   _____

   _____

3. Name two negative pressure ventilators.

   _____

4. How does an IAPV operate?

   _____

5. Describe how a pneumobelt operates.

   _____

   _____

   _____

   _____

   _____

   _____

   _____

6. The motorized bed that moves continuously in a longitudinal plane from the Trendelenburg position to the reverse Trendelenburg position is known as a

   _____.

7. How does NPPV operate?

   _____

   _____

   _____

8. List at least six clinical benefits of NPPV in the acute care setting.

   _____

   _____

   _____

   _____

   _____

9. List at least three clinical benefits of NPPV in the chronic care setting.

   _____

   _____

   _____

10. What are the two most significant benefits of NPPV in the acute care setting?

    _____

    _____

11. How does the use of NPPV in acute respiratory failure improve gas exchange?

    _____

12. What are the benefits of using NPPV with a face mask instead of invasive mechanical ventilation in the treatment of acute respiratory failure caused by COPD?

    _____

    _____

13. What types of NPPV have proved effective in patients with cardiogenic pulmonary edema who do not respond to conventional pharmacological and oxygen therapy?

    _____

    _____

14. The clinical disorders that manifest in chronic respiratory failure requiring NPPV as supportive therapy are _____.

15. List the five symptoms of chronic hypoventilation.

    _____

    _____

    _____

16. How many hours must a patient with chronic hypo-ventilation use NPPV to achieve clinical benefits?

_____

_____

17. The use of NPPV only at night or intermittently during the day for patients with neuromuscular disorders has what clinical benefits?

_____

_____

_____

18. What are the criteria for using NPPV in patients who have chronic stable COPD?

_____

_____

_____

19. What role does NPPV play in the treatment of advanced cystic fibrosis?

_____

_____

20. What therapy is indicated if a patient with OSA continues to hypoventilate and experience nocturnal desaturation while receiving CPAP?

_____

_____

21. What are the benefits of reducing the number of days a patient is ventilated invasively?

_____

_____

22. What can NPPV do for a patient who shows fatigue after extubation?

_____

_____

23. What role does NPPV play in end-of-life situations?

_____

_____

_____

24. List nine indications for the use of NPPV in adult patients with acute respiratory failure.

_____

_____

_____

_____

_____

_____

25. Name three signs of moderate to severe dyspnea that are selection criteria for NPPV.

_____

_____

26. The physiological criteria for use of NPPV in adult patients with acute respiratory failure include what two factors?

_____

_____

27. List the eight exclusion criteria for NPPV.

_____

_____

_____

_____

_____

_____

28. What are the physiological criteria for institution of NPPV in a chronic care setting in patients with restrictive thoracic disorders?

_____

_____

_____

29. The physiological criteria for institution of NPPV in a chronic care setting for patients with severe stable COPD include the following:

_____

_____

_____

_____

_____

30. The physiological criteria for institution of NPPV in a chronic care setting for patients with nocturnal hypoventilation include _____

_____.

31. How do portable pressure-targeted ventilators maintain pressure levels and flush exhaled gases from the circuit?

_____

_____

_____

32. What are the trigger, limit, and cycle variables for bilevel CPAP ventilators?

_____

_____

33. What are the inspiratory and expiratory settings called on bilevel CPAP ventilators?

_____

34. The typical ranges for the inspiratory and expiratory settings on bilevel CPAP ventilators are _____

_____ and

_____.

35. Most PTVs offer what modes of ventilatory support?

_____

36. What determines the patient's V_T with a PTV?

_____

_____

_____

37. What is the source of nonintentional leaks in a PTV?

_____

38. Why are PTVs able to flow trigger even though intentional and nonintentional leaks are present in the system?

_____

_____

39. Patient-ventilator synchronization has been improved in the newer PTV units with the addition of

_____.

40. What four factors cause variation of the F_IO_2 with a portable PTV?

_____

_____

_____

_____

41. How does an inadequate continuous flow from a PTV affect the patient?

_____

_____

42. The flow of gas through the leak port of a PTV depends on what settings?

_____

43. How can CO_2 rebreathing be minimized with a PTV?

_____

_____

_____

44. What advantage does a new generation portable volume ventilator (e.g., Pulmonetics LTV 900) have over a portable PTV?

_____

_____

_____

45. What are the advantages and disadvantages of using an adult acute care ventilator for noninvasive ventilation?

Advantages	Disadvantages
_____	_____
_____	_____
_____	_____
_____	_____
_____	_____
_____	_____
_____	_____
_____	_____

46. What mode will make the patient most comfortable when an adult acute care ventilator is used for NPPV and why?

_____

_____

47. Why is it important for heated humidity to be added during NPPV?

_____

_____

48. What type of heated humidifier is recommended for NPPV?

_____

49. Which type of NPPV/CPAP interface is most widely used?

_____

50. What advantages does the nasal mask have over the full face mask for administration of NPPV?

51. What are the two most common disadvantages of the nasal mask?

_____

_____

_____

_____

52. What type of NPPV interface should be used when a patient has large air leaks through the mouth?

_____

53. What are the major disadvantages to using the full face mask and total face mask for administration of NPPV?

_____

_____

_____

54. What are the advantages of using a mouthpiece or lip seal over a nasal mask?

_____

_____

55. List the steps involved in the initiation of NPPV.

_____

_____

_____

_____

_____

_____

_____

_____

_____

_____

_____

_____

_____

56. What clinical indicators demonstrate improvement in patient comfort?

_____

_____

57. What measures can be taken to ensure patient comfort when the clinical indicators are absent?

_____

_____

_____

58. What V_T range should be used with NPPV?

_____

59. Failure of NPPV to alleviate respiratory distress can be noted by what clinical manifestations?

_____

_____

_____

_____

_____

60. Clinical improvement should be noticeable when the patient can tolerate how much time on NPPV?

_____

61. Lack of improvement with NPPV may be due to what factors?

_____

_____

62. Complications from NPPV are usually due to what three factors?

_____

63. What causes eye irritation with NPPV and what can be done to alleviate it?

_____

_____

_____

_____

64. What causes pressure sores on the nasal bridge and what can be done to alleviate this problem?

_____

_____

_____

65. When a mouthpiece or lip seal is used, what may be done to reduce leakage of air from the nose?

_____

66. What can be done to reduce gastric insufflation?

_____

67. List the five most serious complications of NPPV.

_____

_____

_____

68. What is the most common method of weaning a patient from NPPV?

_____

Critical Thinking Questions

1. What situation would cause a noninvasive positive pressure ventilator _not_ to trigger from EPAP to IPAP or cycle from IPAP to EPAP?

_____

_____

_____

2. What factors lead to patient noncompliance with NPPV and how can these problems be resolved?

_____

_____

_____

_____

3. Describe how placement of the leak port and oxygen bleed-in affects the F_IO_2 delivered to the patient through NPPV.

_____

_____

_____

_____

_____

_____

_____

_____

Case Studies

Case Study #1

A 62-year-old male is seen in the emergency department for what appears to be an exacerbation of congestive heart failure. He is oriented × 3 but very anxious. Physical examination reveals the following: pulse = 129 and thready, BP = 108/64 mm Hg, T = 37° C, respirations = 28 breaths/min, shallow, and labored with accessory muscle use. Auscultation reveals bilateral decreased breath sounds with diffuse coarse crackles on inspiration. The patient has no cough and is diaphoretic. The respiratory therapist decides to use a nonrebreathing mask for treatment and draws an ABG sample 15 minutes later. The ABG results are these: pH = 7.31; $PaCO_2$ = 49 mm Hg; PaO_2 = 53 mm Hg; SaO_2 = 86%; HCO_3^- = 23 mEq/L.

1. Does this patient meet the selection criteria for NPPV? Why or why not?

_____

_____

_____

_____

2. If NPPV is appropriate, what settings should be used? If not, what other respiratory therapy should be initiated?

_____

_____

_____

_____

After 3 hours of treatment, the patient becomes agitated, confused, and uncooperative.

3. What action should be taken at this time?

_____

_____

Case Study #2

A 75-year-old man with a long history of COPD and a past smoking history of 114 pack-years is is brought to the emergency department with shortness of breath; a productive cough with green, purulent sputum; and cyanosis. He has had two previous hospitalizations for acute infective exacerbations of COPD within the past year. He has no comorbidities or occupational exposure. Physical examination reveals the following: pulse = 105 and regular; BP = 140/85 mm Hg; respirations = 30 breaths/min with prolonged expiration and use of accessory muscles; percussion is hyperresonant; breath sounds are reduced bilaterally with prolonged expiratory wheezes. The WBC count is 11,500 cells/mm^3. ABG values on room air are these: pH = 7.3, $PaCO_2$ = 55 mm Hg, PaO_2 = 53 mm Hg, HCO_3^- = 32 mEq/L.

1. Analyze this situation and identify and explain five presenting problems.

_____

_____

_____

_____

_____

_____

_____

2. What treatment recommendations should be suggested for this patient at this time?

_____

_____

_____

A repeat ABG analysis after appropriate therapy reveals the following: pH = 7.19, $PaCO_2$ = 67 mm Hg, PaO_2 = 60 mm Hg.

3. What is the most appropriate treatment option at this time? _____

NBRC–Style Questions

1. Symptoms of chronic hypoventilation include which of the following?
   I. Fatigue
   II. Morning headache
   III. Hypoxemia
   IV. Insomnia
   a. I and II
   b. II and III
   c. III and IV
   d. I and IV

2. A 5′ 10″ male patient with COPD has been placed on NPPV with an IPAP of 8 cm H_2O and an EPAP of 4 cm H_2O. The patient's measured exhaled volume is 350 mL, and the ABGs on this setting are pH = 7.27, $PaCO_2$ = 77 mm Hg, PaO_2 = 50 mm Hg and base excess of +7. The most appropriate action is which of the following?
   a. Increase EPAP to 6 cm H_2O
   b. Increase IPAP to 10 cm H_2O
   c. Decrease IPAP to 6 cm H_2O
   d. Bleed in 4 L/min of oxygen

3. The target V_T for a patient receiving NPPV with an ideal body weight of 58 kg is which of the following?
   a. 250 mL
   b. 350 mL
   c. 500 mL
   d. 700 mL

4. The respiratory therapist notes that the $V_T$exh of a patient receiving NPPV has dropped. The most appropriate action to take is which of the following?
   a. Increase the IPAP
   b. Decrease the EPAP
   c. Adjust the interface
   d. Change the tubing

5. A patient with chronic hypercapnic respiratory failure is currently using NPPV only at night, with the following parameters: assist mode, IPAP = 9 cm H_2O and EPAP = 4 cm H_2O. The patient is noted to be short of breath, with a spontaneous rate of 25 breaths/min. The action that will alleviate this problem is which of the following?
   a. Switch to the control mode
   b. Increase the IPAP % to 35%
   c. Reduce the EPAP to 2 cm H_2O
   d. Increase the IPAP to 11 cm H_2O

6. Which of the following situations will provide the highest oxygen concentration to a patient using a portable PTV?
   a. Low IPAP and EPAP settings
   b. High IPAP and EPAP settings
   c. Leak port and oxygen bleed-in at the mask
   d. Leak port and oxygen bleed-in in the circuit

7. The most appropriate type of humidifier to use with NPPV is which of the following?
   a. Wick-type humidifier
   b. Heat and moisture exchanger
   c. Heated bubble humidifier
   d. Heated passover–type humidifier

8. Which of the following can reduce a significant air leak through the mouth of a patient receiving NPPV via a nose mask?
   a. Using a chin strap
   b. Adding a forehead spacer
   c. Switching to nasal pillows
   d. Tightening the headgear straps

9. A patient is receiving mask CPAP with 8 cm H_2O and 80% oxygen. The ABG values on this setting are as follows: pH = 7.37, $PaCO_2$ = 37 mm Hg, and PaO_2 = 55 mm Hg. The most appropriate recommendation is which of the following?
   a. Increase the F_IO_2 to 0.9
   b. Intubate and mechanically ventilate the patient
   c. Increase CPAP to 12 cm H_2O
   d. Switch to bilevel positive pressure ventilation

10. A patient with which of the following problems should be excluded from a trial of NPPV?
    a. Amyotrophic lateral sclerosis
    b. Cardiogenic pulmonary edema
    c. Hemodynamically unstable ARDS
    d. Community-acquired pneumonia

Helpful Internet Sites

- American Sleep Apnea Association: Choosing a mask and head gear. Available at www.sleepapnea.org/mask.htm
- Rowley JA, Lorenzo N: Obstructive sleep apnea: hypopnea syndrome. Available at www.emedicine.com/neuro/topic419.htm
- Scharf T: The pneumobelt: part of my noninvasive ventilation system. Available at www.post-polio.org/ivun/val_18-4c.html#the
- Sharma S: Noninvasive ventilation. Available at http://www.emedicine.com/med/topic3371.htm
- Zoidis JD: Alternatives to invasive mechanical ventilation, *RT*, February 2004. Available at www.rtmagazine.com/Articles.ASP?articleid=R0402F01

Discontinuation of and Weaning from Mechanical Ventilation

Learning Objectives

Upon completion of this chapter the reader will be able to do the following:

1. List weaning parameters and the acceptable values for ventilator discontinuation.
2. Compare the three standard modes of weaning in relation to their success in discontinuing ventilation.
3. Define the closed loop modes of weaning described in the chapter.
4. Recognize appropriate clinical use of closed loop modes of weaning from a description of a clinical setting.
5. Identify assessment criteria for discontinuing a spontaneous breathing trial in a clinical situation.
6. Describe the criteria used to determine whether a patient is ready for extubation.
7. Recognize postextubation difficulties from a clinical case description.
8. Recommend appropriate treatment for postextubation difficulties.
9. State the first recommendation for weaning a patient from mechanical ventilation established by the task force formed by the American College of Chest Physicians, the Society of Critical Care Medicine, and the American Association for Respiratory Care.
10. Describe an appropriate treatment for a patient with an irreversible respiratory disorder that requires long-term ventilation.
11. Name the parameter used as the primary index of drive to breathe.
12. Suggest adjustments in ventilator settings during use of a standard weaning mode based on patient assessment.
13. Explain the appropriate procedure for management of a patient who has failed a spontaneous breathing trial.
14. Describe the effect of sedatives on the respiratory system.
15. Defend the use of nonphysician protocols as key components of efficient and effective patient weaning.
16. Describe the types of patients who might benefit from a tracheostomy.
17. Explain the function of long-term care facilities in the management of ventilator-dependent patients.
18. Assess data to establish the probable cause of failure to wean.

Key Terms Crossword Puzzle

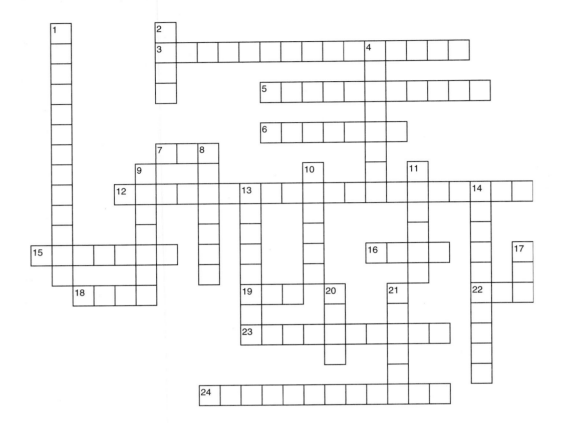

Across

3 This is added to spontaneous breaths to reduce the work of breathing (two words)
5 Type of breathing in which the chest wall moves in during inspiration and out during exhalation
6 Sound caused by 24 across
7 Trial of sustained breathing without mechanical support (abbreviation)
12 Sign of respiratory muscle fatigue (two words)
15 Type of epinephrine used to treat 24 across
16 Index of potential respiratory muscle overload and fatigue (abbreviation)
18 Patients who lie passively in bed have a high _____ factor
19 This is designed specifically to reduce the work associated with ET resistance (abbreviation)
22 Patient-centered method of closed loop mechanical ventilation (abbreviation)
23 Removal of the artificial airway
24 Problem that may be caused by extubation (two words)

Down

1 Type of blockade
2 The opposite of IPPV (abbreviation)
4 An explicit, detailed plan
8 Patients who are optimistic about their illness and are motivated to recover have a high _____ factor
9 Gradual reduction of ventilatory support in a patient who is improving
10 Adapter used for a trial
11 A low-density gas
13 A balance that must be maintained (two words)
14 Foreign material in the airway
17 Closed loop method of weaning (abbreviation)
20 Index for ventilatory muscle capability (abbreviation)
21 Type of trial

Review Questions

1. Define the term *weaning*.

   _____

   _____

2. Name three types of patients who do not require a slow withdrawal process from mechanical ventilation.

   _____

   _____

3. Name four potential risk factors that can be avoided by discontinuing mechanical ventilation as soon as possible.

   _____

   _____

4. List four potential hazards of halting ventilation prematurely or removing an airway too soon.

   _____

   _____

5. Name three traditional weaning methods that involve a gradual reduction in mechanical support, which progressively allows the patient to do more of the work of breathing.

   _____

6. Which of the three methods in question 5 requires the most time to liberate the patient from mechanical ventilatory support?

   _____

7. What should be the primary factor in determining whether a patient is ready to be weaned from mechanical ventilation?

   _____

8. How does SIMV help facilitate weaning of a patient from mechanical ventilation?

   _____

   _____

   _____

9. Why should PS be added during SIMV?

   _____

   _____

10. PSV is _____ triggered, _____ limited, and _____ cycled.

11. What parameters are within the patient's control during PSV?

    _____

12. Name the most practical method of establishing a PS level.

    _____

    _____

13. What are considered acceptable ranges for the V_T and respiratory rate in a patient receiving PSV?

    _____

    _____

14. Give the signs and symptoms that would indicate an inappropriately set PS level.

    _____

    _____

    _____

15. When the inspiratory pressure is titrated during PSV, what level is not high enough to contribute significantly to ventilatory support of the patient?

    _____

16. How is weaning from mechanical ventilation by T-piece trials accomplished?

    _____

    _____

    _____

17. What is the major disadvantage of T-piece weaning?

    _____

    _____

18. (a) What mode of mechanical ventilation can be used as a substitute for T-piece weaning?

    _____

    (b) What is the major advantage of using this mode instead of a T-piece trial?

    _____

19. Name four types of patients who are less likely to tolerate T-piece weaning.

    _____

    _____

    _____

20. Name five advanced closed loop techniques that have been used for weaning.

_____

_____

_____

_____

21. In the following list, match the description with the appropriate weaning mode.

Weaning Mode	Description
____ ATC	(a) Allows spontaneous breathing between mechanical breaths
____ Volume	(b) Similar to a T-piece with alarm support capability
____ MMV	(c) Compensates for increased resistance and WOB through an ET
____ ASV	(d) Adjusts the PS level or mode based on measured parameters
____ KBS	(e) Allows patient control of the rate, time, and depth of each breath
____ SIMV	(f) Provides pressure-limited breaths that target a volume and rate
____ PSV	(g) Maintains a consistent minimum $\dot{V}_E$
____ CPAP	(h) Delivers a set VT in a pressure mode of ventilation

22. List 10 physical signs and measurements of an increase in WOB.

_____

_____

_____

_____

_____

_____

_____

23. Identify seven assessment criteria for discontinuation of a SBT.

_____

_____

_____

_____

_____

_____

_____

24. According to the ACCP/SCCM/AARC task force, what is the first recommendation for weaning a patient from mechanical ventilation?

_____

_____

25. List four criteria for determining the potential for extubation.

_____

_____

_____

_____

_____

26. List eight psychological factors that may adversely affect the weaning process.

_____

_____

_____

27. Describe how underfeeding or overfeeding affects the patient's ability to be weaned from mechanical ventilation.

(a) Underfeeding:

_____

_____

(b) Overfeeding:

_____

_____

28. Describe the procedure for a cuff leak test.

_____

_____

_____

29. In a cuff leak test, what does the measured volume that escapes from around a deflated cuff indicate?

_____

_____

30. Why is vital capacity not considered a good indicator for discontinuation of ventilator support?

_____

_____

31. What parameter is a primary index of the inspiratory drive to breathe?

_____

32. The parameter in question 31 may reflect both the

drive to breathe and _____.

33. A _____ (high; low) oxygen cost

of breathing and a (an) _____

(increased; decreased) metabolic rate may result in

increased WOB.

34. (a) What index is used to assess the potential for respiratory muscle overload and fatigue?

_____

(b) What four components does this index measure?

_____

_____

_____

_____

35. (a) Calculate the CROP index using these data: C_D = 20 mL/cm H_2O, P_{Imax} = 25 cm H_2O, PaO_2 = 70 mm Hg, P_AO_2 = 100 mm Hg, rate = 18 breaths/min.

_____

_____

_____

_____

(b) Does this value indicate the possibility of successful ventilator withdrawal? Give your reasons.

_____

_____

36. How long must a patient tolerate an SBT to be considered ready for ventilator discontinuation and extubation?

_____

37. (a) Write the formula for the RSBI.

_____

_____

(b) Calculate the RSBI, given the following values: V_T = 600 mL, rate = 26 breaths/min.

_____

(c) Does the RSBI indicate that weaning will be successful? Why or why not?

_____

_____

38. What two criteria must be met before a decision is made on whether to remove an artificial airway?

_____

_____

39. List four factors that indicate that extubation will be successful.

_____

_____

_____

40. List three patient conditions in which an artificial airway cannot be removed after weaning from mechanical ventilation.

_____

_____

41. List three risks associated with prolonged intubation.

_____

42. (a) How does administration of heliox aid the treatment of partial airway obstruction and stridor caused by postextubation glottic edema?

_____

_____

_____

_____

_____

(b) How is heliox therapy administered in this situation?

_____

43. List six factors that may increase the risk of aspiration after extubation.

_____

_____

_____

_____

_____

44. What is the primary indication for NPPV after extubation?

_____

_____

45. List five benefits of using NPPV after extubation.

_____

_____

_____

_____

46. List the criteria for instituting NPPV when an extubated patient is unable to sustain adequate ventilation.

_____

_____

_____

_____

_____

47. List four types of medication that can depress the central ventilatory drive.

_____

_____

48. Referring to question 47, why would CMV, SIMV, and MMV be the preferred ventilator modes for postoperative patients or patients receiving the medications listed?

_____

_____

_____

49. Explain the advantages of TDPs for both patients and hospital staff.

_____

_____

_____

50. Patients who may benefit from tracheostomy include those _____

_____

_____

_____

_____

_____.

51. List five beneficial outcomes for tracheostomy.

_____

_____

_____

52. What would be the most important beneficial outcome from tracheostomy?

_____

53. What alternative sites are available to patients who fail multiple weaning attempts in the ICU and are medically stable?

_____

_____

_____

54. List five goals for weaning in long-term care facilities.

_____

_____

_____

_____

_____

Critical Thinking Questions

For questions 1 and 2, refer to the following scenario:

A patient is successfully weaned from mechanical ventilatory support. A leak test is performed before extubation, and the measured volume is 80 mL.

1. What can the respiratory therapist conclude from this finding?

2. What should the respiratory therapist recommend before extubation?

3. Ten minutes after a patient was extubated, the respiratory therapist observes marked stridor, increased WOB, intercostal retractions, and a 20% drop in the SpO_2. An aerosolized racemic epinephrine treatment is given, but no effect is noted. What should the therapist recommend?

Case Studies

Case Study #1

While monitoring a patient 10 minutes after initiation of a T-piece trial, the respiratory therapist observes increased restlessness, an increase in the respiratory rate from 16 to 36 breaths/min with paradoxical chest movement and use of accessory muscles, and an increase in the heart rate from 80 to 120 beats/min.

1. What may be the primary reason for this patient's failed weaning attempt?

2. What would be the most appropriate action to take at this time?

Case Study #2

A 45-year-old male trauma patient has been maintained on volume-controlled ventilation for approximately 3 weeks. The patient's overall condition is improving, but he is not totally alert, and he has periods of apnea. The physician would like to start weaning the patient from the ventilator.

1. What weaning modalities should the therapist recommend and why?

Case Study #3

A 65-year-old patient who suffered a myocardial infarction several days ago is being ventilated in a volume control mode at a set rate of 12 breaths/min and a V_T of 800 mL. The patient currently is stable, and his overall condition is improving. The physician asks the respiratory therapist to initiate a weaning trial; the results are as follows:

Mode	SIMV
Mandatory rate	6 breaths/min
Mandatory V_T	800 mL
Spontaneous rate	35 breaths/min
Spontaneous V_T	185 mL

1. What is the cause of the high spontaneous respiratory rate?

2. What are the therapist's options at this point?

NBRC–Style Questions

1. In the assessment of a patient's respiratory rate, which of the following values would indicate the highest probability that the patient will be able to maintain spontaneous ventilation?
   a. <45 breaths/min
   b. <40 breaths/min
   c. <30 breaths/min
   d. <25 breaths/min

2. Which of the following drugs is used most often to treat postextubation glottic edema?
   a. Racemic epinephrine
   b. IV steroids
   c. Albuterol via MDI
   d. Cromolyn sodium

3. Which of the following is the minimal acceptable range for maximal inspiratory pressure when assessing ventilatory muscle strength?
   a. -5 to -10 cm H_2O
   b. -10 to -15 cm H_2O
   c. -20 to -30 cm H_2O
   d. -40 to -50 cm H_2O

4. A patient is being weaned from mechanical ventilation. The ventilator settings and ABG results are as follows:

Mode	SIMV
Set rate	8 breaths/min
V_T	650 mL
F_IO_2	0.35
PS	25 cm H_2O
pH	7.44
$PaCO_2$	34 mm Hg
PaO_2	96 mm Hg

   Based on this information, what should the respiratory therapist recommend?
   a. Increase the SIMV rate
   b. Reduce the PS level
   c. Reduce the V_T
   d. Reduce the F_IO_2

5. Which of the following statements is true?
   a. In SIMV all breaths are spontaneously triggered.
   b. In the A/C mode every patient effort delivers the set V_T.
   c. In SIMV all breaths deliver the same V_T.
   d. PS can be used to augment the V_T in A/C.

6. A patient is being weaned in the MMV mode. The MMV is set at 7 L, and the patient is breathing at a rate of 14 breaths/min with a spontaneous V_T of 600 mL. How much ventilatory assistance is the ventilator providing?
   a. $\dot{V}_E$ of 4 L
   b. No assistance is required.
   c. Respiratory rate of 8 breaths/min
   d. $\dot{V}_E$ of 7 L

7. Which of the following would indicate a successful weaning trial and extubation?
   I. PaO_2 ≥ 60 mm Hg on F_IO_2 ≤ 0.4
   II. PaO_2/F_IO_2 ratio ≤ 150 to 200 mm Hg
   III. Dopamine >5 $\mu g/kg/min$ to maintain BP
   IV. pH ≥ 7.25
   a. I
   b. II, III, and IV
   c. I and IV
   d. I, II, III, and IV

8. Which of the following modes of mechanical ventilation automatically adjusts ventilatory parameters based on continuous monitoring of compliance and airway resistance?
   I. Proportional assist ventilation
   II. Pressure-regulated volume control
   III. Adaptive support ventilation
   IV. Airway pressure release ventilation
   a. I and II
   b. I and III
   c. I, II, and IV
   d. I, II, III, and IV

9. Which of the following should be required *before* an SBT?
   I. The patient should be given a sedative.
   II. The patient should be able to maintain an adequate PaO_2 and $PaCO_2$ during spontaneous breathing.
   III. The patient should be hemodynamically stable.
   IV. The patient's P_{Imax} should be ≥ 50 mm Hg.
   a. I
   b. I, II, and III
   c. I, II, III, and IV
   d. II and III

10. Which of the following parameters indicate that an SBT will be successful?
    a. $\dot{V}_E$ of 14 L
    b. PaO_2 of 55 mm Hg on an F_IO_2 of 0.5
    c. V_D/V_T ratio of 0.7
    d. PaO_2/F_IO_2 ratio of 180 mm Hg

Helpful Internet Sites

- Perkal MF: Discontinuation of mechanical ventilation. *Clinical Window*, International Web Journal for Medical Professionals. Highlighting Critical Care, Issue 18, March 2005. Available at www.datex-ohmeda.com/clinical/cw_issue_18_article1.htm#
- Frutos-Vivar F, Esteban A: When to wean from a ventilator: an evidenced-based strategy. *Cleveland Clinic J Med* 70: May 2003. Available at www.ccjm.org/pdffiles/Frutos-Vivar503.pdf
- Wesley Ely E: Weaning from mechanical ventilation: acute and chronic management. Lesson 10, vol 15. Pulmonary and Critical Care Update (ACCP Education Website). Available at www.chestnet.org/education/online/pccu/vol15/lessons9_10/lesson10.php
- Allà I, Esteban A: Weaning from mechanical ventilation. *Critical Care Forum*. Available at http://ccforum.com/content/4/2/072

CHAPTER 21

Long-Term Ventilation

Learning Objectives

Upon completion of this chapter the reader will be able to do the following:

1. Recognize realistic goals of home mechanical ventilation.
2. List criteria for selection of patients suitable for successful home care ventilation.
3. Name factors used to estimate cost of home mechanical ventilation.
4. Describe facilities used for the care of patients requiring extended ventilator management in terms of type of care provided and cost.
5. Identify factors used when considering selection of a ventilator for home use.
6. Compare criteria for discharging a child versus discharging an adult who is ventilator dependent.
7. Explain the use of the following noninvasive ventilation techniques: pneumobelt, chest cuirass, full-body chamber (tank ventilator), and body suit (jacket ventilator).
8. List follow-up assessment techniques used with home-ventilated patients.
9. Describe some of the difficulties families experience when caring for a patient in the home.
10. Identify pieces of equipment that are essential to accomplishing intermittent positive pressure ventilation in the home.
11. Name the specific equipment needed for patients in the home who cannot be without ventilator support.
12. Name the appropriate modes used with first-generation portable/home care ventilators.
13. On the basis of a patient's assessment and ventialtor parameters, name the operational features required for that patient's home ventilator and any additional equipment needed.
14. Discuss the instructions given to the patient and caregivers when preparing a patient for discharge home.
15. List the items that should appear in a monthly report of patient on home mechanical ventilation.
16. Describe patients who would benefit from continuous positive airway pressure by nasal mask or pillows.
17. Recommend solutions to potential complications and side effects of nasal mask continuous positive airway pressure.
18. Recognize from a clinical example a potential complication of negative pressure ventilation.
19. Name three methods of improving secretion clearance besides suctioning.
20. List the advantages of using mechanical insufflation exsufflation in conjunction with positive pressure ventilation.
21. List five psychological problems that can occur in ventilator-assisted individuals.
22. Explain the procedure for accomplishing speech in ventilator-assisted individuals.
23. Compare the functions of the Portex and the Pittsburg speaking tracheostomy tubes.
24. Name one essential step required by the respiratory therapist when settling up a speaking valve for a ventilator-assisted individual.
25. List six circumstances in which speaking devices may be contraindicated.

Key Terms Crossword Puzzle

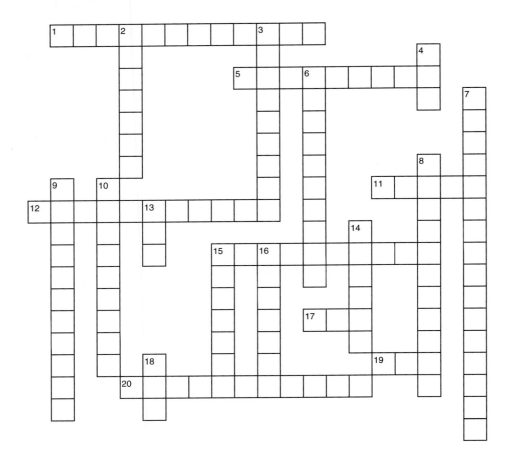

Across

1 Easy to understand and manipulate (two words)
5 Reflux can cause this to erode
11 Failure of appropriate forward movement of bowel contents
12 Removal of the tracheostomy tube
15 Producer of speech (two words)
17 Home care equipment supplier (abbreviation)
19 Mechanical cough machine (abbreviation)
20 Type of tube that goes into the stomach

Down

2 Temporary relief for the caregiver
3 Type of planning team
4 Type of sleep disorder (abbreviation)
6 Intermittent abdominal pressure ventilator
7 Type of breathing used to assist patients with poor respiratory muscle strength
8 Type of TT with an extra opening
9 Surgical opening between the jejunum and the surface of the abdominal wall
10 Type of speaking valve (two words)
13 Opposite of PPV (abbreviation)
14 Name of a speaking TT
15 Home care disinfectant
16 A type of ventilation indicated in 13 down
18 Ventilator-assisted individuals (abbreviation)

Review Questions

1. List the overall goals of long-term home mechanical ventilation.

   _____

   _____

   _____

   _____

2. When is improvement seen in the psychosocial well-being of a patient on long-term ventilation?

   _____

   _____

3. What are the criteria for classifying a patient as chronically ventilator dependent?

   _____

   _____

4. What are the two general categories of patients who require long-term mechanical ventilation?

   _____

   _____

5. List the three factors that are assessed when a patient is evaluated for home mechanical ventilation.

   _____

   _____

6. As part of the health care team, the respiratory therapist must evaluate what information before making recommendations prior to discharge?

   _____

   _____

7. What factors must be considered for a patient to be considered for long-term mechanical ventilation in the home?

   _____

   _____

   _____

   _____

   _____

   _____

   _____

   _____

8. A patient who has required mechanical ventilation for longer than 30 days and who suffers from cardiovascular instability would best be treated in which type of facility?

   _____

9. Name the factors that must be considered in estimating the cost to the patient of home mechanical ventilation.

   _____

   _____

10. In order of cost (most expensive to least expensive), list the possible locations for patients requiring long-term ventilatory care.

    _____

    _____

    _____

11. List the five primary factors in choosing a ventilator for home use.

    _____

    _____

12. What backup equipment should be available for a patient requiring long-term mechanical ventilation at home? Give the rationale for each item.

Backup Equipment	Rationale
_____	_____
_____	_____
_____	_____
_____	_____

13. List four criteria besides clinical stability and adequate financial support for considering a child for home mechanical ventilation.

    _____

    _____

    _____

    _____

14. Why is the ventilatory status of children maintained on mechanical ventilation at home followed up and evaluated more often than that of adults?

    _____

    _____

15. Identify the three classifications of ventilator-dependent patients.

_____

_____

16. Identify the psychosocial factors that must be addressed to ensure a successful transition home for the ventilator-dependent patient.

_____

_____

17. What factors must be addressed in the evaluation of the home environment before discharge of a patient requiring mechanical ventilation?

_____

_____

_____

18. Discuss the difficulties family members face in caring for a patient in the home.

_____

_____

19. In addition to the mechanical ventilator, list some of the equipment and supplies needed to support a patient receiving mechanical ventilation in the home.

_____

20. List the three electrical power sources used by home ventilators.

_____

21. Complete the following table, which compares the three types of NPVs.

Ventilator	Advantages	Disadvantages
Iron lung	_____	_____
	_____	_____
	_____	_____
	_____	_____
Chest cuirass	_____	_____
	_____	_____
	_____	_____
Body suit	_____	_____

22. List the four contraindications to use of an NPV.

_____

_____

23. What is the main disadvantage of placing a patient in the IMV mode when using an earlier model (first-generation) home care ventilator?

_____

24. Explain why a patient receiving mechanical ventilation with oxygen and PEEP in the home may have difficulty triggering the ventilator.

_____

_____

25. What are some of the advantages of providing home mechanical ventilation with the newer (second generation) portable home care ventilators?

   _____

   _____

   _____

   _____

26. What three complications are common to both long-term and critically ill patients who require mechanical ventilation?

   _____

   _____

27. Fifteen minutes after initiating PEEP in a patient supported by a home care ventilator, the respiratory therapist observes that the patient's respiratory rate has doubled, V_T has dropped significantly, and the ventilator's low pressure alarm has been activated. What is the probable cause of this problem?

   _____

   _____

28. List the four most common gastrointestinal disorders associated with patients receiving long-term mechanical ventilation.

   _____

   _____

   _____

   _____

29. Of patients who transfer to a chronic care facility, a _____ disorder generally is the main cause of their _____.

30. List the seven most common factors that contribute to the psychological problems of patients requiring long-term mechanical ventilation.

   _____

   _____

   _____

31. Explain how the rocking bed and the pneumobelt support spontaneous ventilation.

   _____

   _____

32. Use of a rocking bed or pneumobelt is contraindicated under what three circumstances?

   _____

   _____

33. What two types of patients may benefit from a rocking bed or pneumobelt?

   _____

   _____

34. In what type of therapy is the phrenic nerve stimulated through surgically implanted electrodes?

   _____

35. What form of respiratory therapy is most often used to treat OSA?

   _____

36. Patients with OSA become _____ and _____ during sleep. CPAP is used to alleviate _____ and _____.

37. List the goals of CPAP therapy for OSA.

   _____

   _____

   _____

38. What are the two most common methods of delivering CPAP therapy?

   _____

   _____

39. List two major advantages of the newer home CPAP units.

   _____

   _____

40. List the three important complications associated with CPAP therapy.

   _____

   _____

41. The most common patient complaint with the use of CPAP is _____ or _____ from high airflows, which can be alleviated by increasing _____ or _____.

42. What are the physical requirements for performing glossopharyngeal breathing?

_____

_____

_____

43. What are the minimum VC and PCEF required to produce an effective cough?

_____

44. List three techniques that aid secretion management in patients with neuromuscular disease.

_____

_____

45. Assisted coughing is the technique of applying

_____ and/or

_____ to the patient's

anterior chest wall to increase _____.

46. What are the advantages of MI-E compared with tracheal suctioning?

_____

_____

47. In what type of patients is MI-E contraindicated?

_____

_____

48. What type of tracheostomy tube should a therapist recommend for a patient who is unable to speak and who is at risk of aspiration?

_____

49. What type of tracheostomy tube should a therapist recommend for a patient who has no trouble swallowing and who can breathe spontaneously for long periods?

_____

50. Why is evaluation of language and vocal skills in children with tracheostomies important?

_____

_____

51. Besides cuff deflation, what ventilator parameters can be adjusted to help produce speech or improve the quality of a patient's speech?

_____

52. What are the potential hazards of cuff deflation in VAIs?

_____

_____

53. Before a cuff is deflated to allow for speaking, patients

need to be evaluated for their ability to _____

and _____ their airway to avoid the risk of

_____.

54. List three possible complications associated with the use of speaking tracheostomy tubes.

_____

_____

_____

55. How does a Passy-Muir speaking valve allow for speech in a patient with a tracheostomy who is mechanically ventilated?

_____

_____

56. List the circumstances in which use of speaking devices may be contraindicated.

_____

_____

_____

_____

57. What is the most cost-effective disinfecting solution available for home care ventilation equipment?

_____

58. How long must water be boiled before it can be used in a humidifier?

_____

59. List the steps a respiratory therapist must take before attaching a speaking valve.

_____

_____

_____

_____

60. List the primary skills the respiratory therapist must teach the patient, family, and others involved in home care before a patient is discharged.

_____

_____

_____

61. What components must be included in a written monthly report on a home visit?

_____

_____

_____

_____

Critical Thinking Questions

For questions 1 and 2, refer to the following scenario.

After undergoing a sleep study, a patient diagnosed with OSA is prescribed CPAP via nasal mask. During a follow-up visit by the respiratory therapist, the patient states that his sleep is not improving and his eyes are irritated.

1. What could be the cause of the patient's problem?

_____

_____

_____

_____

2. What steps can the therapist take to solve the problem?

_____

_____

_____

_____

3. A ventilator-dependent patient in a long-term care facility is being maintained on PSV. The respiratory therapist is asked to evaluate the patient to see whether she can tolerate a speaking valve. After cuff deflation and before the valve is attached, the patient suddenly becomes short of breath and her heart rate increases. What could have caused the sudden onset of respiratory distress?

_____

_____

_____

Case Studies

Case Study #1

A patient in the early stages of a neuromuscular disease complains to his physician that he is having difficulty sleeping. He also has headaches and becomes increasingly tired toward the end of the day.

1. What are the possible causes of this patient's symptoms?

_____

_____

2. What type of therapy should the respiratory therapist recommend for this patient?

_____

_____

3. What would be the goals of the recommended therapy?

_____

_____

_____

4. How would the effectiveness of the therapy be evaluated?

_____

_____

_____

Case Study #2

A 70-year-old woman had spent 1 month in the hospital for exacerbation of COPD. Numerous attempts at weaning failed, and the patient received a tracheotomy. After careful evaluation, the patient was discharged home on continuous ventilatory support. A follow-up visit was made 2 weeks after discharge. The respiratory therapist found that the patient was febrile, auscultation revealed rhonchi in the right upper and middle lobes, and the patient was suctioned for a moderate amount of yellow sputum. The patient was admitted to the hospital and diagnosed with pneumonia.

1. Why do you think this patient developed a pulmonary infection so soon after discharge and what recommendations, if any, would you make?

_____

_____

_____

NBRC–Style Questions

1. If a home care ventilator does not have an F_IO_2 control, what is the most common means by which oxygen can be delivered to the patient?
   a. External blender
   b. Microprocessor-controlled proportioning valve
   c. Mixing of air and oxygen cylinders to approximate the desired F_IO_2
   d. Bleeding of oxygen into the system through the inspiratory limb

2. In the home setting, how long should suction catheters be soaked in a disinfectant solution?
   a. At least 2 minutes
   b. At least 5 minutes
   c. At least 10 minutes
   d. At least 25 minutes

3. Which of the following represents the range of CPAP available on most home care units?
   a. 0 to 2 cm H_2O
   b. 2.5 to 20 cm H_2O
   c. 25 to 35 cm H_2O
   d. 35 to 45 cm H_2O

4. All of the following patient conditions can be treated with NPV *except*
   a. Excessive secretions
   b. Neuromuscular disease
   c. Spinal cord injuries
   d. Central hypoventilation syndromes

5. During a follow-up visit with a patient recently started on CPAP therapy by nasal mask, the patient complains of nasal dryness and congestion. Which of the following recommendations would help remedy the problem?
   a. Reduce the flow rate
   b. Reduce the CPAP level
   c. Add humidification or recommend use of a nasal spray
   d. Adjust the mask to correct for any leaks

6. Which of the following is *not* generally part of a monthly home evaluation?
   a. Vital signs
   b. Pulse oximetry
   c. Bedside pulmonary function studies
   d. ABG analysis

7. Contraindications to long-term home mechanical ventilation include which of the following?
   a. F_IO_2 requirement >0.4
   b. PEEP >10 cm H_2O
   c. Need for continuous invasive monitoring
   d. All of the above

8. Which of the following conditions allow(s) patients certain periods of spontaneous breathing during the day and generally require(s) only nocturnal ventilatory support?
   I. Myasthenia gravis
   II. End-stage COPD
   III. Kyphoscoliosis
   IV. Multiple sclerosis
   a. I
   b. III and IV
   c. I, III, and IV
   d. I, II, III, and IV

9. Patient assessment before decannulation includes which of the following?
   I. Airway patency
   II. Sufficient muscle strength to generate a cough
   III. Volume and thickness of secretions
   IV. Sleep studies
   a. I
   b. I and IV
   c. I, II, and III
   d. I, II, III, and IV

10. All of the following are realistic goals of home mechanical ventilation *except*
    a. To reverse the disease process
    b. To improve quality of life
    c. To prolong life
    d. To reduce the number of hospitalizations

Helpful Internet Sites

- American College of Chest Physicians: *Mechanical ventilation beyond the ICU.* Available at www.chestnet.org/patients/guides/mech_vent/p3.php
- International Ventilator Users Network: Available at www.post-polio.org/ivun/index.html
- Passy-Muir: Available at www.passy-muir.com/

Neonatal and Pediatric Mechanical Ventilation

Learning Objectives

Upon completion of this chapter the reader will be able to do the following:

1. Identify the primary and secondary goals of ventilatory support of newborn and pediatric patients.
2. Explain some key areas of assessment that affect the decision on whether to initiate ventilatory support.
3. Discuss the guidelines for the use of CPAP in newborn and pediatric patients.
4. Recognize the indications, goals, limitations, and potentially harmful effects of CPAP in a clinical case.
5. Describe the basic design of nasal devices used to deliver CPAP to an infant.
6. Compare and contrast a mechanical ventilator equipped with a CPAP delivery system to a mechanical ventilator equipped with a freestanding CPAP system.
7. From patient data, recognize the need for mechanical ventilatory support in newborn and pediatric patients.
8. Identify the essential features of an infant ventilator.
9. Explain how nonessential features of a ventilator enhance its usefulness over a wide range of clinical settings.
10. Summarize the historical development of mechanical ventilators for newborns and explain how time-cycled flow controllers became the standard.
11. Relate the use of time-cycled, pressure-limited ventilation (TCPL) to the basic circuit design of a typical infant ventilator.
12. Distinguish demand flow from continuous flow and discuss other modifications that have been made to the basic infant ventilator.

13. Select appropriate ventilator settings for TCPL, given the patient's weight, diagnosis, and clinical history: also, discuss strategies and rationale for ventilator settings.
14. Discuss newborn and pediatric applications, technical aspects, patient management, and cautions for the following ventilatory modes: pressure control ventilation, volume ventilation, volume-cycled intermittent mandatory ventilation/synchronized intermittent mandatory ventilation, pressure-regulated volume contol ventilation, assist/contol in infants, volume support ventilation, mandatory minute ventilation, and pressure support ventilation.
15. Discuss the rationale and indications for high-frequency ventilation in newborns and pediatric patients.
16. Identify the contraindications and complications of high-frequency ventilation from patient information.
17. Compare the characteristics and basic delivery systems of the following high-frequency ventilation techniques: high-frequency positive pressure ventilation, high-frequency jet ventilation, high-frequency flow interruption, high-frequency percussive ventilation, and high-frequency oscillatory ventilation.
18. Explain the physiological and theoretical mechanisms of gas exchange in high-frequency ventilation, and defend the mechanism believed to be most correct.
19. Explain how settings of a given high-frequency technique are initially adjusted, the effect of individual controls on gas exchange, and strategies of patient management.
20. Discuss the characteristics of artificial surfactants.
21. Describe the dosing procedure for Survanta.

Key Terms Crossword Puzzle

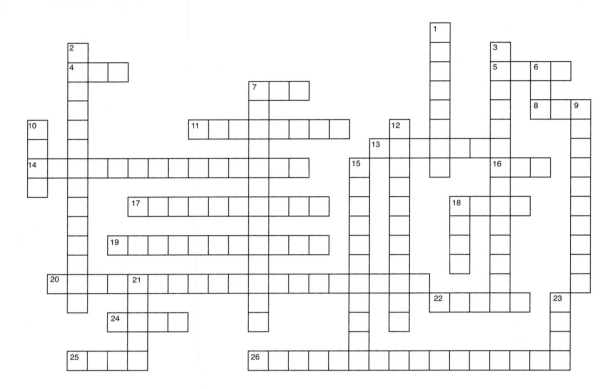

Across

4   Condition that is responsive to 24 across (abbreviation)
5   Type of ventilation that uses the highest rates (8 to 20 Hz) (abbreviation)
7   Pulmonary disease of infants of which high airway resistance is a major component (abbreviation)
8   Neonatal problem commonly treated with methyl-xanthines (abbreviation)
11 Type of aspiration syndrome that occurs in term or postterm neonates
13 Abnormal tubelike passage between the trachea and the esophagus
14 A deficiency in the cartilage around of a bronchus leading to atelectasis
16 Infant who weighs 1500 to 2500 g (abbreviation)
17 Type of heart disease that is present at birth
18 Mode that is unique to infant mechanical ventilation (abbreviation)
19 Congenital split of the roof of the mouth (two words)
20 Incomplete embryological formation of the diaphragm leads to this (two words)
22 Type of hemoglobin present in a fetus
24 Noninvasive method of increasing FRC and improving lung compliance
25 Mode of ventilation used to percuss the chest to remove secretions (abbreviation)
26 Structure that may remain open after birth (two words)

Down

1   Brand of surfactant replacement
2   Softening of the cartilages of the trachea
3   Failure of the nasopharyngeal septum to rupture causes this malformation (two words)
6   This is usually treated by 24 across. (abbreviation)
7   Viral infection that causes inflammation, swelling, and airway obstruction
9   Exchange of gas between lung units with different time constants
10 Infant weighing less than 1500 g (abbreviation)
12 Used to improve pulmonary blood flow and enhance arterial oxygenation (two words)
15 Interface most often used for application of 24 across (two words)
18 Historically, the mode most often used for infants (abbreviation)
21 Mode that uses frequencies up to 150 breaths/min (abbreviation)
23 An invasive life support procedure (abbreviation)

Review Questions

1. Name the three basic types of devices involved in the mechanical ventilation of newborn and pediatric patients.

   _____

   _____

2. Name the goals of mechanical ventilatory support in newborn and pediatric patients.

   _____

   _____

   _____

3. What is the goal of mechanical ventilatory support for premature infants who have adequate spontaneous ventilation, oxygenation, and lung volumes but have periods of apnea?

   _____

   _____

4. What laboratory data define respiratory failure in newborns?

   _____

5. The minimum acceptable pH for a premature or term

   newborn is _____.

6. What factors must be weighed against each other in the decision on whether to intubate and ventilate a newborn infant?

   _____

   _____

   _____

   _____

7. What laboratory data define respiratory failure in pediatric patients?

   _____

8. How can tissue oxygenation be assessed physically?

   _____

   _____

   _____

   _____

9. In what way can oxygen delivery and tissue perfusion be evaluated clinically?

   _____

   _____

   _____

10. When maximum oxygen delivery to the tissues is critical, why is fetal hemoglobin not desirable?

    _____

    _____

11. What are the most common uses for CPAP in pediatric patients?

    _____

    _____

12. CPAP is usually recommended for a pediatric or newborn patient with what condition?

    _____

    _____

13. Name the three methods of delivering CPAP to newborns.

    _____

14. What six factors constitute the physical examination indicators for the use of CPAP?

    _____

    _____

    _____

    _____

15. The blood gas values that indicate a need for CPAP

    are _____

    _____

    _____.

16. Chest radiographic indications for the use of CPAP include what two findings?

    _____

    _____

17. List the seven conditions that are thought to respond to CPAP and are associated with one or more of the previously listed clinical presentations.

_____

_____

_____

_____

18. CPAP may be used as a method of early intervention for what type of neonate? ·

_____

_____

19. Describe how some infants with certain congenital heart diseases may benefit from the use of CPAP.

_____

_____

_____

_____

_____

20. What are the contraindications to the use of CPAP?

_____

_____

_____

21. The most commonly used interface for the application of CPAP is _____.

22. The most critical facts concerning the application of CPAP interfaces are _____

_____.

23. How is the CPAP apparatus stabilized?

_____

_____

24. CPAP stabilizing equipment should be checked periodically for what?

_____

_____

_____

25. Describe how a nasopharyngeal tube is inserted.

_____

_____

_____

_____

_____

_____

_____

26. List four problems that improper positioning of the NP tube can cause.

_____

27. Why are improvised CPAP systems not the safest method of CPAP administration?

_____

_____

_____

_____

28. What is the initial pressure setting for CPAP and how should the CPAP level be adjusted?

_____

_____

29. What is considered an adequate level of CPAP?

_____

30. List ten possible complications of CPAP.

_____

_____

_____

_____

_____

_____

_____

31. nSIMV is most effectively delivered with which type of triggering device?

_____

32. Complete the following table.

Disorder	CPAP Application Device
Four-year-old with juvenile spinal muscle atrophy (Kugelberg-Welander disease)	_____
One-year-old with progressive spinal muscular atrophy of infants (Werdnig-Hoffmann paralysis)	_____
Ten-year-old with OSA	
Three-year-old with bronchomalacia	_____

33. List the major categories of indications for mechanical ventilation in the neonate.

   _____

   _____

   _____

   _____

   _____

   _____

   _____

   _____

34. Respiratory failure in a neonate is characterized by what laboratory and clinical data?

   _____

   _____

   _____

35. What neurological problems can compromise the central drive of a newborn?

   _____

   _____

36. List seven diseases/syndromes that can reduce lung compliance and/or increase airway resistance in a neonate.

   _____

   _____

   _____

37. List four diseases/syndromes that impair the cardiovascular function of a neonate.

   _____

   _____

   _____

   _____

38. What are the indicators of respiratory failure in pediatric patients?

   _____

   _____

39. List four neuromuscular/hypotonic disorders that are indicators for mechanical ventilation of pediatric patients.

   _____

   _____

   _____

40. List the essential features of an infant ventilator.

   _____

   _____

   _____

   _____

   _____

   _____

   _____

   _____

41. How do nonessential features enhance a ventilator's usefulness over a wide range of clinical settings?

   _____

   _____

42. The modality that was used more than any other to ventilate infants in the past was _____.

43. Why were flow controllers so popular in the past?

   _____

   _____

The following figure is referred to in questions 44-46.

(Redrawn from Betit P, Thompson JE, Benjamin PK: Mechanical ventilation. In Koff P, Gitzman D, Neu J: *Neonatal and pediatric respiratory care,* ed 2, St Louis, 1993, Mosby.)

44. Label the parts in the figure and explain the phase of ventilation represented.

   A _____ E _____

   B _____ F _____

   C _____ G _____

   D _____

45. Explain what will happen with the ventilator represented in the previous figure when the inspiratory phase begins.

   _____

   _____

   _____

46. Explain what will happen during the pressure-limiting phase of inspiration in previous figure.

   _____

   _____

   _____

   _____

   _____

47. Discuss the difference between continuous flow and demand flow for spontaneous breaths.

   _____

   _____

   _____

   _____

   _____

48. In an infant ventilator, what type of trigger avoids breath stacking and asynchrony?

   _____

49. Describe how PIP can be optimized during manual ventilation.

   _____

   _____

   _____

   _____

   _____

   _____

50. What is the target V_T range for TCPL?

   _____

51. What is the purpose of PEEP when used in newborns?

   _____

52. What guideline is used to set the flow rate for most newborn patients?

   _____

   _____

53. What are the signs of insufficient flow for spontaneous and mandatory breaths?

   _____

   _____

   _____

   _____

54. (a) Calculate the time constant when Raw = 45 cm/H_2O/L/sec and $C_L = 0.004$ L/cm H_2O.

   _____

   _____

   (b) What T_I should be set for this time constant?

   _____

55. (a) Calculate the time constant when Raw = 30 cm/H_2O/L/sec and $C_L = 0.002$ L/cm H_2O.

   _____

   _____

   (b) What T_I should be set for this time constant?

   _____

56. What can be done to reduce the potential for ventilator-induced hyperinflation in patients with bronchopulmonary dysplasia or meconium aspiration?

   _____

   _____

57. Calculate the estimated V_T when $T_I = 0.5$ second and the flow rate = 4 L/min.

   _____

58. Calculate the percent leak when $V_T$insp = 67 mL and $V_T$exh = 55 mL.

   _____

   _____

   _____

   _____

59. Calculate the T_I setting for a respiratory rate of 40 breaths/min at an I:E ratio of 1:2.

_____

_____

_____

60. Mean airway pressures greater than _____ have been associated with lung injury in neonates.

61. What is the major difference between PCV and TPTV?

_____

_____

62. Explain mixed-mode ventilation and its advantages with newborn and pediatric patients.

_____

_____

_____

_____

_____

63. Specify the values for PaO_2/F_IO_2, PIP, and PEEP that, in a child weighing more than 10 kg or in an older pediatric patient, indicate the need for PCV.

_____

_____

64. The recommended V_T values for PCV are

_____.

65. What is meant by the term *flow chop*?

_____

_____

_____

_____

_____

66. What factors determine T_I when VV is used?

_____

_____

67. What types of pediatric patients respond well to VV with SIMV?

_____

_____

_____

68. What advantage does VSV have over PSV in the administration of surfactant replacement therapy to an infant?

_____

_____

_____

69. How is weaning accomplished in infants with the A/C option?

_____

_____

70. What types of lung-protective strategies may be used during ventilation of neonatal and pediatric patients?

_____

_____

_____

_____

71. What do preparations of exogenous surfactant typically contain?

_____

_____

72. Describe the dosing procedure for exogenous surfactant.

_____

_____

_____

_____

_____

73. What is the recommended therapeutic range for NO concentrations?

_____

_____

74. Name the two types of toxicity that have been reported with application of inhaled NO.

_____

_____

75. When should high-frequency ventilation be considered in an infant's clinical course?

_____

_____

_____

_____

76. List three complications from HFV.

_____

77. Complete the following table.

HFV Type	Definition (including frequencies)	Uses

78. Explain the physiological mechanism of gas exchange in HFV.

_____

_____

79. List the preparations that should be completed before a patient is placed on HFV.

_____

_____

_____

80. What is the general goal for all types of HFV?

_____

_____

Critical Thinking Questions

1. A pediatric patient with a 4-mm ET is receiving PSV. The respiratory therapist notes that inspiration seems to exceed 1 second. What is the most likely cause of this problem and how can it be corrected?

_____

_____

2. VSV has what advantage over PSV during surfactant replacement therapy?

_____

_____

3. An infant receiving nasal CPAP is crying, and each time the infant's mouth opens, the CPAP level on the pressure manometer drops significantly. Why is the pressure dropping and what can be done to correct it?

_____

_____

_____

_____

Case Studies

Case Study #1

A 29 weeks' gestation, 2-hour old infant is in the neonatal ICU in an oxyhood with an F_IO_2 of 0.5. Physical examination reveals intercostal and substernal retractions, a respiratory rate of 68 breaths/min, and a pulse of 145. The ABG values are as follows: pH = 7.21, $PaCO_2$ = 70 mm Hg, PaO_2 = 41 mm Hg. Manual ventilation of this patient demonstrates bilateral chest movement and aeration at 25 cm H_2O.

1. The most appropriate PIP setting for this patient is

_____.

During mechanical ventilation, the patient's pressure-volume loop changes from that shown in Figure A to that shown in Figure B.

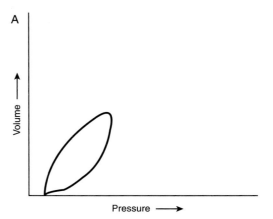

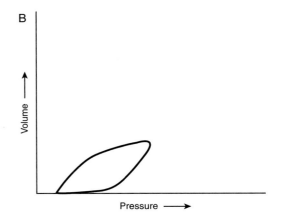

2. What is the most likely cause of this change?

_____

The patient receives Survanta at 2 mL/kg. During this time the ventilator F_IO_2 is increased to 1. Each partial dose is followed by a 30-second period on the ventilator. The pressure-volume loop then takes on the shape shown in Figure C.

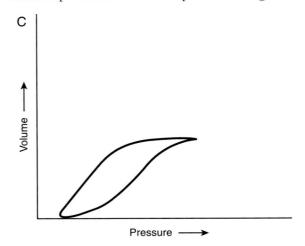

3. What is the most likely cause of this change?

_____

Case Study #2

A newborn male infant weighing 1275 g and approximately 28 weeks' gestation currently is intubated and receiving mechanical ventilation with TCPL at these settings: rate = 40 breaths/min, PIP = 24 cm H_2O, PEEP = 4 cm H_2O, F_1O_2 = 0.75. The patient received Survanta about 1 hour ago. The ABG results after surfactant therapy were these: pH = 7.36, $PaCO_2$ = 38 mm Hg, PaO_2 = 80 mm Hg. The infant is pink and active; the pulse oximeter reads 96%.

1. What would be the most appropriate action in this situation?

_____

Over the next 2 hours the patient's oxygen saturations begin to decline and his oxygen requirements increase. Breath sounds are bilaterally diminished, the pulse oximeter reading is 86% with an F_1O_2 of 0.55, and the patient is agitated. The respiratory therapist suctions the patient, but no improvement is noted.

2. Name the two most likely causes of this patient distress.

_____

_____

3. What is the most appropriate action at this time?

_____

Case Study #3

A 24 weeks' gestation neonate weighing 730 g had no signs of respirations and had central cyanosis at birth. He was intubated in the delivery room and transported to the neonatal ICU. He had poor gas exchange during manual resuscitation, and the decision was made to place him on HFOV.

1. What should be the setting for the mean airway pressure?

_____

2. The initial frequency setting should be _____ Hz.

3. How should the initial pressure gradient be set?

_____

NBRC–Style Questions

1. Which of the following is the best method of ensuring an effective CPAP system?
   a. Use of audible and visual alarm systems
   b. Incorporation of F_1O_2 and pressure monitors
   c. Careful monitoring of the patient's WOB and oxygenation status
   d. Use only of a mechanical ventilator with continuous flow capability

2. The type of CPAP delivery system that produces vibrations that may have a beneficial effect is which of the following?
   a. Bubble CPAP
   b. Freestanding CPAP device
   c. Mechanical ventilators with CPAP settings
   d. Improvised freestanding CPAP delivery device

3. The safest and most effective method of CPAP delivery to a newborn is with which of the following?
   a. Vapotherm
   b. Hamilton Arabella
   c. Fisher & Paykel Bubble CPAP
   d. Improvised freestanding CPAP device

4. In newborns PEEP is used to accomplish which of the following?
   I. Recruit alveoli
   II. Prevent atelectasis
   III. Decrease compliance
   IV. Establish functional residual capacity
   a. I and III
   b. I and II
   c. III and IV
   d. II and IV

5. The disease state that prolongs time constants is which of the following?
   a. Acute lung injury
   b. Apnea of prematurity
   c. Bronchopulmonary dysplasia
   d. Respiratory distress syndrome

6. The tip of an NP tube is palpated in the posterior oropharynx. How far back should the tube be pulled before stabilization?
   a. 0.5 to 1 cm
   b. 1.5 to 2 cm
   c. 2 to 2.5 cm
   d. 2.5 to 3 cm

7. A newborn is currently in an oxygen hood with an F_1O_2 of 0.7. The patient's ABG values are these: pH = 7.31, $PaCO_2$ = 49 mm Hg, PaO_2 = 50 mm Hg. The most appropriate action is to initiate which of the following?
   a. PSV
   b. CPAP
   c. TPV
   d. SIMV

8. A neonate receiving nasal CPAP of 8 cm H_2O with an F_IO_2 of 0.65 has the following ABG values: pH = 7.2, $PaCO_2$ = 69 mm Hg, and PaO_2 = 48 mm Hg. The most appropriate action is which of the following?
   a. Increase the F_IO_2 to 0.75
   b. Increase CPAP to 10 cm H_2O
   c. Change to nasopharyngeal CPAP
   d. Intubate and mechanically ventilate with TPTV

9. Before an infant is put on TPTV, the PIP should be determined by which of the following methods?
   a. Estimate the PIP for the patient, set the value at a level higher than this, and adjust downward
   b. Compare chest movement and bilateral aeration to the PIP during manual ventilation
   c. Estimate the PIP for the patient, set the value at a level lower than this, and adjust upward as needed
   d. Set the PIP to a safe level, attach the patient to the ventilator, and monitor for improvement in overall appearance and oxygen saturation

10. Calculate the patient's estimated V_T in TPTV when T_I is 0.5 second and flow is 8.75 L/min.
    a. 54 mL
    b. 62 mL
    c. 73 mL
    d. 95 mL

11. V_T is increased during PCV by which of the following?
    a. Increasing PIP
    b. Increasing PEEP
    c. Decreasing flow rate
    d. Increasing T_I

12. Which of the following must be monitored during administration of surfactant replacements?
    I. Heart rate
    II. Oxygenation
    III. Temperature
    IV. Airway patency
    a. I, II, and IV
    b. II, III, and IV
    c. I and III
    d. I, II, III, and IV

Helpful Internet Sites

- Virtual Children's Hospital, Iowa Neonatology Handbook: Management strategies with high frequency ventilation in neonates using the SenorMedics 3100A HFO ventilator. Available at www.vh.org/pediatric/provider/pediatrics/iowaneonatologyhandbook/pulmonary/practicalaspectsof.html
- Auckland City Hospital, Newborn Services Clinical Guideline: Basic principles and guidelines for conventional ventilation. Available at www.adhb.govt.nz/newborn/TeachingResources/Ventilation/VentilationBaics.htm
- Oregon Health and Science University: Mechanical ventilator simulator. Available at www.ohsu.edu/academic/picu/medialab/vent/

CHAPTER 23

Special Techniques in Ventilatory Support

Learning Objectives

Upon completion of this chapter the reader will be able to do the following:

1. Discuss the benefits and disadvantages of airway pressure-release ventilation (APRV) compared with other forms of ventilation.
2. Recommend initial settings for APRV in patients with acute lung injury/acute respiratory distress syndrome.
3. Describe one method for weaning a patient from APRV.
4. Explain how the controls operate with the SensorMedics 3100B oscillator.
5. Recommend initial ventilator settings for an adult with the 3100B unit.
6. Describe the function of each of the valves on the 3100B circuit.
7. Name the control that governs piston displacement in the 3100B unit.
8. List types of medications that may be used in transitioning from volume-targeted continuous mandatory ventilation (VC-CMV) to high-frequency oscillatory ventilation (HFOV) in an adult.
9. Explain how the chest wiggle factor is influenced by HFOV settings.
10. Describe the physical characteristics of helium.
11. Name pulmonary pathologies in which heliox therapy may be beneficial.
12. Compare the difference between set V_T, monitored V_T, and actual V_T delivery during heliox therapy

provided by a critical care ventilator such as the Servo 300, the Puritan Bennett 840, or the Dräger Dura 2.

13. Describe how heliox used with a mechanical ventilator may affect pressures and F_IO_2 monitoring and delivery.
14. Explain how to set up heliox cylinders with a mechanical ventilator.
15. Name a circumstance in which heliox therapy should not be used.
16. List surgical procedures in which lung isolation and independent lung ventilation (ILV) are used.
17. Compare synchronous with dyssynchronous ventilation when using two ventilators for ILV.
18. Describe the procedure for measuring the lower inflection point and upper inflection point using a slow flow inflection maneuver (SFIM) for each lung during ILV.
19. Define expiratory inflection point.
20. Explain how appropriate PEEP levels are established during ILV.
21. Provide ventilator settings for performing an SFIM to a single lung and to both lungs.
22. List the types of therapy that can be provided by the Percussionator IPV-1 unit.
23. Describe the characteristics of the Percussionator IPV-1 unit.
24. Identify from a clinical description, the effects a Percussionaire IPV-1 unit has during VC-CMV.

Key Terms Crossword Puzzle

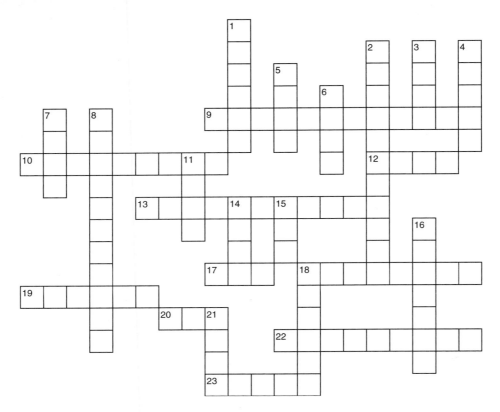

Across

9 Region of the lung receiving the most ventilation
10 HFOV control that influences $PaCO_2$
12 Mode of ventilation with two levels of CPAP (abbreviation)
13 Factor observed from the level of the clavicle to the midthigh during HFOV (two words)
17 HFOV's equivalent to PEEP (abbreviation)
18 First parameter set in starting HFOV (two words)
19 Helium-oxygen mixture
20 Technique that allows the gas flow to each lung to be controlled separately (abbreviation)
22 Region of the lung receiving the best blood flow
23 A property of helium

Down

1 Forward and backward excursion of this helps determine V_T
2 Type of breathing allowed during biphasic CPAP
3 Type of flow waveform produced by HFOV
4 Cycles per minute
5 HFOV is used in the management of this pulmonary problem (abbreviation)
6 HFOV control that directly affects PaO_2 (abbreviation)
7 Heart-lung bypass machine (abbreviation)
8 Brief interval at P_{low} (two words)
11 Type of ET used to accomplish 20 across (abbreviation)
14 Repair of this may cause unilateral lung injury (abbreviation)
15 Applies internal percussion to the lungs (abbreviation)
16 Biphasic CPAP on the Puritan Bennett 840 (two words)
18 Biphasic CPAP on the Servo^i (two words)
21 This can be avoided by starting HFOV early in patients with severe ALI/ARDS (abbreviation)

Review Questions

1. Define *APRV*.

   _____

   _____

   _____

2. Refer to the APRV waveform in the following figure.

Time (seconds)

(Modified from MacIntyre NR, Branson RO: Mechanical ventilation, Philadelphia, 2001, WB Saunders.)

   (a) What is the P_{low}? _____

   (b) What is the P_{high}? _____

3. In APRV, the trigger and cycle variables when the patient does not breathe are _____.

4. Give two other names for APRV that are used in the United States.

   _____

   _____

5. List the physiological and hemodynamic advantages of APRV compared with other forms of ventilation.

   _____

   _____

   _____

   _____

   _____

6. List the main disadvantages of APRV.

   _____

   _____

   _____

   _____

7. Calculate the APRV respiratory rate that would deliver a P_{low} for 0.75 second and a P_{high} for 4.75 seconds.

   _____

   _____

   _____

8. In APRV, $\dot{V}_E$ depends on what two factors?

   _____

   _____

9. The range for the P_{high} setting is _____.

10. The range for the P_{low} setting is _____.

11. The range for the T_{high} setting is _____.

12. The P_{low} setting that allows unimpeded expiratory gas flow and a rapid drop in pressure is _____.

13. How should the T_{low} setting be chosen?

   _____

   _____

   _____

14. For a patient with ARDS the typical range for the T_{low} setting is _____.

15. Ventilation and $PaCO_2$ are determined by what three factors?

   _____

   _____

   _____

16. Describe one method of weaning a patient from APRV.

   _____

   _____

   _____

17. HFOV oscillates the lungs at what rates?

   _____

18. What creates the high-frequency oscillations in the SensorMedics 3100B?

   _____

19. What type of flow waveform is created during HFOV?

   _____

20. What determines V_T during HFOV?

   _____

   _____

21. What determines the appropriateness of the power setting?

   _____

   _____

22. Increasing the HFOV frequency does what to patient ventilation? Why?

_____

23. Reducing the HFOV frequency does what to patient ventilation? Why?

_____

24. What does the $T_I\%$ represent on the SensorMedics 3100B?

_____

_____

25. How does the bias flow setting influence the patient's $PaCO_2$?

_____

_____

_____

26. Complete the following HFOV table.

Control	Brief Description	Typical/Initial Setting
mPaw	_____	_____
	_____	_____
	_____	_____
	_____	_____
	_____	_____
Amplitude	_____	_____
	_____	_____
	_____	_____
	_____	_____
Frequency	_____	_____
$T_I\%$	_____	_____
	_____	_____
Bias flow	_____	_____
	_____	_____
	_____	_____
F_IO_2	_____	_____

27. Describe the function of each of the valves on the SensorMedics 3100B.

_____

_____

_____

28. List the indications for HFOV in adults.

_____

_____

_____

_____

29. What is the one exclusion criterion for use of the SensorMedics 3100B?

_____

30. List the types of medications that may be used in transitioning from VC-CMV to HFOV in an adult.

_____

_____

31. A patient on HFOV may be checked for a return to conventional ventilation when what two parameters have been reached?

_____

32. What two ventilator modes are favored for returning a patient to conventional ventilation after HFOV?

_____

33. Describe the physical characteristics of helium.

_____

_____

34. List the pulmonary pathologies that may be treated with heliox therapy.

_____

_____

35. At what generation bronchi does turbulent flow transition to laminar flow?

_____

36. Calculate the actual flow reading for an 80:20 heliox mixture with a displayed flow rate of 6 L/min.

_____

_____

37. Complete the following table, which compares volumes delivered during heliox therapy provided by critical care ventilators.

Ventilator	Volume with Heliox
VIASYS Avea	_____
	_____
Hamilton Veolar and Galileo	_____
Puritan Bennett 7200	_____
Puritan Bennett 840	_____
Servo 300	_____
Servo^i	_____
Dräger Dura 2	_____
Dräger E-4	_____

38. How is heliox connected to a mechanical ventilator

_____

_____

39. How does the use of heliox with a mechanical ventilator affect F_IO_2 monitoring?

_____

_____

_____

_____

_____

40. How does the use of heliox with a mechanical ventilator affect pressures?

_____

_____

41. Name a circumstance in which heliox therapy should not be used.

_____

_____

42. What is *independent lung ventilation* and how is it accomplished?

_____

_____

_____

43. List the surgical procedures in which lung isolation and ILV are used.

_____

_____

_____

44. Give two nonsurgical indications for ILV.

_____

_____

45. Compare synchronous with dyssynchronous ventilation when two ventilators are used for ILV.

_____

_____

_____

_____

_____

_____

46. Describe the procedure for measuring the lower inflection point and the upper inflection point using a slow flow inflection point maneuver for each lung during ILV.

_____

_____

_____

_____

_____

_____

_____

47. Define *EIP*.

_____

_____

_____

48. What should the mode, rate, and V_T be for performing a slow flow inflection maneuver to one lung? To both lungs?

_____

_____

49. How are appropriate levels of PEEP established for each lung during ILV?

_____

_____

_____

50. List the types of therapy that can be provided by the IPV-1 unit.

_____

_____

51. Describe the characteristics of the IPV-1 unit.

_____

_____

_____

52. How does use of a Percussionaire IPV-1 alter VC-CMV?

_____

_____

_____

_____

Critical Thinking Questions

1. What ventilator settings are represented by the following pressure-time graph?

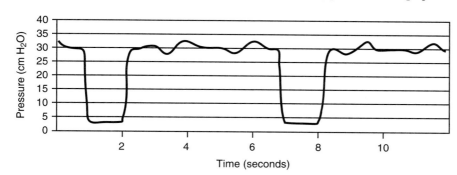

_____

_____

2. After an adult patient is placed on HFOV, a chest radiograph shows the diaphragm in the midclavicular line at the level of the sixth posterior rib. Which ventilator parameter, if any, needs to be changed and why?

_____

_____

For questions 3 through 5, refer to the pressure-volume curve for a slow flow inflection maneuver displayed in the following figure.

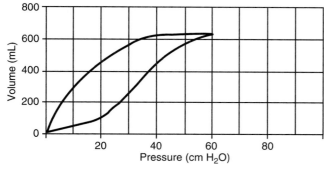

3. Plot the lower inflection point and the upper inflection point for the static pressure-volume loop.

_____

4. PEEP should be set at what level?

_____

5. What V_T should be used to ventilate this patient?

_____

Case Studies

Case Study #1

A patient is ventilated with APRV at the following settings: P_{high} = 20 cm H_2O, P_{low} = 2 cm H_2O, T_{high} = 4 seconds, T_{low} = 1 second, F_IO_2 = 0.4. The patient's spontaneous rate is 12 breaths/min. The current ABG values include a PaO_2 of 86 mm Hg and a $PaCO_2$ of 68 mm Hg.

1. Calculate the current ventilator rate.

_____

_____

2. Which parameter needs to be changed to correct this patient's problem?

_____

3. State the reason for changing that parameter.

_____

_____

Case Study #2

A patient currently is ventilated with APRV at the following settings: P_{high} = 35 cm H_2O, P_{low} = 5 cm H_2O, T_{high} = 7 seconds, T_{low} = 0.5 second, F_IO_2 = 0.3. The patient's spontaneous rate is 14 breaths/min. The current ABG values include a PaO_2 of 58 mm Hg and a $PaCO_2$ of 42 mm Hg.

1. Which parameter needs to be changed to correct this patient's problem?

_____

2. State the reason for changing that parameter.

_____

_____

3. If changing the above parameter does not correct this patient's problem, what other change could be made?

_____

_____

Case Study #3

A 6'2" male patient who weighs 81 kg underwent thoracoabdominal surgical repair of an aortic aneurysm and has been brought to the SICU. He is intubated with a double lumen ET tube, and two ventilators are ready at the bedside.

1. Which lung will have sustained injury as a result of the surgery? Why?

_____

_____

_____

2. What volume should be used in this patient to perform a single lung slow inflation maneuver to determine inflection points?

_____

3. If the right lung's lower inflection point is 6 cm H_2O and the left lung's lower inflection point is 18 cm H_2O, what is the appropriate PEEP level for each lung?

_____

_____

NBRC–Style Questions

1. The advantages of APRV over other forms of conventional ventilation are mainly the result of which of the following?
   a. Preservation of spontaneous breathing
   b. Reduced risk of VILI
   c. Reduced risk of VAP
   d. Reduced need for patient sedation and paralysis

2. Which of the following are the most appropriate APRV settings for an ARDS patient who is receiving VC-CMV at these settings: rate = 12 breaths/min, V_T = 600 mL, F_IO_2 = 1, PEEP = 10 cm H_2O, PIP = 32 cm H_2O, $P_{plateau}$ = 25 cm H_2O?
   a. P_{high} = 42 cm H_2O; P_{low} = 10 cm H_2O; T_{high} = 2 seconds; T_{low} = 2 seconds
   b. P_{high} = 25 cm H_2O; P_{low} = 10 cm H_2O; T_{high} = 4 seconds; T_{low} = 2 seconds
   c. P_{high} = 25 cm H_2O; P_{low} = 0; T_{high} = 4 seconds; T_{low} = 1 second
   d. P_{high} = 15 cm H_2O; P_{low} = 0; T_{high} = 6 seconds; T_{low} = 1.5 seconds

3. The parameter that can generally improve oxygenation during APRV is which of the following?
   a. P_{high}
   b. P_{low}
   c. T_{high}
   d. T_{low}

4. Calculate the APRV ventilator rate when T_{high} is 12 seconds and T_{low} is 2 seconds.
   a. 4 cycles/min
   b. 6 cycles/min
   c. 9 cycles/min
   d. 12 cycles/min

5. The first parameter set when starting HFOV is which of the following?
   a. $T_I\%$
   b. Frequency
   c. Amplitude
   d. Bias flow

6. A decrease in chest wiggle during HFOV may be caused by which of the following?
   - I. Pneumothorax
   - II. ET obstruction
   - III. Increased $PaCO_2$
   - IV. Patient improvement
   - a. I and II
   - b. II and III
   - c. IV
   - d. I and III

7. An ARDS patient is receiving HFOV at the following settings: $\overline{P}aw$ = 28 cm H_2O, frequency = 6 Hz, bias flow = 30 L/min, ΔP = 7 (amplitude 60 cm H_2O), $T_1\%$ = 33, F_1O_2 = 0.8. The patient's PaO_2 on these settings is 75 mm Hg. Which of the following is the most appropriate action in this case?
   - a. Increase the F_1O_2 to 0.9
   - b. Reduce the control to 5
   - c. Reduce the frequency to 5 Hz
   - d. Increase the $\overline{P}aw$ to 30 cm H_2O

8. With HFOV, the first step in reducing an adult patient's $PaCO_2$ is which of the following?
   - a. Increase the $T_1\%$
   - b. Reduce the frequency
   - c. Increase the amplitude
   - d. Increase the cuff leak

9. To achieve a flow of 8 L/min for a 70:30 heliox mixture, the oxygen flowmeter should be set at which of the following?
   - a. 5 L/min
   - b. 8 L/min
   - c. 11 L/min
   - d. 14 L/min

10. During ventilation with heliox mixtures, most ventilators have which of the following problems?
    - I. Inaccurate PEEP measurements
    - II. Discrepancies in flow measurements
    - III. Discrepancies between the set and actual F_1O_2
    - IV. Nonlinear relationship between $V_T$set and $V_T$del
    - a. I and II
    - b. II and III
    - c. III and IV
    - d. I and IV

11. An adult patient has had a severe asthmatic episode and requires intubation. The most appropriate type of ventilation for this patient is which of the following?
    - a. ILV
    - b. APRV
    - c. IPV
    - d. PCV with heliox

12. An adult patient has a left-sided flail and underlying left lung contusions from a motor vehicle accident. The most appropriate type of ventilation for this patient is which of the following?
    - a. ILV
    - b. APRV
    - c. HFOV
    - d. PCV with heliox

13. With HFOV, volume delivery from the oscillator is determined by all of the following *except*
    - a. $T_1\%$
    - b. Oscillator displacement
    - c. ET tube size
    - d. Patient's ability to trigger the ventilator

14. When heliox concentrations $\geq$50:50 are used, the effect on the delivery of albuterol from an MDI during mechanical ventilation, compared with the effects of oxygen or air, is which of the following?
    - a. Delivery of albuterol is reduced by at least 25%.
    - b. Delivery of albuterol is reduced by at least 50%.
    - c. Delivery of albuterol is increased by at least 25%.
    - d. Delivery of albuterol is increased by at least 50%.

Helpful Internet Sites

- Puritan Bennett: BiLevel clinical brochure. Available at www.puritanbennett.com/_Catalog/PDF/Product/BilevelClinicalBrochure.pdf
- Putensen C, Zech S, Wrigge H, et al: Long-term effects of spontaneous breathing during ventilatory support in patients with acute lung injury. The PedsCCM Evidence-Based Journal Club, Article Review, *Am J Respir Crit Care Med* 164:43, 2001. Available at http://pedsccm.wustl.edu/EBJ/THERAPY/ Putensen-APRV.html
- VIASYS Healthcare: 3100B control PowerPoint presentations. Available at www.viasyshealthcare.com/powerpoint/DOCUMENTS/SMC/3100B_Controls.ppt and www.viasyshealthcare.com/powerpoint/DOCUMENTS/SMC/Adult_HFOV.ppt#256,1,3100B Ventilator
- GE Healthcare: AptaÈr heliox delivery system. Available at www.gehealthcare.com/usen/respiratory_care/docs/hx4629a.pdf
- Percussionaire Corp: *Clinical resources manual*. Available at http://web.inetba.com/percussionaire/eduforum.htm

Answer Key

Chapter 1, Oxygenation and Acid-Base Evaluation
Answers to Key Terms Crossword Puzzle

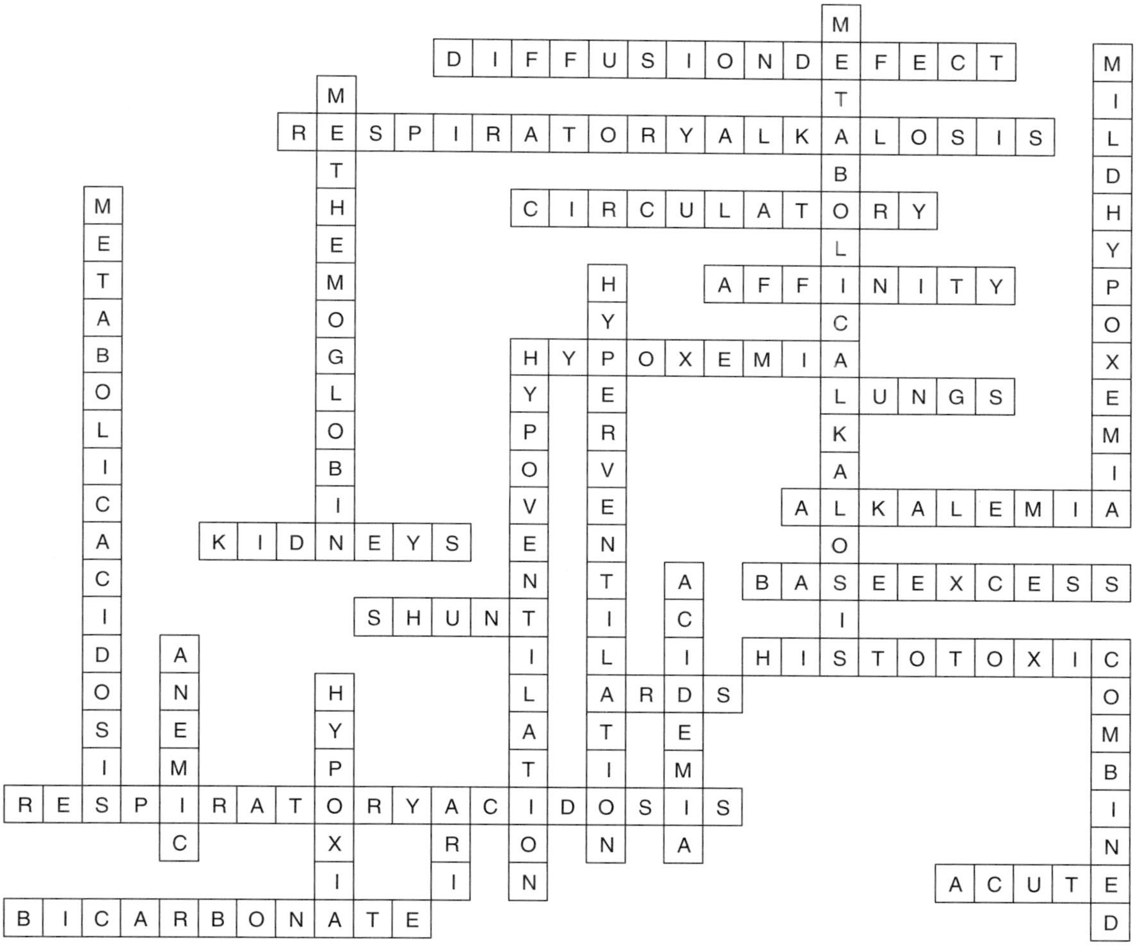

The completed crossword puzzle contains the following answers:

- DIFFUSIONDEFECT
- RESPIRATORYALKALOSIS
- CIRCULATORY
- AFFINITY
- HYPOXEMIA
- LUNGS
- ALKALEMIA
- KIDNEYS
- BASEEXCESS
- SHUNT
- HISTOTOXIC
- ARDS
- RESPIRATORYACIDOSIS
- ACUTE
- BICARBONATE
- METABOLICACIDOSIS (down)
- METHEMOGLOBINBI (down)
- MILDHYPOXEMIA (down)
- HYPOVENTILATION (down)
- ANEMIC (down)
- HYPHPXIA
- METABOLICALKALOSIS
- HYPERVENTILATION
- ACIDEMIA
- RECOMBINED

Answers to Review Questions

1. 1.2 mmol/L
2. 1.5 mmol/L
3. 24 mmol/L, 27.1 mmol/L
4. 25.2, 28.6
5. 40 mm Hg, 46 mm Hg
6. 7.40, 7.37
7. 24, 21
8. ±2
9. 90, 40
10. 97%, 75%
11. 0.3, 0.12
12. 19.5 vol%

13. 14.7 vol%

14. 19.8 vol%, 14.8 vol%

15.
Age	Estimated PaO_2 (mm Hg)
24	99
32	97
40	95
48	93
56	91
60	90
68	88
76	86
84	84

16. The PaO_2 is affected by altitude because as altitude increases, the barometric pressure decreases, thereby decreasing the P_IO_2 at above sea level altitudes.

17. 55.5 mm Hg

18. 22.4 mm Hg

19. 57.5 mm Hg

20. hypoxemic hypoxia (altitude hypoxia)

21. Hypoxia refers to decreased oxygen levels within the tissues or alveoli. Hypoxemia refers to a lower than normal partial pressure of oxygen in the blood.

22. c, a, b, e, d

23. a. WNL; b. mild hypoxemia; c. mild hypoxemia; d. moderate hypoxemia; e. moderate hypoxemia; f. severe hypoxemia; g. severe hypoxemia

24. $P(A\text{-}a)O_2 = P_AO_2 - PaO_2$; PaO_2/P_AO_2; PaO_2/F_IO_2

25. $P(A\text{-}a)O_2$ 5 to 10 mm Hg on 21%, 30 to 60 mm Hg on 100%; PaO_2/P_AO_2 0.8 to 1.0; PaO_2/F_IO_2 380 to 476

26. $P(A\text{-}a)O_2 = 235 - 155 = 80$ mm Hg on 40%; $PaO_2/P_AO_2 = 155/235 = 0.66$; $PaO_2/F_IO_2 = 155/0.4 = 388$. The alveolar/arterial difference is elevated, meaning that an oxygenation problem is present even though the PaO_2 is high. This may be caused by a V/Q abnormality, shunt, or diffusion defect. The PaO_2/P_AO_2 ratio correlates with the A − a gradient. However, the PaO_2/F_IO_2 is within normal limits.

27. $P(A\text{-}a)O_2 = 67 - 58 = 9$ mm Hg on 21%; $PaO_2/P_AO_2 = 58/67 = 0.86$; $PaO_2/F_IO_2 = 58/0.21 = 276$. The moderate hypoxemia in this patient is caused by the elevated CO_2 level (66 mm Hg) because both the $P(A\text{-}a)O_2$ and the PaO_2/P_AO_2 are within normal limits. The PaO_2/F_IO_2 is low, however, because of the low PaO_2.

28. $P(A\text{-}a)O_2 = 183 - 99 = 84$ mm Hg on 30%; $PaO_2/P_AO_2 = 99/183 = 0.54$; $PaO_2/F_IO_2 = 99/0.3 = 330$. The alveolar/arterial gradient is elevated and the PaO_2/P_AO_2 is low. Oxygenation is compromised because of a V/Q abnormality, shunt, or diffusion defect.

29. $P(A\text{-}a)O_2 = 673 - 98 = 575$ mm Hg on 100%; $PaO_2/P_AO_2 = 98/673 = 0.15$; $PaO_2/F_IO_2 = 98/1.0 = 98$. The alveolar/arterial gradient is very high and the PaO_2/P_AO_2 is very low. Both indicate an oxygenation problem caused by a V/Q abnormality or shunt. A diffusion defect can be ruled out because the F_IO_2 is 100%. The PaO_2/F_IO_2 indicates ARDS.

30. $P(A\text{-}a)O_2 = 282 - 84 = 198$ mm Hg on 50%; $PaO_2/P_AO_2 = 84/282 = 0.30$; $PaO_2/F_IO_2 = 84/0.5 = 168$. The elevated $PaCO_2$ is not the cause of this patient's oxygenation problem because the alveolar/arterial gradient is elevated and the PaO_2/P_AO_2 is low, both pointing to a V/Q abnormality or shunt. The PaO_2/F_IO_2 indicates ARDS.

31. Hyperthermia; hypercapnia; alkalosis; decreased 2,3, DPG; abnormal hemoglobin

32. Hypothermia; hypocarbia; alkalosis; decreased 2,3, DPG; carbon monoxide poisoning; fetal hemoglobin

33. P_{50} is the partial pressure of oxygen at 50% saturation. The normal P_{50} is 27 mm Hg.

34. a. left shift; b. right shift; c. right shift; d. right shift; e. left shift

35. $CaO_2 = (Hb \times \%sat \times 1.34) + (PaO_2 \times 0.003)$
$CaO_2 = (9 \times 0.98 \times 1.34) + (95 \times 0.003) = 11.82 + 0.29 = 12.11$ vol%

36. $CaO_2 = (15 \times 0.92 \times 1.34) + (78 \times 0.003) = 18.49 + 0.23 = 18.72$ vol%

37. $CaO_2 = (18 \times 0.90 \times 1.34) + (52 \times 0.003) = 21.71 + 0.16 = 21.87$ vol%

38. $CaO_2 = (11 \times 0.70 \times 1.34) + (45 \times 0.003) = 10.32 + 0.14 = 10.46$ vol%

39. If cardiac output is low, less fresh oxygen is available to the tissues. As blood passes by the tissues, oxygen is taken up. If blood is moving by slowly, the tissues will draw more oxygen out of the slowly moving blood, thereby lowering the mixed venous PO_2.

40. Pulmonary shunt is the amount of blood that passes through the lungs to the left side of the heart without taking on any "fresh" oxygen from the alveoli.

41. $(CcO_2 - CaO_2)/(CcO_2 - CvO_2) = Q_S/Q_T$; assume $CcO_2 \approx C_AO_2$, then:
$C_xO_2 = (Hb \times S_xO_2 \times 1.34) + (P_xO_2 \times 0.003)$, where x = A, a, or $\bar{v}$
$C_AO_2 = (12 \times 1.00 \times 1.34) + (673 \times 0.003) = 16.08 + 2.02 = 18.10$ vol%
$CaO_2 = (12 \times 0.99 \times 1.34) + (98 \times 0.003) = 15.92 + 0.29 = 16.21$ vol%
$C\bar{v}O_2 = (12 \times 0.73 \times 1.34) + (35 \times 0.003) = 11.74 + 0.11 = 11.85$ vol%
$(C_AO_2 - CaO_2)/(C_AO_2 - C\bar{v}O_2) = Q_S/Q_T$
(18.10 vol% − 16.21 vol%)/(18.21 vol% − 11.85 vol%) = 1.89/6.25 = 30% shunt

42. As a patient's total arterial oxygen content falls the percent shunt will rise.

43. Atelectasis; pulmonary edema; pneumonia; pneumothorax; complete airway obstruction

44. An alveolar ventilation of 4 to 5 L/min provides enough gas to keep ABG values within normal range.

45. When alveolar ventilation decreases, P_ACO_2 rises and P_AO_2 falls. According to Figure 1-3 in the text, the P_AO_2 would be 70 mm Hg and the P_ACO_2 would also be 70 mm Hg.

46. P_ACO_2 changes affect PaO_2 levels because as CO_2 levels increase, the CO_2 molecules displace the oxygen molecules trying to enter the alveolus from the atmospheric air. Thus the alveolar PO_2 decreases and less oxygen is available to diffuse across the alveolar/capillary membrane.

47. 140 mm Hg

48. P_AO_2 120 mm Hg, P_ACO_2 20 mm Hg

49. $PaCO_2 \approx 0.863 \times \dot{V}/\dot{V}_A$
a. $PaCO_2 \approx 0.863 \times 100/3 = 0.863 \times 33.33 = 29$ mm Hg
b. $PaCO_2 \approx 0.863 \times 175/3.5 = 0.863 \times 50 = 43$ mm Hg
c. $PaCO_2 \approx 0.863 \times 200/5 = 0.863 \times 40 = 34$ mm Hg
d. $PaCO_2 \approx 0.863 \times 275/5.5 = 0.863 \times 50 = 43$ mm Hg

50. **Acid/Base Balance (Acute or Chronic?)**   **Oxygenation Status**

a. compensated respiratory alkalosis (chronic alveolar hyperventilation) — no hypoxemia

b. uncompensated respiratory alkalosis (acute alveolar hyperventilation) — no hypoxemia

c. acute on chronic respiratory acidosis — severe hypoxemia

d. uncompensated respiratory alkalosis (acute alveolar hyperventilation) — uncorrected, moderate hypoxemia

e. uncompensated metabolic acidosis (acute metabolic acidosis) — corrected hypoxemia

f. compensated respiratory alkalosis (chronic) — uncorrected, mild hypoxemia

g. partially compensated metabolic acidosis (chronic) — no hypoxemia

h. compensated respiratory acidosis (chronic) — uncorrected, moderate hypoxemia

51. Simplified Henderson-Hasselbalch equation is $[H^+] = (24 \times PaCO_2)/HCO_3^-$

	PaCO$_2$ (mm Hg)	HCO$_3^-$ (mEq/L)	[H$^+$] nmol/L	Approximate pH
a.	25	19	$(24 \times 25)/19 = 600/19 = 32$	7.50
b.	15	10	$(24 \times 15)/10 = 360/10 = 36$	7.45
c.	35	17	$(24 \times 35)/17 = 840/17 = 49$	7.30
d.	48	26	$(24 \times 48)/26 = 1152/26 = 44$	7.35
e.	55	33	$(24 \times 55)/33 = 1320/33 = 40$	7.40
f.	65	31	$(24 \times 65)/31 = 1536/31 = 50$	7.30
g.	55	21	$(24 \times 55)/21 = 1320/21 = 63$	7.20
h.	20	5	$(24 \times 20)/5 = 480/5 = 96$	7.00

52. $HCO_3^- = (24 \times PaCO_2)/[H^+]$ when the pH is 7.40, $[H^+]$ = 40 nmol/L. If the $PaCO_2$ is 70 mm Hg, the HCO_3^- = $(24 \times 70)/40 = 42$ mEq/L. If the $PaCO_2$ is 50 mm Hg, the $HCO_3^- = (24 \times 50)/40 = 30$ mEq/L. And, if the $PaCO_2$ is 30 mm Hg, the $HCO_3^- = (24 \times 30)/40 = 18$ mEq/L.

53. 10 mm Hg, 2 mEq/L

54. 10 mm Hg, 1 mEq/L

55. HCO_3^- should increase to 26 mEq/L

56. HCO_3^- should decrease to 22 mEq/L

57. pH should rise to 7.60

58. pH should drop to 7.30

59. pH should fall from 7.30 to 7.20

60. The RT should anticipate a bicarbonate value of 28 mEq/L. $\Delta HCO_3^- = 0.1 \times \Delta PaCO_2$. So $0.1 \times 40 = 4$ and $24 + 4 = 28$.

Answers to Critical Thinking Questions

1. The patient's hemoglobin level should be reviewed so the arterial oxygen content can be assessed. This allows an assessment of how much oxygen is being carried on the hemoglobin.

2. No, because fewer hemoglobin molecules are available to carry the oxygen in the blood.

3. Patients with COPD compensate for their chronic low levels of oxygen by eventually increasing the production of red blood cells. Polycythemia is a common compensation mechanism for these patients.

4. The mixed venous PO_2 should be lower than normal for a patient with circulatory hypoxia because more oxygen will be extracted by the tissues from slow-moving blood. The slower the blood moves the more time is available for oxygen to be extracted by the tissues it is perfusing.

5. Fetal hemoglobin causes a left shift in the oxyhemoglobin dissociation curve. Therefore the P_{50} of a newborn should be lower than that of an adult.

Answers to Case Studies

Case Study #1

1. Partially compensated metabolic acidosis

2. No supplemental oxygen is necessary at this time.

3. Diabetic ketoacidosis

Case Study #2

1. Compensated respiratory alkalosis

2. Severe hypoxemia; the arterial oxygen content is low and tissue hypoxia is possible.

3. Chronic; the kidneys require 2 to 3 days to compensate.

4. Oxygen therapy, aerosolized bronchodilator (possibly continuous nebulization), IV fluids, and IV corticosteroids.

5. Improvement in the oxygen status of the patient; the rise in the pH to 7.44 suggests that the oxygen therapy corrected the lactic acidosis.

Case Study #3

1. Partially compensated respiratory alkalosis

2. No hypoxemia

3. Hemoglobin of 6 gm% changes the patient's oxygen status to anemic hypoxemia. The $CaO_2 = (0.98 \times 6 \times 1.34) + (95 \times 0.003) = 7.88 + 0.29 = 8.17$ vol%. This value is severely low. The patient's respiratory alkalosis is caused by the anemia. Oxygen therapy will not correct this problem.

Answers to NRBC-Style Questions

1. d	6. a	11. d
2. c	7. d	12. d
3. c	8. d	13. b
4. a	9. c	14. b
5. a	10. b	15. b

Chapter 2, Basic Terms and Concepts of Mechanical Ventilation
Answers to Key Terms Crossword Puzzle

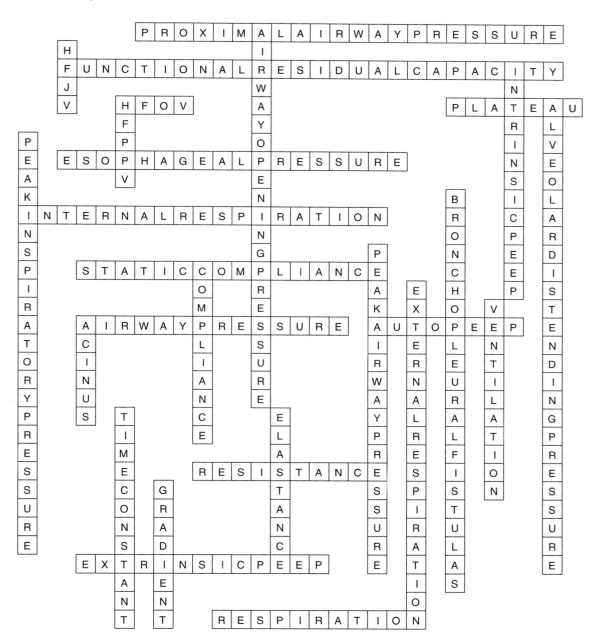

Answers to Review Questions

1. Ventilation refers to the movement of gas into and out of the lungs. Respiration is the movement of gas molecules across a cell membrane.

2. external respiration, internal respiration

3. The pressure at point A needs to be higher than the pressure at point B to create a pressure gradient.

4.

a. $\dfrac{1\text{ mm Hg}}{X} = \dfrac{1.36\text{ cm H}_2\text{O}}{25\text{ cm H}_2\text{O}}, 25 = 1.36X,$

$X = \dfrac{25}{1.36} = 18.34\text{ mm Hg}$

b. $\dfrac{1\text{ mm Hg}}{X} = \dfrac{1.36\text{ cm H}_2\text{O}}{40\text{ cm H}_2\text{O}}, 40 = 1.36X,$

$X = \dfrac{40}{1.36} = 29.41\text{ mm Hg}$

c. $\dfrac{1\text{ mm Hg}}{15\text{ mm Hg}} = \dfrac{1.36\text{ cm H}_2\text{O}}{X}, 15 \times 1.36 = 20.40\text{ cm H}_2\text{O}$

d. $\dfrac{1\text{ mm Hg}}{47\text{ mm Hg}} = \dfrac{1.36\text{ cm H}_2\text{O}}{X}, 47 \times 1.36 = 63.92\text{ cm H}_2\text{O}$

e. $\dfrac{1\text{ kPa}}{7.5\text{ mm Hg}} = \dfrac{X}{40\text{ mm Hg}}, \dfrac{40}{7.5} = X, X = 5.33\text{kPa}$

f. $\dfrac{1}{7.5} = \dfrac{X}{95}, \dfrac{95}{7.5} = X, X = 12.67\text{ kPa}$

g. $\dfrac{760\text{ mm Hg}}{X} = \dfrac{1}{2}, 760 \times 2 = X, X = 1520\text{ mm Hg}$

h. $1\text{ ATM} = 760\text{ mm Hg}, \dfrac{X}{760\text{ mm Hg}} = \dfrac{1\text{ kPa}}{7.5\text{ mm HG}},$

$7.5X = 760, X = 101.3\text{ kPa}$

i. $1\text{ kPa} = 7.5\text{ mm Hg} = 10.2\text{ cm H}_2\text{O},$

$\dfrac{1\text{ kPa}}{15\text{ kPa}} = \dfrac{10.2\text{ cm H}_2\text{O}}{X}, X = 153\text{ kPa}$

j. $\dfrac{1034\text{ cm H}_2\text{O}}{2068\text{ cm H}_2\text{O}} = \dfrac{1\text{ ATM}}{X}, 1034X = 2068, X = 2\text{ ATM}$

5. intrapleural pressure, $-5\text{ cm H}_2\text{O}$, $-10\text{ cm H}_2\text{O}$

6. a. A, P_{aw}; B, P_{bs}; C, P_{pl}; D, P_A.

   b. P_M, P_{aw}, proximal airway pressure, mask pressure, or upper airway pressure

7. P_{pl} is estimated by using P_{ES}. P_{ES} is obtained by placing a balloon in the esophagus and monitoring pressure changes in the balloon.

8. P_{TA}, conductive airways, $P_{TA} = P_{aw} - P_A$

9. P_W, $P_W = P_A - P_{bs}$

10. P_L, $P_L = P_A - P_{pl}$

11. P_{TR}, $P_{TR} = P_{aw} - P_{bs}$

12. Point A represents P_{aw}, Point B represents P_{bs}, Point C represents P_{pl}, and Point D represents P_A.

    a. $P_{aw} - P_{bs} = P_{TR}$

    b. $P_A - P_{bs} = P_W$

    c. $P_A - P_{pl} = P_L$

    d. $P_{aw} - PA = P_{TA}$

13.

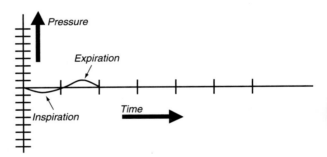

14. The individual's body is encased in an air-tight container subjected to a pressure less than atmospheric pressure (negative pressure). The negative pressure is transmitted across the chest wall into the intraalveolar space. This creates a pressure gradient (P_{TA}) between the alveoli and the mouth and causes air to move into the lungs.

15. No artificial airways such as an ET are necessary; patients are able to eat and speak; fewer physiological disadvantages exist than are associated with PPV.

16. $P_{TA} = P_M - P_A$; $25\text{ cm H}_2\text{O} - 5\text{ cm H}_2\text{O} = 20\text{ cm H}_2\text{O}$

17.

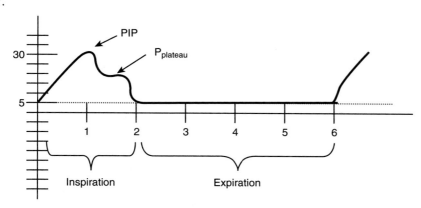

18.

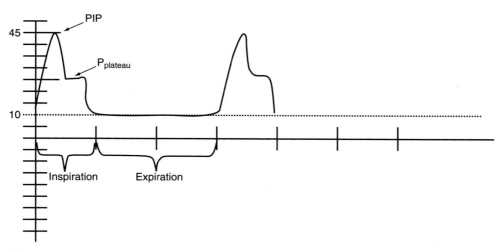

19. PIP, peak airway pressure

20. baseline pressure

21. PEEP

22. $P_{plateau}$, selecting inspiratory pause or inflation hold maneuver

23. elastic, frictional forces

24. compliance, elastance

25. change in volume that corresponds to the change in pressure, $C = \Delta V/\Delta P$

26. 0.1 L/cm H_2O or 100 mL/cm H_2O, 0.05 L/cm H_2O to 0.17 L/cm H_2O

27. 40 to 50 mL/cm H_2O, 35 to 45 mL/cm H_2O

28. $C_S = \Delta V/(P_{plateau} - EEP)$

29. When more pressure is required to deliver a specific volume, the lung compliance is decreasing.

30. $C_S = 750$ mL/$(27 - 10$ cm $H_2O) = 4$ mL/cm H_2O

31. $C_S = 575$ mL/$(35 - 5$ cm $H_2O) = 19$ mL/cm H_2O

32. $C_S = 650$ mL/$(18 - 0$ cm $H_2O) = 36$ mL/cm H_2O

33. As the lungs become harder to ventilate, PIP will increase. As the lungs become harder to ventilate, lung compliance will decrease.

34. Resistance is defined as frictional forces associated with ventilation.

35. Raw = (PIP $- P_{plateau}$)/flow (L/sec)

36. At flow rates of 0.5 L/sec, Raw is 0.6 to 2.4 cm H_2O/L/sec.

37. Emphysema can cause increased compliance from tissue destruction and loss of elastic recoil as well as airway resistance from airway inflammation, small airway obstruction, and bronchospasm.

38. $P_{TA} = PIP - P_{plateau}$, 27 cm H_2O − 20 cm H_2O = 7 cm H_2O

39. The amount of pressure needed to overcome airway resistance or the amount of pressure lost to airway resistance is equal to the P_{TA}. P_{TA} = 30 cm H_2O − 20 cm H_2O = 10 cm H_2O

40. 5 cm H_2O

41. Raw = $(PIP - P_{plateau})$/flow (L/sec)
    = (48 − 30 cm H_2O)/(40 L/60 sec)
    = 18 cm H_2O/0.67 L/sec
    Raw = 27 cm H_2O/L/sec

42. flow rate 60 L/min = 1 L/sec; Raw = (25 − 15 cm H_2O)/1 L/sec
    Raw = 10 cm H_2O/L/sec

43. The characteristics of the lung are not homogeneous because each acinus may have entirely different values for compliance and resistance.

44. A low compliance unit, because it is stiff, will receive less volume than a normal unit, but it will fill and empty more rapidly than the normal unit. A unit with high airway resistance will fill slowly and take longer to empty than a normal lung unit. The faster the respiratory rate the less volume will enter a unit with high airway resistance.

45. The movement of structures—including the lungs, abdominal organs, rib cage, and diaphragm—and gas viscosity, gas density, the length and diameter of the airways, and the flow rate of the gas are all factors that contribute to airway resistance.

46. Clinical factors that contribute to airway resistance include bronchospasm, airway secretions, mucosal edema, small ETs, and airway inflammation.

47. $C_S \times Raw$ = time constant;
    25 mL/cm H_2O = 0.025 L/cm H_2O;
    0.025 L/cm H_2O × 30 cm H_2O/L/sec = 0.75 second

48. *Step 1*: Calculate C_S. C_S = 0.6 L/24 cm H_2O = 0.025 L/cm H_2O
    Step 2: Calculate Raw. First convert L/min to L/sec: 60 L/min = 1 L/sec.
    Then calculate the resistance: Raw = (30 − 24 cm H_2O)/1 L/sec = 6 cm H_2O/L/sec.
    Step 3: The product of Raw and C_S is the time constant: 6 cm H_2O/L/sec × 0.025 L/cm H_2O = 0.15 second.

49. 1. 63%; 2. 86%; 3. 95%; 4. 98%; 5. 100%

50. The time constant for patient 1 is very short, meaning that this patient's lungs are noncompliant or stiff. Patient 1 would receive less volume than normal lungs. The time constant for patient 2 is very long, meaning increased airway resistance is present. This patient's lungs will fill very slowly and will receive less volume than a normal lung unless slower rates are used. Patient 3 has a normal time constant and will receive the most volume of the three patients.

51. 0.055 L/cm H_2O × 6 cm H_2O/L/sec = 0.33 second

52. The third time constant will have 95% of the volume emptied. So 0.33 × 3 = 0.99 second.

53. Patients with increased airway resistance will have longer time constants. This means that their lungs will take longer to fill and empty. Rapid respiratory rates will decrease the expiratory time, causing gas to remain in the lungs. The patient will not be able to exhale fully. This incomplete emptying of the lungs will increase the FRC (air trapping) and cause auto-PEEP.

54. C_S = 0.7 L/(18 − 5 cm H_2O) = 0.054 L/cm H_2O
    Raw = (45 − 18 cm H_2O)/(60 L/60 seconds) = 27 cm H_2O/L/sec
    Time constant = 0.054 L/cm H_2O × 27 cm H_2O/L/sec = 1.46 seconds

55. Figure A represents a normal lung unit. Figure B represents a lung unit with increased airway resistance. Given the same inspiratory time, the unit with increased airway resistance will receive less volume because it has a longer time constant.

56. Figure A represents a normal lung unit. Figure B represents a lung unit with low compliance. The low compliance lung unit has a shorter time constant and will therefore fill faster, but with less volume than the normal lung unit.

Answers to Critical Thinking Questions

1. PIP represents the amount of pressure required to overcome both the resistance of the airways and the elastic resistance of the alveoli and ventilator circuitry. Therefore, $PIP - P_{plateau}$ equals the amount of pressure to overcome airway resistance, in this case 43 − 18 = 25 cm H_2O.

2. ARDS causes the lung compliance to decrease, which will shorten time constants.

3. Emphysema is characterized by dilation and destruction of lung units from the terminal bronchioles to the alveoli. This tissue destruction causes a loss of elastic recoil and thereby an increase in lung compliance. This lengthens fill and empty time, which is represented by a long time constant.

4. At 30 weeks of gestation respiratory distress syndrome is a significant risk because of pulmonary immaturity. Insufficient pulmonary surfactant production will lead to low lung compliance and therefore short time constants.

Answers to Case Studies

Case Study #1

1. $PIP - P_{plateau}$ = pressure required to overcome airway resistance (P_{TA})

Time	PIP	$P_{plateau}$	P_{TA}
0800	18 cm H_2O	10 cm H_2O	**8 cm H_2O**
1000	24 cm H_2O	12 cm H_2O	**12 cm H_2O**
1200	35 cm H_2O	11 cm H_2O	**24 cm H_2O**

2. $Raw = P_{TA}/flow$ (L/sec)

Time	P_{TA}	Flow (L/sec)	P_{TA}/Flow = Raw
0800	8 cm H_2O	45 L/ 60 seconds = 0.75 L/sec	8/0.75 = **10.7 cm H_2O/L/sec**
1000	12 cm H_2O	45 L/60 seconds = 0.75 L/sec	12/0.75 = **16 cm H_2O/L/sec**
1200	24 cm H_2O	45 L/60 seconds = 0.75 L/sec	24/0.75 = **32 cm H_2O/L/sec**

3. $C_S = V_T/(P_{plateau} - PEEP)$

Time	V_T	$P_{plateau}$ – PEEP	C_S
0800	600 mL	10 cm H_2O – 5 cm H_2O = 5 cm H_2O	600 mL/5 cm H_2O = **120 mL/cm H_2O**
1000	600 mL	12 cm H_2O – 5 cm H_2O = 7 cm H_2O	600 mL/7 cm H_2O = **85.7 mL/cm H_2O**
1200	600 mL	11 cm H_2O – 5 cm H_2O = 6 cm H_2O	600 mL/6 cm H_2O = **100 mL/cm H_2O**

4. Time constant = $Raw \times C_S$

Time	Raw	C_S	Time Constant
0800	10.7 cm H_2O/L/sec	120 mL/cm H_2O	**1.28 seconds**
1000	16 cm H_2O/L/sec	85.7 mL/cm H_2O	**1.38 seconds**
1200	32 cm H_2O/L/sec	100 mL/cm H_2O	**3.20 seconds**

5. There is a significant rise in both the P_{TA} and the airway resistance from 0800 to 1200, along with an increased time constant. This is indicative of clinical manifestations such as bronchospasm, increased secretions, and mucus plugging. Because a single time constant has increased to 3.2 seconds, incomplete time will be available for inspiration and expiration. Therefore until corrected air trapping or auto-PEEP is very likely.

Case Study #2

1. 40 L/min = 40 L/60 seconds = 0.67 L/sec; 60 L/min = 1 L/sec

Time	P_{TA}	Raw	C_S	Time Constant
1000	40 – 28 = **12 cm H_2O**	12 cm H_2O/0.67 L/sec = **17.9 cm H_2O/L/sec**	0.550 L/(28 – 0) = **0.0196 L/cm H_2O**	17.9 × 0.0196 = **0.35 seconds**
1200	47 – 37 = **10 cm H_2O**	10 cm H_2O/0.67 L/sec = **14.9 cm H_2O/L/sec**	0.550 L/(37 – 5) = **0.0172 L/cm H_2O**	14.9 × 0.0172 = **0.26 seconds**
1400	54 – 43 = **11 cm H_2O**	11 cm H_2O/0.67 L/sec = **16.4 cm H_2O/L/sec**	0.550 L/(43 – 7) = **0.0153 L/cm H_2O**	16.4 × 0.0153 = **0.25 seconds**
1600	55 – 33 = **12 cm H_2O**	12 cm H_2O/1L/sec = **12 cm H_2O/L/sec**	0.550 L/(33 – 12) = **0.0214 L/cm H_2O**	12 × 0.0214 = **0.26 seconds**

2. The rising PIP between 1000 and 1400 hours is caused by a decrease in static compliance. The decrease in compliance is caused by a rise in plateau pressure from 28 cm H_2O at 1000 hours to 37 cm H_2O at 1200 hours to 43 cm H_2O at 1400 hours. This rise demonstrates stiffening of the lungs. The plateau pressure, and therefore static compliance, dropped at 1600 hours.

3. Minimum inspiratory time should be 3 time constants, which correspond to 95% filling of the lungs. Therefore at 1600 hours the inspiratory time should be 0.26 second × 3 = 0.78 second.

Answers to NBRC-Style Questions

1. c	5. a	9. c
2. c	6. a	10. b
3. d	7. c	
4. b	8. c	

Chapter 3, How Ventilators Work

Answers to Key Terms Crossword Puzzle

PNEUMATIC CIRCUIT / P

V A   M   I

O T   V   MICROPROCESSOR

L I   T

USER INTERFACE   SOLENOID

M N   I   N O

E T   N   U

F   C O M P R E S S O R G   B

L   I   E O C L

C O N T R O L S Y S T E M E P L E

W   C   L   C E O C

C   U   E   I N S T

F L O W I   S C I S S O R V A L V E R

N   T   T   C O D C

T   R   U O L U

D R I V E M E C H A N I S M I P O I

O   C   T   O T

L   P N E U M A T I C   P

                L

Answers to Review Questions

1. Electrically powered; pneumatically powered; combined powered
2. Pneumatic power
3. Electric power
4. Electric power
5. Combined power
6. Electric power
7. Pneumatic power
8. An open loop system is an unintelligent system in which the ventilator delivers what is set by the operator but does not have the ability to automatically change its operation.
9. A closed loop system is called an intelligent system because it has the ability to compare a set of control variables and make adjustments to the system.
10. Ventilators cause air to move into the lungs by altering the transrespiratory pressure (P_{TR}).
11. Negative pressure ventilators cause air to move into the lungs by causing a negative pleural pressure that increases the pressure gradient between the airway opening and the alveoli, causing air to flow into the lungs. Positive pressure ventilators increase the same pressure gradient but achieve it by increasing the pressure at the airway opening.
12. user interface (control panel)
13. internal pneumatic circuit
14. external (pneumatic) circuit (patient circuit)
15. single circuit
16. double circuit
17. Main inspiratory line connecting the ventilator output to the patient connector; patient adapter or Y-connector; expiratory tubing that takes gas away from the patient to the exhalation valve; an expiratory valve that conducts the patient's exhaled gas from the expiratory tubing to the room

18. A. Internally mounted exhalation valve
    B. Main expiratory line
    C. Main inspiratory line
    D. Patient connector (Y-connector)

19. Older ventilators used externally mounted exhalation valves. These valves had a separate exhalation valve line that powered the exhalation valve. When inspiration began, gas flowed through the main inspiratory tube and also through the separate exhalation valve line. The gas in the exhalation valve line closed the exhalation valve. During exhalation the flow from the ventilator to the main inspiratory tube and to the exhalation valve line stopped. This allowed the patient to exhale passively through the expiratory port.

20. Proportional solenoid valves; stepper motors with valves; digital valves with on-off configurations

21. The *proportional solenoid valve* has a plunger, a valve seat, an electromagnet, a diaphragm, a spring, and two electrical contacts. When an electrical current flows, the electromagnet creates a magnetic field that pulls the plunger and opens the valve. The amount of electrical current determines the strength of the magnetic field and thereby the position of the plunger. The *stepper valve* is an electronically operated scissor valve that can open and close rapidly. *Digital valves* are grouped together, opening or closing specifically sized openings. The amount of flow can be varied depending on which valves are open.

22. drive mechanism

23. Piston; rotating blades (vanes); moving diaphragms; bellows

24. An adjustable spring is attached to the top of a bellows where it applies pressure to force the gas mixture (air and oxygen) out of the ventilator and to the patient. The tighter the spring, the greater the force and the greater the pressure.

25. The Servo 900C ventilator has a spring-loaded bellows.

26. A linear drive piston uses an electrical motor connected by special gearing (rack and pinion) to a piston rod. The rod moves the piston forward, pushing volume to the patient.

27. The Puritan Bennett 740 ventilator uses a linear drive piston.

28. A rotating wheel is connected to a rod and piston. An electric motor rotates the drive wheel, causing the gas to flow to the patient, slowly at first and reaching its greatest speed at mid-inspiration and then tapering off at end inspiration. This pattern is called a sinusoidal waveform.

29. The Puritan Bennett Companion 2801 home care ventilator uses a rotary drive piston.

30. Today's ventilators are microprocessor controlled, closed looped, single circuit, PPVs.

31. A pneumatically controlled fluidic ventilator uses the Coanda effect.

Answers to Critical Thinking Questions

1. An open loop system can sound an alarm when apnea is detected. A closed loop system can sound an alarm and switch to a type of mode that will provide full ventilatory support for the patient.

2. Inspiratory gas flow would not go to the patient. The flow would bypass the patient, taking the course of least resistance into the room.

3. pneumatic (or fluidic)

Answers to Case Studies

Case Study #1

DC battery powered or pneumatically powered

Case Study #2

This would be a closed loop system because the ventilator detects the period of apnea and is able to make an adjustment to how it functions by switching to full ventilatory support.

Answers to NBRC-Style Questions

1. a	5. d	9. a
2. a	6. a	10. c
3. c	7. b	
4. c	8. c	

Chapter 4, How a Breath Is Delivered

Answers to Key Terms Crossword Puzzle

Answers to Review Questions

1. Muscle pressure and ventilator pressure

2. flow

3. Muscle pressure + Ventilator pressure = (Volume/compliance) + (Resistance/flow)

4. The left side of the equation of motion represents the two forces that can provide ventilation: the patient's muscles or the ventilator. The result of this work is represented on the right side of the equation as flow and volume delivery. In this equation both compliance and resistance stay constant during any single breath.

5. Volume-targeted ventilation, volume-limited ventilation, and volume-controlled ventilation

6. Pressure-targeted ventilation, pressure-limited ventilation, and pressure-controlled ventilation

7. Pressure, volume, and flow

8. the control variable

9. The volume and flow will vary with the patient's lung characteristics during pressure-controlled ventilation.

10. The pressure will vary with the patient's lung characteristics during volume-controlled ventilation.

11. The volume will remain unchanged, but the pressure will vary with the patient's lung characteristics during flow-controlled ventilation.

12. time control

13. high-frequency jet ventilators and oscillators control time

14. Flow = Volume change per unit of time (L/min)

15. The flow waveform is established and will remain consistent.

16. at the upper, or proximal, airway where the patient is connected to the ventilator, internally near where the main circuit lines connect to the ventilator, and near the exhalation valve

17. assisted breath

18. mandatory

19. spontaneous

20. Change from exhalation to inspiration; inspiration; change from inspiration to exhalation; exhalation

21. trigger variable

22. Time triggered

23. mandatory

24. control mode

25. Approximately −1 cm H_2O

26. If the ventilator is too sensitive it will trigger on its own without the patient making an effort.

27. Baseline flow − Flow sensitivity = Flow sensed at exhalation by the ventilator to trigger a breath; 8 L/min − 2 L/min = 6 L/min

28. Volume triggering occurs when the ventilator detects a small drop in volume in the patient circuit during expiratory time.

29. Control mode (controlled ventilation)

30. 3 seconds

31. 1 second

32. Time trigger

33. Time trigger

34. Patient trigger

35. Assist/control mode

36. Pressure, flow, and volume

37. volume trigger

38. limit variable

39. assisted

40. assisted

41. mandatory

42. spontaneous

43. assisted

44. less

45. Flow triggering

46. The maximum safety pressure should be set at 10 cm H_2O above the average PIP during volume or pressure ventilation.

47. The ventilator will alarm, pressure will be limited, and inspiration will end.

48. Most ICU ventilators measure the gas flow that has left the ventilator over a specific time and convert it to a volume reading (flow × inspiratory time = V_T).

49. 2 to 3 mL/cm H_2O

50. When volume cycling, less volume may return from the patient because of tubing compressibility and system leaks.

51. The ventilator will time cycle between 3 and 5 seconds.

52. flow cycled

53. A pressure-cycled ventilator can be used for short-term ventilation of patients with stable lung conditions, such as the postoperative patient.

54. Inspiratory time will increase and expiratory time will decrease during an inflation hold.

55. expiratory time

56. baseline pressure

57. PEEP

58. High-frequency oscillatory ventilator

59. expiratory hold (end-expiratory pause); auto-PEEP

60. Flow-time curve

61. Measure auto-PEEP; observe the flow-time curve; put a respirometer in line between the ventilator Y-connector and the ET and observe for continued movement at the beginning of inspiration (patient is still exhaling when the next mandatory breath occurs).

62. Ventilator circuits, expiratory valves, and bacterial filters

63. increased resistance to exhalation

64. CPAP

65. PEEP

66. CPAP or bilevel positive pressure

67. When inspiratory flow drops to a certain point, which is a set parameter on some ventilators and constant on others, the ventilator will end inspiration. The set parameter for flow termination is a percentage of the peak inspiratory flow.

Answers to Critical Thinking Questions

1. Pressure is the limit.

2. Pressure control or pressure support.

3. Flow is the trigger mechanism.

4. Flow is the cycling mechanism.

5. The trigger for A is time.

6. The trigger for B is patient (pressure).

7. The P_{TA} is 35 − 20 = 15 cm H_2O.

8. The baseline is 5 cm H_2O.

Answers to Case Studies

Case Study #1

1. The primary area of concern for this patient is hypoxemia. While receiving oxygen from a nonrebreathing mask the patient only has a PaO_2 of 42 mm Hg. The patient's acid-base status is acceptable at this time.

2. The most appropriate type of support at this time is CPAP by mask with supplemental oxygen.

3. The patient is receiving mechanical ventilatory support with volume control.

4. The limit variables are volume and flow.

5. The trigger variable being used at this time is patient (pressure).

6. Yes, the pressure-time curve.

7. The patient is pulling too hard to trigger the ventilator. The pressure-time curve shows that the patient has to deflect from a PEEP of +10 cm H_2O down to approximately +3 cm H_2O. That means that the machine is not sensitive enough to the patient's effort.

8. The RT must adjust the sensitivity to approximately 1 cm H_2O below the baseline of 10 cm H_2O.

Case Study #2

1. V_T, ventilator rate, F_IO_2, baseline, flow rate, and sensitivity

2. Set the maximum safety pressure at 38 cm H_2O.

3. to prevent excessive amounts of pressure from building up in the lungs

4. The maximum safety pressure, when reached, will cycle the ventilator, thereby stopping the ventilator from delivering all the set volume. Reaching the maximal safety pressure may be caused by excessive mucus, bronchospasm, tension pneumothorax, stiffening lungs, and so forth.

5. loss of volume from tubing compressibility, a leak in the system, or air trapping

Answers to NBRC-Style Questions

1. b
2. c
3. a
4. d
5. b
6. c
7. a
8. b
9. b
10. a
11. a
12. b
13. c

Chapter 5, Establishing the Need for Mechanical Ventilation

Answers to Key Terms Crossword Puzzle

Across answers include: SUPRACLAVICULAR, HYPOXIC, RESPIROMETER, HOMEOSTASIS, PEFR, COMA, MYASTHENIA GRAVIS, CHEYNE STOKES, EMPYEMA, ASYNCHRONOUS, SOMNOLENCE, ACUTE LUNG INJURY, GUILLAIN BARRE, SEPSIS

Answers to Review Questions

1. Acid-base balance; oxygen; carbon dioxide

2. to support or manipulate pulmonary gas exchange (oxygen and carbon dioxide), increase lung volume, and reduce the WOB

3. Reverse acute respiratory failure; reverse respiratory distress; reverse hypoxemia; prevent or reverse atelectasis and maintain FRC; reverse respiratory muscle fatigue. These three answers are also correct: permit sedation or paralysis; reduce systemic or myocardial oxygen consumption; minimize associated complications and reduce mortality rate.

4. Tachypnea; nasal flaring; diaphoresis; accessory muscle use; retractions of suprasternal, supraclavicular, and intercostal spaces; paradoxical or abnormal movement of thorax and abdomen; abnormal breath sounds; tachycardia; arrhythmia; hypotension

5. ARF

6. hypoxic respiratory failure, lung failure

7. oxygen alone, PEEP/CPAP

8. hypercapneic respiratory failure, ventilatory pump failure

9. respiratory muscles, thoracic cage nerves, nerve centers that control ventilation

10. Brain or brainstem lesions such as stroke, head or neck trauma, cerebral hemorrhage, or spinal cord injury; depressant drugs; hypothyroidism; central sleep apnea; inappropriate oxygen therapy

11. Myasthenia gravis; Guillain-Barré syndrome; poliomyelitis; muscular dystrophy; amyotrophic lateral sclerosis. These answers are also correct: tetanus; botulism.

12. Flail chest; rib fracture; kyphoscoliosis; obesity

13. Asthma, emphysema, chronic bronchitis, croup, acute epiglottitis, and acute bronchitis

14. Level of consciousness, presence of cyanosis or diaphoresis, respiratory rate, heart rate, blood pressure, and temperature

15. Tachycardia and tachypnea

16. Cheyne-Stokes breathing, Biot's breathing

17. Every 2 to 4 hours

18. VC equal to or less than 10 to 15 mL/kg and a MIP of 0 to –20 cm H_2O

19. Respiratory muscle fatigue

20. Tachypnea; increased depth of respiration; paradoxical breathing

21. 20 seconds

22. –50 to –100 cm H_2O

23. 65 to 75 mL/kg

24. 10 L/min

25. FEV_1, less than 10mL/kg

26. peak expiratory flow rate, less than 75 to 100 L/min

27. $PaCO_2$

28. 0.3, 0.4, greater than 0.6

29.

Measurement	Normal Range	Critical Value
$P(A\text{-}a)O_2$	2 to 30 mm Hg on room air	Greater than 450 mm Hg on supplemental oxygen
PaO_2/P_AO_2	0.75 to 0.95	Less than 0.15
PaO_2/F_1O_2	475	Less than 200

30. Patients with acute-on-chronic respiratory failure

31. Intubate and mechanically ventilate the patient

32. CPAP or PEEP

33. 28%

34. Apnea; acute respiratory failure; impending respiratory failure; refractory hypoxic respiratory failure with an increased WOB or ineffective breathing pattern

35. Intubation would be contraindicated when it is contrary to the patient's wishes, medically pointless, and futile.

36. Respiratory arrest; cardiac arrest; nonrespiratory organ failure; upper airway obstruction; inability to protect airway or high risk of aspiration. These two answers are also correct: inability to clear secretions; facial/head surgery or trauma.

37. This patient is hypoxemic with a nonrebreather mask and is unable to move an adequate amount of air. The pink frothy sputum is pulmonary edema and the hypotension is caused by cardiogenic shock. This is a medical emergency and the patient requires intubation, mechanical ventilation, and PEEP.

38. Oxygen therapy would be most appropriate for this patient. If the patient wishes further intervention, ABG and other diagnostic tests may be performed.

39. Aggressive bronchodilator therapy (continuous), corticosteroids, oxygen therapy, and close monitoring of this patient are required. If the bronchospasm does not respond to aggressive therapy, intubation and mechanical ventilation may be necessary.

40. This patient requires oxygen and bronchodilator therapy. The patient's $PaCO_2$ reveals that he is able to move air and therefore does not require any mechanical ventilation at this time.

41. This patient is developing acute respiratory failure and meets some of the criteria for mechanical ventilatory support (pH, 7.21; $PaCO_2$ greater than 55 and rising, PaO_2/F_1O_2 less than 200). This patient should be intubated and mechanical ventilatory support begun. This patient's head trauma makes NPPV an absolute contraindication.

42. $CaO_2 = [Hb \times 1.34 \times SaO_2] + [PaO_2 \times 0.003]$
    $= [12 \times 1.34 \times 0.91] + [59 \times 0.003]$
    $= 14.63 + 0.18$
    $= 14.81$ vol%

43. $CaO_2 = [Hb \times 1.34 \times SaO_2] + [PaO_2 \times 0.003]$
    $= [8 \times 1.34 \times 0.9] + [58 \times 0.003]$
    $= 9.65 + 0.17$
    $= 9.82$ vol%

44. $CaO_2 = [Hb \times 1.34 \times SaO_2] + [PaO_2 \times 0.003]$
    $= [17 \times 1.34 \times 0.79] + [48 \times 0.003]$
    $= 18.00 + 0.14$
    $= 18.14$ vol%

45. $P_AO_2 = [F_IO_2 (P_{bs} - PH_2O)] - [PaCO_2/R]$
    $= [0.7(760 - 47)] - [48/0.8]$
    $= [0.7 \times 713] - 60 = 499 - 60 = 439$ mm Hg
    $PaO_2 = 50$ mm Hg
    $P_AO_2 - PaO_2 = 439 - 50 = 389$ mm Hg

46. $PaO_2/P_AO_2 = 50$ mm Hg/439 mm Hg = 0.11
    Of the oxygen available to the alveolus, only 11% is getting into the artery. Yes, 0.11 is a critical value.

47. $PaO_2/F_IO_2 = 50$ mm Hg/0.70 = 71.43. Yes, this is a critical value indicating the need for mechanical ventilatory support.

48. $P_AO_2 = [F_IO_2 (P_{bs} - PH_2O)] - [PaCO_2/R]$
    $= [0.21(760 - 47)] - [55/0.8]$
    $P_AO_2 = 150 - 69 = 81$ mm Hg, $P_AO_2 - PaO_2 = 81 - 51 = 30$ mm Hg. This value is within the normal range.

49. $PaO_2/P_AO_2 = 51$ mm Hg/81 mm Hg = 0.63. This is not a critical value.

50. $PaO_2/F_IO_2 = 51/0.21 = 243$. This is not a critical value.

Answers to Critical Thinking Questions

1. A rapid physical assessment of a trauma patient should include checking for a patent airway, respirations, chest auscultation, patient appearance, pulse, blood pressure, temperature, chest inspection, chest palpation, chest percussion, and patient sensorium.

2. The diagnostic evaluations that should be done to assess the need for mechanical ventilation include ABGs, chest radiograph, and pulse oximetry.

3. The patient would be quite anxious looking, be flushed and sweating, leaning forward in a tripod position, using accessory muscles, and be cyanotic or pale.

4. The patient requiring oxygen therapy only will present with hypoxic respiratory failure as evidenced by a PaO_2 level below predicted normal for the patient's age. This patient will have a normal $PaCO_2$ level. A patient requiring mechanical ventilation will be one that has both hypoxic respiratory failure and hypercapneic respiratory failure.

Answers to Case Studies

Case Study #1

1. Hypoxemia is the cause of the patient's tachycardia.

2. The patient's PaO_2 of 48 mm Hg on 40% oxygen and the PaO_2/F_IO_2 value of 120 are critical. However, both the $P(A-a)O_2$ and PaO_2/P_AO_2 are outside the normal range but not at critical levels.

3. This patient is having an acute asthma episode. At the onset of an asthma episode the patient will hyperventilate. A normal $PaCO_2$, in this situation, indicates a severe episode (stage III) and impending respiratory failure.

4. Continuous bronchodilator therapy would be appropriate. However, if little or no improvement occurs, ventilatory support will be necessary.

Case Study #2

1. The patient's oxygenation status is not at a critical level. The alveolar-arterial oxygen gradient is wider than normal, at 42.5 mm Hg, but not critical. The arterial/alveolar PO_2 at 0.59 is lower than normal, but also not critical. And the PaO_2/F_IO_2 is lower than normal but again not critical.

2. The patient's pH and $PaCO_2$ are both within normal limits. The patient is not weak enough to require mechanical ventilatory intervention at this time.

3. The patient should be closely monitored for acute ventilatory failure by measuring MIP and VC in addition to ABG for $PaCO_2$ changes. Medical treatment of myasthenia gravis includes an anticholinesterase medication. The patient may benefit from low-flow oxygen, approximately 2 L/min by nasal cannula.

Case Study #3

1. The alveolar-arterial oxygen gradient is increased (315 mm Hg) but not critical. However, the PaO_2 (41 mm Hg), the PaO_2/P_AO_2 (0.13) and the PaO_2/F_IO_2 (68) indicate hypoxemic respiratory failure.

2. The $PaCO_2$ is markedly elevated and the pH is very low. This is an indication that the patient is in acute respiratory failure.

3. This patient requires intubation on the basis of the deteriorating ABG.

Answers to NBRC-Style Questions

1. a	5. c	9. b
2. b	6. c	10. a
3. d	7. c	
4. d	8. b	

Chapter 6, Selecting the Ventilator and the Mode
Answers to Key Terms Crossword Puzzle

Crossword answers include: RESPIRATORY ALKALOSIS, APRV, SPONTANEOUS BREATHS, PRESSURE, PCIRV, CONTROL VENTILATION, FULL VENTILATORY SUPPORT, DYSSYNCHRONY, CMV, PRESSURE SUPPORT, MANDATORY, VOLUME VENTILATION, SENSITIVITY, ASSIST/CONTROL, CONTROLLER, ARTIFICIAL, ASSISTED BREATHS

Answers to Review Questions

1. Indication; pathology; goals; interface; location; length of time; staff familiarity

2. d   NPV
   a, b, c, e   CPAP
   a, e   PPV
   b, c   NPPV

3. improving oxygenation, OSA

4. bilevel positive airway pressure

5. NPPV

6. Full ventilatory support has the ventilator providing all the energy necessary to maintain the patient's effective alveolar ventilation. Partial ventilatory support has the patient participating in the WOB to help maintain effective alveolar ventilation.

7. 8 breaths/min, 6 to 12 mL/kg IBW

8. 6 breaths/min

9. Full ventilatory support while allowing the ventilatory muscles to rest while supplying all the necessary ventilation

10. a. Assisted breath because flow initiates (patient) and set pressure is reached and held until a set time is reached (ventilator). b. Mandatory breath because time initiates (ventilator) and when set volume is reached inspiration ends (ventilator). c. Assisted breath because pressure initiates (patient) and set pressure is reached and held until a set time is reached (ventilator). d. Spontaneous breath because flow initiates (patient) and set pressure is reached but patient's flow ends inspiration.

11. The main advantage of volume ventilation is that it guarantees a specific volume delivery and minute ventilation regardless of changes in lung compliance and resistance or patient effort.

12. a. The PIP will rise any time there is an increase in airway resistance, such as with bronchospasm. b. The amount of volume will remain constant because it is the set variable.

13. decrease

14. **Advantages**

    Avoidance of complications associated with artificial airways; flexibility in initiating and removing mechanical ventilation; reduced requirements for heavy sedation; preservation of airway defense, speech, and swallowing mechanism; reduced need for invasive monitoring

    Disadvantages

    Gastric distention, skin pressure lesions, facial pain, dry nose, eye irritation, discomfort, claustrophobia, poor sleep, mask leaks

15. increase, hyperinflation, less

16. Inappropriate sensitivity settings will increase the work to trigger inspiration and may cause patient-ventilator dyssynchrony.

17. When targeting pressure as the control variable, volume will vary with changing lung characteristics.

18. decrease, hypoventilation, more

19. | Type of Ventilation | Advantages | Disadvantages |
| --- | --- | --- |
| Volume ventilation | Delivers specific volume regardless of lung characteristics. Improved lung conditions generate less pressure in lungs.

Most practitioners are comfortable with this type of ventilation. | Deteriorating lung conditions cause increased P_A and overdistention. Flow delivery may be fixed and not meet patient demand, causing patient-ventilator dyssynchrony. |
| Pressure ventilation | Decreased risk of overdistention of the lungs. Descending flow pattern better matches patient's needs, decreasing the patient's WOB. May be more comfortable for spontaneously breathing patients. | Clinicians are less familiar with this type of ventilation. Variability of volume delivery. Lung deterioration decreases V_T and minute volume. |

20. Pressure ventilation demonstrates more benefit for spontaneously breathing patients because it may lower the WOB and improve comfort.

21. CMV; SIMV; spontaneous modes

22. a. controlled mechanical ventilation; b. continuous mechanical ventilation; c. assist/control ventilation

23. When a ventilator is in the control mode the time trigger is utilized.

24. Controlled ventilation is appropriate for patients who are obtunded because of drugs; are sedated and paralyzed; have cerebral malfunction, spinal cord, or phrenic nerve injury; or have motor nerve paralysis with no voluntary efforts.

25. Sedation and paralysis may be necessary for uncontrolled seizure activity, tetanic contractions, during the use of inverse ratio ventilation or permissive hypercapnia.

26. Iatrogenic hyperventilation may benefit patients with closed-head injury or who are recovering from neurosurgery because respiratory alkalosis will decrease intracranial pressure.

27. The patient will be "locked out" and be unable to trigger a breath.

28. Time-trigger; pressure-trigger; flow-trigger

29. An increased ventilatory drive will increase patient triggering. This will cause hyperventilation and respiratory alkalosis.

30. The patient may contribute 33% to 50% of the work of inspiration in this situation.

31. In the PC-CMV mode the control variables are time or patient trigger, pressure limit, and time cycle.

32. maximum pressure limit, +10 cm H_2O, inspiration

33. PC-CMV

34. PCIRV is appropriate when a patient with very stiff lungs is not successfully ventilated with VC-CMV and PEEP or PC-CMV and PEEP.

35. IMV differs from CMV in that IMV allows the patient to breathe spontaneously between mandatory breaths. In CMV all breaths are machine breaths.

36. With SIMV the mandatory breaths may be patient triggered. When the operator-selected time interval is reached the ventilator waits for the next patient inspiratory effort. When this effort is sensed the ventilator synchronously delivers a mandatory breath (assisted breath).

37. Spontaneous breathing through a ventilator circuit may be obtained from a continuous gas flow or a demand valve.

38. PSV

39. Assist/control advantages: guaranteed minimum minute ventilation, can provide synchronous patient breaths, patient can set rate, guaranteed volume or pressure breath with each breath. Assist/control risks and disadvantages: respiratory alkalosis if rate is too high; high airway pressures and associated complications; excessive work if flow or sensitivity is not set correctly; may be poorly tolerated in awake, non-sedated patients; may cause or worsen auto-PEEP; and possible respiratory muscle atrophy.

40. IMV/SIMV advantages: can be used for weaning, may reduce respiratory alkalosis associated with assist/control, prevents respiratory muscle atrophy, lower airway pressure. IMV/SIMV risks and disadvantages: excessive WOB if flow and sensitivity are not set correctly, hypercapnia, fatigue and tachypnea if rate is set too low, demand valve WOB with older ventilators, and increased WOB for spontaneous breaths unless PSV is added.

41. spontaneous breathing, CPAP, PSV

42. Advantages to using a ventilator as a T-piece include the monitoring capabilities of the ventilator plus the ability of the ventilator to alarm if something undesirable occurs. The disadvantage is that some ventilator valve systems require more work than others to open up for the patient to receive gas flow.

43. The appropriate type of patient for PSV is one that has a consistent spontaneous respiratory pattern.

44. inspiratory pressure, expiratory pressure (PEEP), sensitivity

45. In PSV, the V_T is determined by the pressure gradient, lung compliance, airway resistance, and patient effort.

46. A leak in the circuit will cause a ventilator in PSV to time cycle because inspiratory time would reach the maximum inspiratory time setting.

47. Patient coughing or forcible exhalation will cause a ventilator to pressure cycle in the PSV mode. For an adult patient this pressure cycle level is set 1.5 to 2 cm H_2O above the set pressure support level.

48. Overcoming the WOB for spontaneously breathing patients, by using CPAP or SIMV, imposed by the demand valve system, ventilator circuit, and ET. Decreasing the WOB in the CPAP or SIMV mode further by setting the pressure level higher than is required to overcome system resistance. Providing full ventilatory support while maintaining spontaneous breathing (PSmax).

49. rise time (also known as flow acceleration percent, inspiratory rise time, inspiratory rise time percent, and slope adjustment)

50. pressure cycle (premature end to inspiration)

51. flow

52. Time trigger and patient trigger

53. Flow cycle or time cycle

54. PAug, PRVC, VS

55. Each breath in PAug is patient triggered and pressure targeted, such as a pressure-supported breath. However, PAug guarantees that at least the volume set on the control panel is delivered for each breath.

56. If the set volume is achieved before flow cycling, the breath will be volume cycled.

57. If the set volume is not reached before flow drops to the set level, the ventilator will maintain the flow at its set value until the volume is delivered (volume cycled).

58. The patient can receive more volume than set in PAug when the patient's inspiratory flow demand is high enough to prevent the maintenance of the set pressure level. This will cause the ventilator to provide additional flow to the patient.

59. PCRV is patient or time triggered, pressure limited (targeted), and time cycled.

60. The ventilator will not allow the pressure to rise higher than 5 cm H_2O below the upper pressure limit setting. Therefore 35 cm H_2O would be the level to activate the alarm.

61. Patient triggered (pressure or flow triggered), pressure limited (targeted), and flow cycled.

62. With PRVC inspiration can be either time triggered or patient triggered. In VS, inspiration is only patient triggered. A PRVC breath is time cycled and a VS breath is usually flow cycled (it may pressure cycle if pressure rises too high or time cycle if inspiratory time is extended for some reason).

63. MVV

64. In MVV, the high-rate alarm and the low V_T alarm must be set to protect against rapid shallow breathing by the patient.

65. APRV

66. time constant

67. stiff lungs

68. Pressure, flow, and volume delivery

69. In PAV, the amount of pressure produced by the ventilator depends on the patient's demand for inspiratory flow and volume and the amplification setting selected by the clinician.

70.

Advantages	**Disadvantages**
Inability to track changes in patient effort	PAV only provides for assisted ventilation, cannot compensate for system leaks, and may be more difficult for the patient to trigger in the presence of auto-PEEP.

Answers to Critical Thinking Questions

1. The patient's use of accessory muscles and the presence of diaphoresis are manifestations of acute respiratory distress. Patient-ventilator asynchrony can also be a sign of acute respiratory distress. The use of the accessory muscles and diaphoresis shows that the patient is working to breathe. However, there are no assisted breaths. This situation could be caused by an improper sensitivity setting. If the setting is too insensitive, the patient will have inspiratory efforts but will be unable to trigger assisted breaths from the ventilator. Make sure that sensitivity is set so that the patient is able to trigger the ventilator without auto-triggering.

2. When a patient's ventilatory drive is increased during VC-CMV the patient's assist rate will increase. Because every breath will be a machine breath at the set volume this can easily lead to a decreased $PaCO_2$ or respiratory alkalosis. Identification of the source of the increased drive (fever, sepsis, etc.) and correction of this is the best way to control the respiratory alkalosis. However, because this may take some time, sedatives, paralytic agents, or switching to SIMV with similar settings may be tried.

3. Central sleep apnea occurs when the brain fails to send the appropriate signals to the breathing muscles to initiate breathing. It is characterized by apneic events during sleep with no associated ventilatory effort. The apnea will cause hypoxemia and hypercapnia. Because bilevel positive airway pressure creates a pressure gradient between EPAP and IPAP, air is pushed into the lungs. Therefore bilevel PAP would "breathe" for the patient during periods of apnea.

4.

Answer	**Rationale**
d. VC-CMV; 1. intubated with quadriplegia from a spinal cord injury	Patient will most likely be unable to breathe without full ventilatory support.
e. PC-CMV with PEEP; 2. intubated with ARDS	With ARDS, guarding against increasing peak pressures from stiff lungs is important.
a. Nasal mask CPAP; 3. OSA at home	This will keep the upper airways open so the patient may spontaneously breathe.
b. CPAP through ventilator; 4. intubated with spontaneous breathing with ALI	This will improve oxygenation while allowing the patient to be monitored. The patient would also benefit from pressure support.
c. pressure support; 5. intubated with consistent spontaneous respiratory pattern	This will help the patient overcome the resistance from the ET, ventilator circuit, and demand valve system while allowing the patient to be monitored.
a. Nasal mask CPAP; 6. nonintubated spontaneously breathing with refractory hypoxemia	This will improve oxygenation without having to intubate the patient. This will hopefully avoid intubation.
d. VC-CMV; 7. intubated with drug overdose	The patient will require full ventilatory support until the effects of the drugs wear off.

Answers to Case Studies

Case Study #1

1. The ventilator is set to deliver PC-SIMV.
2. The inspiratory time is 1 second.
3. The expiratory time is 3.0 seconds.

Case Study #2

1. Full ventilatory support to ensure adequate ventilation.
2. PC-SIMV with pressure support and PEEP. Pressure control may be necessary to guard against high inspiratory pressures. Pressure support to overcome the airway resistance caused by the small ET and ventilator circuit and PEEP for the refractory hypoxemia. If peak pressures are not an issue, VC-SIMV with pressure support and PEEP may be used.

Case Study #3

1. The scalar represents PSV.
2. The problem is pressure overshoot at the beginning of inspiration.
3. To correct this problem, lower the set flow rate or slow down the rise time.

Answers to NBRC-Style Questions

1. b	5. a	9. b
2. c	6. c	10. d
3. a	7. b	
4. c	8. d	

Chapter 7, Initial Ventilator Settings

Answers to Key Terms Crossword Puzzle

Answers to Review Questions

1. minute ventilation
2. V_T; f; inspiratory gas flow; flow waveform; I:E ratio; pressure limit; inflation hold; PEEP
3. 250 mL/min, 200 mL/min
4. 2.18 m^2
5. 1.74 m^2
6. 1.92 m^2

	Calculations	$\dot{V}_E$
7.	$3.5 \times 1.6 = 5.6$ L/min $+ (5.6 \times 0.18) = 5.6 + 1 =$	6.6 L/min
8.	$4 \times 2.8 = 11.2$ L/min $+ (11.2 \times 0.15) = 11.2 + 1.7 =$	12.9 L/min
9.	$4 \times 2.3 = 9.2$ L/min $+ (9.2 \times 0.1) = 9.2 + 0.9 =$	10.1 L/min
10.	$3.5 \times 1.9 = 6.65$ L/min $+ (6.65 \times 0.2) = 6.65 + 1.33 =$	8.0 L/min

11. 4 to 12 mL/kg IBW

12. 5 to 10 mL/kg IBW

13. IBW = 105 + 5(64 in – 60) = 105 + 20 = 125 lb/2.2 = 57 kg × 4 mL/kg = 228 mL; 57 kg × 12 mL/kg = 684 mL. The range is 228 mL to 684 mL.

14. IBW = 106 + 6(74 in – 60) = 106 + 84 = 190 lb/2.2 = 86 kg × 4 mL/kg = 344 mL; 86 kg × 12 mL/kg = 1032 mL. The range is 344 mL to 1032 mL.

15. The normal range for spontaneous V_T in a human being is 5 to 7 mL/kg.

16. The normal range for spontaneous breathing rate in a human being is 12 to18 breaths/min.

17. The normal minute ventilation is approximately 100 mL/kg IBW.

18. 105 + 5(62 – 60) = 115 lb/2.2 = 52 kg. By using 10–12 mL/kg, V_T should range between 520 mL and 624 mL at a rate between 8 and 12 breaths/min. For example, 600 mL × 10 breaths/min = 6.0 L/min.

19. 106 + 6(71 – 60) = 172 lb/2.2 = 78 kg. By using 8–10 mL/kg, V_T should range between 624 mL and 780 mL at a rate between 8 and 12 breaths/min. For example, 680 mL × 10 breaths/min = 6.8 L/min.

20. 106 + 6(69 – 60) = 160 lb/2.2 = 73 kg. by using 4–8 mL/kg, V_T should range between 292 mL and 584 mL at a rate of 15 to 25 breaths/min. For example, 400 mL × 20 breaths/min = 8.0 L/min.

21. 300 mL/110 cm H_2O = 2.7 mL/cm H_2O

22. 210 mL/115 cm H_2O = 1.8 mL/cm H_2O

23. 28 cm H_2O × 2.5 mL/cm H_2O = 70 mL lost

24. 30 cm H_2O × 1.8 mL/cm H_2O = 54 mL lost. 450 mL – 54 mL = 396 mL delivered.

25. The RT should add the amount of volume lost to the V_T setting.

26.

	V_T	Respiratory Rate	$\dot{V}_E$
a.	750 mL	12 breaths/min	**0.75 L × 12 = 9 L/min**
b.	580 mL	10 breaths/min	**0.58 L × 10 = 5.8 L/min**
c.	**6.9/15 = 0.46 L = 460 mL**	15 breaths/min	6.9 L/min
d.	**8.3/20 = 0.415 = 415 mL**	20 breaths/min	8.3 L/min
e.	460 mL	**5.2/0.46 = 11 breaths/min**	5.2 L/min
f.	660 mL	**9.5/0.66 = 14 breaths/min**	9.5 L/min

27. a. 30 breaths/min: 60 seconds/30 breaths/min = 2 seconds

    b. 15 breaths/min: 60 seconds/15 breaths/min = 4 seconds

    c. 12 breaths/min: 60 seconds/12 breaths/min = 5 seconds

    d. 10 breaths/min: 60 seconds/10 breaths/min = 6 seconds

28. a. $T_I = 1$ second; f = 30; $T_E = TCT - T_I$; 2 seconds – 1 second = $T_E = 1$ second

    b. $T_I = 0.75$ second; f = 15; $T_E = TCT - T_I$; 4 seconds – 0.75 second = $T_E = 3.25$ seconds

    c. $T_I = 1.25$ second; f = 12; $T_E = TCT - T_I$; 5 seconds – 1.25 seconds = $T_E = 3.75$ seconds

    d. $T_I = 2$ seconds; f = 10; $T_E = TCT - T_I$; 6 seconds – 2 seconds = $T_E = 4$ seconds

29. Use the formula I:E = $T_I/T_I:T_E/T_I$.

    a. 1 second/1 second:1 second/1 second = 1:1 ratio

    b. 0.75 second/0.75 second:3.25 seconds/0.75 second = 1:5 ratio

    c. 1.25 seconds/1.25 seconds:3.75 seconds/1.25 seconds = 1:3 ratio

    d. 2 seconds/2 seconds:4 seconds/2 seconds = 1:2 ratio

30. TCT = 60/rate = 60/12 = 5 seconds. Therefore one breath cycle is 5 seconds long and is represented by the rectangle below.

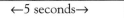

$\leftarrow$5 seconds$\rightarrow$

The I:E ratio shows how much of the rectangle is allotted to inspiratory time and how much to expiratory time. The ratio given is 1:3. That means that 1 part of the rectangle is for inspiration and 3 parts for expiration. If the two numbers from the ratio are added, the sum will show how many equal parts the TCT is divided into.

1.25 seconds	1.25 seconds	1.25 seconds	1.25 seconds

TCT/(I + E) = 1 part of the rectangle. 5 seconds/ (1 + 3) = 5/4 = 1.25 seconds. Each part of the rectangle is equal to 1.25 seconds. Because T_I is one part, it is equal to 1.25 seconds. And T_E = 5 – 1.25 = 3.75 second.

31. TCT = 60/25 = 2.4 seconds.

$\leftarrow$2.4 seconds$\rightarrow$

I:E = 1:2; I + E = 1 + 2 = 3 equal parts. 2.4 seconds/ 3 = 0.8 second.

0.8	0.8	0.8

T_I = 0.8 second and T_E = 1.6 seconds.

32. Flow rate × Inspiratory time = V_T. 50 L/min = 50 L/60 seconds = 0.83 L/sec. 0.83 L/sec × 1 second = 0.83 L, or 830 mL.

33. V_T/Flow rate = Inspiratory time. 0.7 L/0.83 L/sec = 0.84 second.

34. shorten, increase, decrease

35. When slower flow rates are used, the T_I will be longer and the TE will be shorter, causing air trapping and possible cardiovascular side effects. However, PIP may be reduced and gas exchange may be improved.

36. T_I range, 0.8 to 1.2 seconds; I:E ratio, 1:2 to 1:4; and flow rates, 40 to 80 L/min.

37. descending or decelerating waveform

38. sine waveform

39. descending or constant waveforms

40. In patients with hypoxemia and low lung compliance, the descending flow pattern may be beneficial because it keeps PIP low and Paw high, improving gas distribution.

41. The measurement of plateau pressure that helps estimate P_A for the calculation of static compliance.

42. The plateau pressure is unattainable because the patient is actively breathing, which will cause an unstable reading.

43. PC-CMV, bilevel PAP, and PRVC

44. PSV, PC-CMV, bilevel PAP, PAug, PRVC, and VS

45. PSV, bilevel PAP, PAug, and VS

46. PC-CMV and PRVC

47.

Advantages	Disadvantages
Providing flow on demand and limiting pressures to avoid overinflation	Alveolar shearing from rapid initial flows to heterogeneous lungs and the variation in V_T as lung characteristics change

48. Because the elastic recoil of a patient with COPD is weakened, small airways tend to collapse during exhalation because thoracic pressures are greater than intraluminal pressure. Low levels of PEEP will increase the intraluminal pressure and prevent this collapse on exhalation.

49. It is established by the change in pressure between PIP and baseline (PEEP + auto-PEEP).

50. C = $\Delta V/\Delta P$; therefore $\Delta P = \Delta V/C$. Compliance for this patient is 400 mL/18 cm H_2O = 22.2 mL/cm H_2O. ΔP = 750 mL/22.2 mL/cm H_2O = 33.8 cm H_2O. The PIP needs to be increased to 33.8 cm H_2O to achieve the 750 mL.

51. C = $\Delta V/\Delta P$, therefore $\Delta P = \Delta V/C$. Compliance for this patient is 550 mL/14 cm H_2O = 39.3 mL/cm H_2O. ΔP = 800 mL/39.3 mL/cm H_2O = 20.4 cm H_2O. The PIP needs to be increased to 20.4 cm H_2O to achieve the 800 mL.

52. The easiest method for establishing initial levels of pressure support is to use the formula for P_{TA} (PIP – $P_{plateau}$), the values for which are measured during volume ventilation.

53. PTA = PIP – $P_{plateau}$ = 28 cm H_2O – 20 cm H_2O = 8 cm H_2O PS

54. The patient is actively exhaling before flow cycling, which is causing pressure cycling.

55. The flow cycling variable can be adjusted to a higher flow cycling percentage.

56. Flow cycle percentage × Peak inspiratory flow = Flow rate level for cycling: 0.2 × 50 L/min = 10 L/min

57. 0.4 × 50 L/min = 20 L/min

58. The 40% flow cycling percentage will have the shortest inspiratory time because the ventilator will cycle when the peak inspiratory flow drops from its peak at 50 L/min to 20 L/min (rather than 10 L/min caused by the 20% setting).

59. The initial PIP should be set at the $P_{plateau}$ level taken during VV; $P_{plateau}$ is not available, use PIP from VV – 5 cm H_2O as a starting point; if volume settings are not available, use a setting of 10 to 15 cm H_2O with simultaneous volume measurements and adjust appropriately.

60. IPAP 5 to 10 cm H_2O, EPAP 3 to 10 cm H_2O, rate 25 breaths/min or less, and V_T of 7 mL/kg or more; if necessary, 2 L/min oxygen flow added

61. PRVC

62. bronchospasm; increased secretions; pneumothorax; decreased lung compliance (anything that will increase airway resistance or decrease lung compliance)

Answers to Critical Thinking Questions

1. Things to consider before placing a patient on mechanical ventilatory support include the patient's metabolic rate, body surface area, IBW, lung pathology, acid-base balance, oxygenation status, and tubing compliance.

2. The tubing compression factor is the amount of volume lost in the patient circuit per pressure generated during the delivery of the breath. The higher the pressure the more volume will be lost.

3. Pediatric patients and other patients who require low V_T will be affected most by tubing compressibility.

4. Decreasing compliance will cause an increase in pressure ($P_{plateau}$) during VV and cause a decrease in V_T during PV. Improving compliance will decrease pressure during VV and increase V_T delivery during PV.

5. The two PSV safety systems are (1) a maximum safety pressure system that will pressure cycle the ventilator when a sudden rise in pressure occurs (usually with an active exhalation) and (2) a time cycle to prevent increased T_I because of a leak in the system.

Answers to Case Studies

Case Study #1

1. Intubate and place on mechanical ventilation. (The patient has a neuromuscular disorder and is already showing signs of breathing difficulties. She is having difficulty swallowing, which necessitates protection of the airway.)

2. BSA = 1.82 m^2; 1.82 m^2 × 3.5 = 6.4 L/min

3. V_T 10 to 12 mL/kg because the patient has no underlying lung problems. Her IBW is 105 + 5(68 – 60) = 145 lb/2.2 = 66 kg. Therefore V_T range is 660 mL to 792 mL. Set rate should be 10 to 12 breaths/min.

4. volume ventilation because the patient has no underlying pulmonary problems

5. VC-CMV, rate 10 breaths/min, V_T 660 mL (remember minimum minute ventilation should be 6.4 L/min), flow rate to achieve this V_T with T_I = 1 second is 40 L/min

Case Study #2

1. Compliance factor = V_T/(PIP – PEEP). 250 mL/(68 – 3 cm H_2O) = 3.85 mL/cm H_2O

2. 27 cm H_2O × 3.85 mL/cm H_2O = 104 mL lost volume in the circuit.

3. 250 mL – 104 mL = 146 mL is being delivered to the patient.

4. Add the amount lost, 104 mL, to the set volume, 250 mL. The volume set should be 354 mL to compensate for the tubing compliance.

Answers to NBRC-Style Questions

1. a	5. b	9. b
2. c	6. a	10. b
3. b	7. d	
4. b	8. c	

Chapter 8, Final Considerations in Ventilator Setup

Answers to Key Terms Crossword Puzzle

Crossword answers include: FLOW, INOTROPIC, MYASTHENIA GRAVIS, PERMISSIVE, APNEA, BRONCHOSCOPY, BAROTRAUMA, YELLOW, PASSOVER, DYSYNCHRONUS, SIGH, FACEMASK, THAM, CRACKLES, STERILE WATER, DYNAMIC HYPERINFLATION, RATIO ALARM, HYPERRESONANCE, DIURETICS, STATUS ASTHMATICUS, CUSHING RESPONSE, WICK, CARDIOMEGALY, HYDROMETER, CATION, APICAL, HEAT MOISTURE EXCHANGER, PULSUS PARADOXUS

Answers to Review Questions

1. 60 to 100 mm Hg

2. A nasal cannula at 2 L/min is equivalent to approximately 28% oxygen. The ventilator F_IO_2 should therefore be 28%.

3. Desired F_IO_2 = PaO₂ (desired) × [F_IO_2 (known)/PaO₂ (known)]

   Desired F_IO_2 = 90 mm Hg × (0.5/60 mm Hg)

   Desired F_IO_2 = 90 × 0.00833 = 0.75, or 75%

4. 100%

5. More than 92%

6. 10 to 20 minutes after placement on a ventilator

7. absorption atelectasis; oxygen toxicity; intrapulmonary shunting

8. Flow triggering is faster because (1) the exhalation valve does not close, so no time is taken up there, and (2) flow is already present in the system when the patient begins to breathe; this provides immediate flow to the patient.

9. Auto-PEEP makes pressure triggering more difficult because it causes the patient to have to breathe through the amount of auto-PEEP plus the sensitivity setting to trigger the breath. For example, if the auto-PEEP is +8 cm H_2O and the sensitivity setting is −1 cm H_2O, the patient would have to create −9 cm H_2O to trigger a breath.

10. Isothermic saturation boundary, fourth to fifth generation of subsegmental bronchi

11. at least 30 mg H_2O/L, 31° to 35° C

12. A closed system maintains a steadier temperature and reduces the risk of potential contamination because the ventilator circuit does not have to be opened to refill the humidifier.

13. A ventilator circuit that does not have heated wires is exposed to the cooler temperatures of the room and will subsequently cool down heated gas as it travels toward the patient. Because the cooler the gas the less water it can hold, water condensation will form in the tubing.

14. 10 to 14 mg/L of water

15. 22 to 34 mg/L of water

16. Resistance to flow will increase, causing auto-PEEP and an increased WOB

17. The HME should be removed to avoid increasing resistance from the collection of the aerosol within the HME. A circuit adapter that selectively bypasses the HME can be used during aerosol treatments.

18. The MDI with spacer should be placed within the inspiratory limb of the circuit. The HME needs to be removed during the treatment.

19. thick, copious, or bloody secretions; exhaled V_T less than 70% of inhaled V_T; body temperature less than 32° C; spontaneous minute ventilation more than 10 L/min; during aerosol treatments; when V_T is small so as to be compromised by the HME dead space; with large V_T

20. Level 1, immediately life-threatening; level 2, potentially life-threatening; level 3, non–life-threatening but a potential source of patient harm

21. level 2, heater/humidifier malfunction

22. level 1, timing failure

23. level 2, autocycling

24. level 3, auto-PEEP

25. level 1, excessive gas delivery to patient

26. level 2, inappropriate PEEP/CPAP

27. level 1, exhalation valve failure

28. level 2, I:E ratio inappropriate

29. level 1, electrical power failure

30. level 3, changes in lung characteristics

31. level 2, circuit leak

32. level 1, no gas delivery to patient

33. level 2, circuit partially obstructed

34. level 2, inappropriate oxygen level

35. level 3, changes in ventilatory drive

36. Low pressure alarm 20 cm H_2O, high pressure alarm 40 cm H_2O, and low PEEP/CPAP 3 cm H_2O

37. 20 seconds

38. Both sigh maneuvers and lung recruitment strategies attempt to reverse atelectasis; in fact, sighs may be used as a lung recruitment strategy while using lung protective ventilation (especially when V_T is less than 7 mL/kg) with patients who have ARDS.

39. Before and after suctioning; before and after bronchoscopy; during an extubation procedure; during chest physiotherapy; during ventilation with V_T less than 7 mL/kg; as a recruitment maneuver in some patient with ARDS

40. Check ventilator and circuit function for leaks; fill humidifier with sterile water and set appropriate temperature or place an HME in line; place a temperature/monitoring device near patient connector when heated humidifier is used; check F_IO_2; adjust alarms; make sure ECG is connected to the patient; ensure emergency airway equipment is available; provide suction equipment; attach a volume monitoring device and oxygen analyzer if not available on the ventilator; keep a manual resuscitator (and mask) with the ventilator

41. *Modes:* VC-CMV, VC-SIMV or PC-CMV, PC-SIMV, and spontaneous CPAP/PSV; V_T *range:* 100 to 1000 mL; *respiratory rate range:* 1 to 60 breaths/min; *pressure range:* 0 to 100 cm H_2O; *PEEP/CPAP range:* 0 to 30 cm H_2O; *flow rate range:* 10 to 180 L/min; *flow waveforms:* constant and descending; F_IO_2: 21% to 100%; *diagnostic measurements:* inflation hold (to measure C_S) and expiratory pause (to measure auto-PEEP); *alarms:* apnea, power failure, gas source failure, low pressure, high-pressure limit, increased rate, decreased V_T, high and low minute ventilation

42. Patients with COPD have increased airway resistance and may also have increase lung compliance.

43. A respiratory infection superimposed on chronic disease (acute on chronic respiratory failure)

44. Air trapping; nosocomial infections; barotrauma; cardiac problems; aspiration; weaning difficulties

45. bilevel PAP

46. orotracheal

47.

Parameter	Preferred Setting or Range
V_T	8 to 10 mL/kg
Rate	8 to 12 breaths/min
Inspiratory time	0.6 to 1.2 seconds
Flow rate	more than 60 to 100 L/min
Flow waveform	descending ramp
PEEP	5 cm H_2O or less (or approximately 50% of auto-PEEP)
F_IO_2	Maintain PaO_2 55 to 75 mm Hg with F_IO_2 less than 0.5

48. Myasthenia gravis; amyotrophic lateral sclerosis; muscular dystrophy; polio or postpolio syndrome; Guillain-Barré syndrome; tetanus; cervical spinal cord injury; botulism

49. Progressive respiratory muscle weakness leads to problems coughing and clearing secretions and eventually respiratory failure. Also, a weak gag reflex may lead to aspiration.

50. | Parameter | Preferred Setting or Range |
|---|---|
| V_T | 12 to 15 mL/kg |
| Rate | 8 to 12 breaths/min |
| Inspiratory time | 1 second to start |
| Flow rate | 60 L/min or more |
| Flow waveform | constant or descending ramp |
| PEEP | 5 cm H_2O |
| F_IO_2 | 0.21 |

51. The alteration of blood flow through the thorax and heart as a result of dramatic intrapleural pressures changes during the inspiration and expiration of a patient with acute severe asthma.

52. Increased airway resistance and air trapping

53. less than 30 cm H_2O despite the high PIP

54. bicarbonate and tris-hydroxymethyl-aminomethane

55. | Parameter | Preferred Setting or Range |
|---|---|
| V_T | 4 to 8 mL/kg |
| Rate | less than 8 breaths/min |
| Inspiratory time | 1 second or less |
| Flow rate | 80 to 100 L/min |
| Flow waveform | descending ramp |
| PEEP | at approximately 80% of auto-PEEP |
| F_IO_2 | keep PaO_2 between 60 and 100 mm Hg with 0.5 or more |

56. hyperresonance

57. Trauma to the head from falls; automobile accidents and blows to the head; and postcraniotomy, cerebrovascular accident, and postresuscitation hypoxemia

58. CPP = MAP – ICP

59. MAP is 90 to 95 mm Hg, ICP is less than 10 mm Hg, therefore normal CPP is 80 to 85 mm Hg.

60. CPP less than 60 mm Hg

61. Iatrogenic hyperventilation should only be used temporarily for increased ICP by maintaining $PaCO_2$ levels between 25 and 30 mm Hg and gradually allowing it to return to normal levels in 24 to 48 hours.

62. | Parameter | Preferred Setting or Range |
|---|---|
| V_T | 8 to 12 mL/kg while maintaining Palv less than 30 cm H_2O |
| respiratory rate | 15 to 20 breaths/min |
| inspiratory time | 1 second (avoid auto-PEEP) |
| flow rate | more than 60 L/min |
| flow waveform | descending or constant |
| PEEP | 0 to 5 cm H_2O (use PEEP to avoid severe hypoxemia and measure ICP) |
| F_IO_2 | 1.0 initially, titrate PaO_2 to between 70 and 100 mm Hg |

63. The open lung approach uses PEEP levels equal to or exceeding the inflection point on a pressure-volume curve. This helps prevent opening and closing of small airways and alveoli, which may cause shear stress.

64. | Parameter | Preferred Setting or Range |
|---|---|
| V_T | 4 to 8 mL/kg (while maintaining $P_{plateau}$ 30 cm H_2O or less) |
| respiratory rate | 15 to 25 breaths/min |
| inspiratory time | less than 1 second |
| flow rate | more than 60 L/min |
| flow waveform | descending |
| PEEP | high levels more than 15 cm H_2O |
| F_IO_2 | less than 0.5 to 0.6 |

65. pH = 7.20 to 7.40; $PaCO_2$ = 40 to 80 mm Hg; PaO_2 = 60 to 100 mm Hg

66. Sepsis; aspiration of gastric contents; thoracic and nonthoracic trauma; drug overdose; massive blood transfusions; fat emboli; smoke or chemical inhalation injury; burns; pancreatitis; near-drowning; interstitial viral pneumonitis; disseminated intravascular coagulation; oxygen toxicity; prolonged cardiopulmonary bypass

67. PaO_2/F_IO_2 200 or less

68. Diffuse alveolar infiltrates

69. Shunt more than 20%; C_L less than 30 mL/cm H_2O; PCWP less than 15 to 18 mm Hg

70. Acute myocardial infarction; hypertension; rapid heart rates with inadequate filling time; valvular heart disease; fluid overload

71.

Parameter	Preferred Setting or Range
V_T	8 to 10 mL/kg
Respiratory ate	10 or more breaths/min
Inspiratory time	1 to 1.5 seconds
Flow rate	60 L/min or more
Flow waveform	descending or constant
PEEP	5 to 10 cm H_2O
F_IO_2	start at 1.0, then titrate to SpO_2 more than 90% to 92%

Answers to Critical Thinking Questions

1. A deep breath or a sigh is a part of the normal breathing pattern and usually occurs in nonintubated individuals every 6 minutes. A ventilator sigh is usually set at 1.5 to 2 times the V_T set. Sighs are beneficial before and after suctioning of intubated patients and also before and after bronchoscopy. Sighs, however, may cause overdistention when used with larger V_T levels and with CPAP. Recently sighs have become part of lung recruitment strategies during the ventilation of patients with ARDS.

2. On arrival at the emergency department a patient would most likely present with tachycardia and hypertension. The patient would be using accessory muscles during inspiration and possibly expiration. Increased resonance on percussion, bilateral inspiratory and expiratory wheezes, and prolonged expiration would be present. ABGs at that time would show acute alveolar hyperventilation with hypoxemia. If the patient is unresponsive to aggressive bronchodilator therapy and corticosteroids the episode may progress and the ABGs would reveal a $PaCO_2$ of 40 mm Hg or higher and a normal to acidotic pH. Hypoxemia would be moderate to severe with supplemental oxygen. At this point the patient would be exhausted, breath sounds and chest movement would become decreased, and life-threatening arrhythmias may occur. The patient should be intubated before respiratory arrest.

3. PAV may not be appropriate for use in patients with COPD because PSV is flow cycled at set percentages of the patient's inspiratory flow rate. This can lead to longer inspirations than the patient can tolerate. Patients with COPD need to have shortened inspiratory times to allow for longer expiratory times. The patient's active breathing pattern may increase WOB, cause dyssynchrony with the ventilator, and auto-PEEP. PSV may be used in patients with COPD if the ventilator allows for adjustments in the expiratory flow cycle percentage. Higher flow cycle percentages will begin expiration earlier, allowing enough time to exhale all the volume.

4. For flow triggering to work a constant flow of gas must be maintained within the ventilator circuit. This means that the exhalation valve must remain open during this time. The ventilator's computer compares the flow readings from sensors located before the inspiratory limb and after the expiratory limb. When the patient inspires, a portion of the gas from the continuous flow is inhaled. When the amount of gas inhaled by the patient reaches the flow trigger setting, the ventilator will begin inspiration. Therefore, as the breath begins, the patient pulls from the constant flow first and the exhalation valve does not close until the flow trigger threshold is reached.

5. A patient with increased airway resistance requires more time for exhalation. Inadequate expiratory time in these patients leads to air trapping and auto-PEEP.

Answers to Case Studies
Case Study #1

1. Noninvasive mask CPAP would be appropriate at this time. It may improve oxygenation, reduce the $PaCO_2$, reduce the WOB, and reduce myocardial work. This would allow time for pharmacological treatment to become effective.

2. The most appropriate mode would be either VC-CMV or PC-CMV. This patient's BSA is 2.42 m^2, giving him a minute ventilation of 9.7 L/min. The patient's IBW is 84 kg. The guideline for ventilation of patients with CHF recommends a moderate V_T of 8 to 10 mL/kg IBW. This puts the patient's V_T in the range of 672 to 840 mL. The use of 9 mL/kg makes the V_T 760 mL; 9.7 L/min/760 mL = 12.8 breaths/min.

Case Study #2

1. The patient has hypercapnic respiratory failure. This is most likely because of the closed head injury.

2. The patient has acute respiratory acidosis.

3. PC-CMV or VC-CMV would be most appropriate.

4. BSA for this patient is 1.94 m^2, making her minute ventilation 6.8 L/min. The V_T range for closed-head injury is 8 to 12 mL/kg IBW. The patient's IBW is 66 kg. By using 10 mL/kg, the V_T should be 660 mL and the rate would be 10.3 breaths/min. To keep T_I at 1 second, the flow rate needs to be set at 41 L/min. PEEP needs to be kept to a minimum because of the potential to increase ICP.

Case Study #3

1. The ABG results show that the patient is tiring. Acute asthma episodes cause the patient to hyperventilate at first. This will continue until either the episode clears or the patient becomes tired. As the patient tires the $PaCO_2$ rises back to the normal range. Meanwhile, the patient will become hypoxemic. This patient demonstrates acute respiratory acidosis with moderate hypoxemia (the low pH is too low to be caused by the $PaCO_2$; it is most likely caused by lactic acidosis).

2. This patient does require intubation. The patient has already been receiving continuous nebulization of a bronchodilator and oxygen therapy. Despite this she demonstrates fatigue and impending respiratory failure.

3. Full ventilatory support with either VC-CMV or PC-CMV. Pressure may be easier to keep under control with PC-CMV.

4. Keep set PIP less than 30 cmH$_2$O, target V_T at 4 to 8 mL/kg IBW (244 mL to 488 mL) at a rate less than 8 breaths/min, T_I less than 1 second, descending ramp, and only use PEEP to offset auto-PEEP.

5. Patients with increased airway resistance require more than normal time for exhalation. Without this extra time, air trapping (auto-PEEP) will occur. This will increase the patient's WOB and cause dyssynchrony with the ventilator. Auto-PEEP can be a lethal complication.

Answers to NBRC-Style Questions

1. a	5. a	9. b
2. c	6. b	10. a
3. c	7. c	
4. a	8. b	

Chapter 9, Initial Assessment of the Mechanically Ventilated Patient
Answers to Key Terms Crossword Puzzle

Answers to Review Questions

1. Patient's color, respiratory rate, breathing pattern, use of accessory muscles, chest movement, audible breath sounds, WOB, level of consciousness, observation of monitor displays

2. on a regular basis, the ventilator flow sheet

3. an operational verification procedure

4. Before obtaining an ABG; when obtaining a new physician's order; before obtaining hemodynamic or pulmonary function data; when a change in ventilator settings has been made; because of an acute change in the patient's condition; when ventilator performance is questionable

5. 24 hours, continuously

6. −0.1 to −2.0 cm H_2O

7. auto-triggering (too sensitive), increased patient WOB (too insensitive)

8. Air trapping, which results in artificial PEEP

9. Decrease the V_T, decrease the frequency, increase inspiratory flow rate (all of which will increase expiratory time), suction, add mechanical PEEP

10. When the C_T and PIP are known, the volume lost in the circuit is calculated by multiplying the PIP by the compliance factor: 3.25 mL/cm H_2O × 48 cm H_2O = 156 mL.

11. the amount of gas that participates in gas exchange, $VA = V_T − V_{Danat} − V_{Dmech}$

12. An HME would add mechanical dead space, therefore decreasing VA.

13. $VA = V_T − V_{Danat} − V_{Dmech}$ 775 mL − 160 mL − 85 mL = 530 mL

14. Anatomic dead space; mechanical dead space; added mechanical dead space

15. a decrease, an increase

16. An inspiratory pause or hold

17. When a patient is making active respiratory efforts, has a high frequency, or is resisting inspiratory time extension

18. dynamic, static

19. the amount of pressure required to overcome airway resistance, $P_{TA} = PIP - P_{plateau}$

20. an increase in airway resistance

21. The patient requires suctioning or is biting on the tube, the tube is kinked, bronchospasm, or the HME is plugged with moisture or secretions

22. mP_{aw} parallels mean P_A, is important to tissue oxygenation, and affects lung volumes and cardiac output.

23. 10, terminate inspiration

24. Patient coughing, an increase in airway resistance (bronchospasm or the patient requires suctioning), a decrease in compliance (pulmonary edema, pneumonia, pleural effusion), or the patient biting down on the tube

25. 5 to 10, a significant drop in pressure

26. Patient disconnection from the ventilator, leaks around the humidifier or water traps, loose tubing connections

27. manually ventilated

28. The PIP and exhaled volume will be lower than previous. When observing the volume-time waveform, the delivered V_T is larger than the expired V_T.

29. First, listen over the trachea to establish that the cuff is maintaining an adequate seal. Check the circuit by occluding the Y-connector and cycling the ventilator. If the high pressure is not reached, a significant leak is present. Pinch closed the main inspiratory tubing on the distal side of the humidifier. If the peak pressure alarm sounds, no leak is present in the humidifier system between your hand and the ventilator. If the alarm does not sound, the leak is either in the humidifier assembly or where the circuit attaches to the ventilator or humidifier. Tubing connections and water traps should also be checked.

30. The ventilator would stay in inspiration and prevent flow cycling.

31. Severe hypoxemia or hypercapnia, myocardial infarction, hypoxia, drug reactions, anxiety, pain, or elevated temperature

32. Infection, tissue necrosis, late-stage carcinomatosis, Hodgkin's disease, leukemia, and hypothyroidism

33. Metabolic diseases, CNS disorders, drugs (phenothiazines, tricyclic antidepressants, benzodiazepines), and other substances such as alcohol, heroin, and carbon dioxide

34. right arterial pressure, right ventricular end diastolic pressure, and right heart function

35. Critically ill patients who have severe cardiopulmonary complications or problems with fluid management

36. Raw = $(PIP - P_{plateau})$/flow; therefore Raw = $(48 - 30)$/40 Raw = $18/40 = 0.45$ cm H_2O/L/sec

37. 25 mm Hg, tracheal damage, necrosis

38. Hypotensive patients

39. Maintain MLT; establish MLT for which only 50 to 100 mL of V_T is lost; the cuff should require no more than 5 mL for inflation; if a minimal leak cannot be maintained with a cuff volume less than 5 mL, ensure that cuff pressure is less than 25 cm H_2O. If steps 1 to 4 cannot be achieved, patients should be monitored for the presence of tracheal stenosis for at least 1 year after discharge.

40. The cuff and artificial airway have moved up in the patient's airway and reside in the larynx or pharynx, or the ET may be too small for the patient, requiring a large volume to maintain a seal.

41. stopcock, off position, clamp

42. By positioning a three-way stopcock between a blunt-tipped needle inserted into the cut pilot balloon and a syringe, the cuff can be inflated and kept inflated.

43. To avoid pressure injuries to the gums, mouth, or lips from the constant pressure of the tube

44. Air trapping, pulmonary edema, atelectasis, consolidation, pneumonia, pneumothorax, hemothorax, and pleural effusion

45. 70 to 100 mL/cm H_2O

46. V_T will decrease

47. $C_S = V_T/(P_{plateau} - EEP)$

48. decreases, increases

49. $C_D = Volume/P_{Peak}$

50. Peak pressures would increase, but no change in the delivered V_T would occur.

51. 740 mL/(44 cm H_2O − 8 cm H_2O) = 740/36 = 0.02 L/cm H_2O

52. (58 cm H_2O − 51 cm H_2O)/0.5 L/sec = 7 cm H_2O/0.5 L/sec = 14 cm H_2O/L/sec

Answers to Critical Thinking Questions

1. The sensitivity may be set too high. The patient cannot generate the negative inspiratory effort necessary to trigger the ventilator. The sensitivity needs to be adjusted so the patient can trigger a breath with minimal effort. If the sensitivity is set correctly, auto-PEEP is present. The patient is unable to "draw through" the positive pressure in the airway and therefore unable to trigger a breath. If adjustments to increase expiratory time (decrease frequency or V_T, increasing inspiratory flow rate) do not alleviate the problem, the addition of mechanical PEEP may help.

2. The ET is too small for a person of this size. The cuff pressure of 40 cm H_2O needed to maintain a seal will cause tracheal damage. The patient needs to be extubated and a larger size tube inserted.

3. When a set inspiratory pressure is delivered to the airway, V_T depends on lung mechanics. ARDS results in a decrease in C_S. In this case, an inspiratory pressure of 30 cm H_2O delivered V_T between 400 and 450 mL. As the disease process resolves, the elastic recoil of the lung improves. The same delivered pressure resulted in an increased V_T.

4. 43 cm H_2O – 18 cm H_2O – 25 cm H_2O

Answers to Case Studies

Case Study #1

1. Approximately 32 cm H_2O and 42 cm H_2O, 10 cm H_2O above and below the PIP

2. 100 mL below the set V_T

3. Use the inspiratory control with a setting of approximately 0.5 to 1.5 seconds

4. Minimal airway resistance is present

Case Study #2

1. The patient may be biting on the ET, coughing, or not in sync with delivered breaths.

2. When the high-pressure limit is reached, inspiration is prematurely terminated. If the high pressure is constantly activated, the low V_T and low minute volume alarm thresholds will be reached, thus activating both alarms.

3. The patient may be agitated and confused because of pain, and giving a sedative may be appropriate. Agitation and confusion can also be caused by hypoxia, so checking the oxygen saturation and ABGs may also be indicated. Assessment of breath sounds and vital signs is also appropriate to rule out any other undetected problem.

Answers to NBRC-Style Questions

1. c
2. c
3. c
4. b
5. a
6. d
7. c
8. d
9. c
10. d

Chapter 10, Ventilator Graphics

Answers to Key Terms Crossword Puzzle

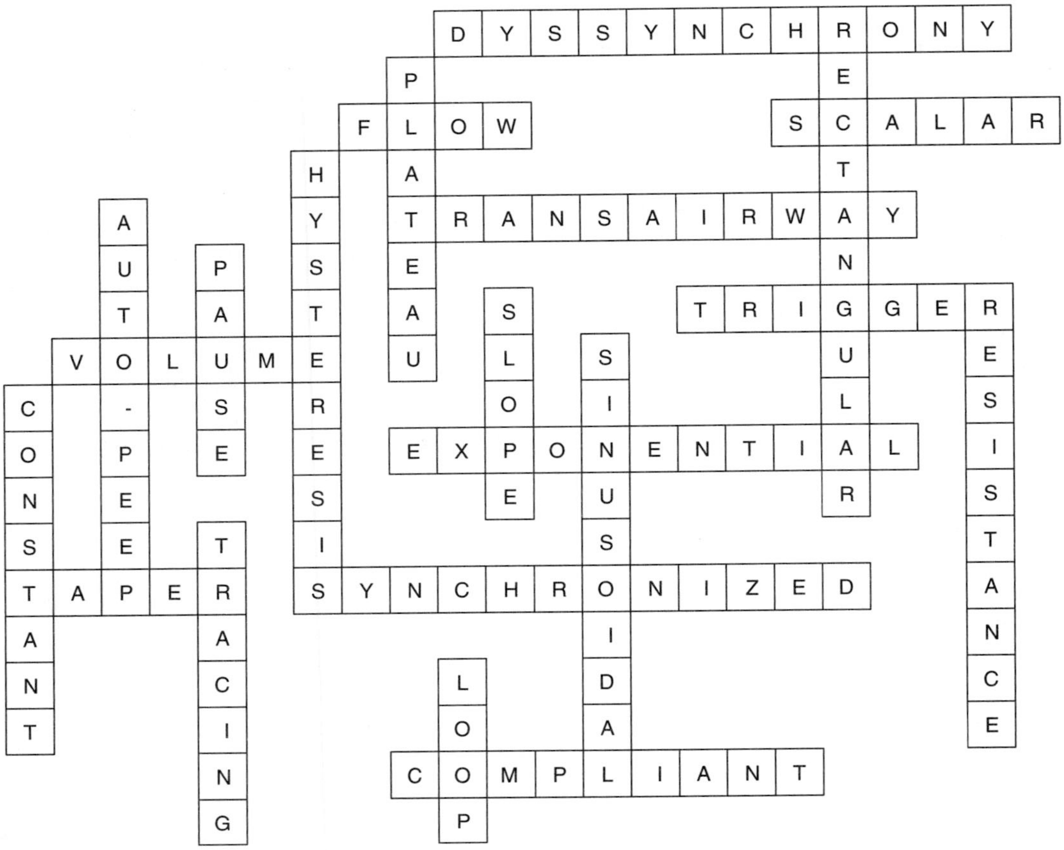
DYSSYNCHRONY
FLOW
SCALAR
TRANSAIRWAY
TRIGGER
VOLUME
EXPONENTIAL
TAPER
SYNCHRONIZED
COMPLIANT
PLATEAU
HYSTERESIS
AUTO-PEEP
PAUSE
RECTANGULAR
SLOPE
SINUSOIDAL
RESISTANCE
CONSTANT
TRACING
LOOP

Answers to Review Questions

1. A. rectangular; B. ascending or accelerating ramp; C. exponential rise; D. descending or decelerating ramp; E. sinusoidal or sine; F. exponential decay
2. Data are obtained from the flow and pressure monitors on the inspiratory side of the ventilator just before where the gas exits the ventilator to go to the patient and from the flow and pressure monitors on the expiratory side of the ventilator just as the gas goes back to the ventilator through the exhalation valve.
3. The ventilator will use the $V = \text{flow} \times T_I$ formula to calculate volume.
4. Gas flow and inspiratory time
5. decrease (or drop), increase (or rise)
6. $P_{TA} + P_A$
7. When the flow is constant
8. T_I = volume/flow. Given that flow of 60 L/min = 60 L/60 sec = 1 L/sec and a volume of 600 mL = 0.6 L, then T_I = 0.6 L/1 L/sec = 0.6 second.
9. $P_A = \Delta V/C_S$ = 800 mL/(25 mL/cm H_2O) = 32 cm H_2O
10. A. inspiration begins; B. inspiration ends; C. maximum or peak expiratory flow
11. Sinusoidal
12. 45 L/min
13. 40 L/min
14. 1 second
15. Air trapping or auto-PEEP
16. An auto-PEEP measurement would not be valid if the patient was actively attempting to take a breath during the maneuver. (An unstable expiratory pause invalidates the measurement.)
17. Auto-PEEP is measured at the end of exhalation.
18. Active inspiration by the patient in a ventilator that responds to patient flow demand
19. 1 to 2 cm H_2O
20. Sensitivity (pressure trigger) and flow settings

21. Changing the flow pattern during volume ventilation will change the pressure patterns.

22. 45 cm H_2O

23. Descending or decelerating ramp, 40 L/min

24. 600 mL

25. $C_S = \Delta V/(P_{plateau} - PEEP) = 600$ mL$/(20 - 0) = 30$ mL/cm H_2O

26. Raw $= (PIP - P_{plateau})/flow = (45 - 20)/0.67$ L/sec $= 37.3$ cm H_2O/L/sec (convert 40 L/min to L/sec)

27. Auto-PEEP is not present.

28. The flow rate drops to zero before the end of inspiration because an inspiratory pause occurs where there is no flow. After the inspiratory pause the gas is exhaled, giving the negative appearance on the graph.

29. During decreases in lung compliance the delivered V_T will decrease in PC-CMV.

30. Flow returns to zero when P_A becomes equal to the set pressure during PC-CMV.

31. Descending ramp or exponential decay, which will vary with the patient's lung characteristics

32. The largest pressure gradient occurs at the beginning of inspiration.

33. Pressure, sensitivity, rise time or slope, and flow-cycle time

34. VC-SIMV (no pressure support). Look closely at the pressure waveform. It has a peak as opposed to a flat top, and the two mechanical breaths do not have the same PIP. This means that the pressure is variable. In volume control the volume is set and the pressure is determined by lung characteristics.

35. PC-SIMV with CPAP and pressure support.

36. **A** is a pressure supported breath with a set pressure of 20 cm H_2O. **B** is a pressure-controlled breath with a set pressure of 38 cm H_2O.

37. During inspiration ATC augments flow. During expiration it provides a slightly negative pressure gradient between the lungs and the upper airways.

38. Peak flow rate × Flow cycling percentage = Flow rate when cycling occurs: 45 L/min × 0.25 = 11 L/min

39. $T_I = 1$ second

40. 45 L/min

41. 10 L/min

42. (Ending flow/Peak inspiratory flow) × 100 = Flow-cycling percentage; therefore (10/45) ×100 = 22%.

43. 40 L/min

44. Patients with COPD have increased airway resistance and therefore need a long expiratory time to exhale. (During normal inspiration flow drops toward the end of inspiration. Percent flow cycling sets up a criterion to determine when inspiration will end for a pressure supported breath. So when inspiratory flow tapers down to that set percentage of the peak inspiratory flow, inspiration will end. Patients with increased airway resistance will require longer times for exhalation. A higher flow cycle percentage will end the inspiration sooner than a lower flow cycle percentage, giving the patient more time for exhalation.)

45. A patient with reduced compliance will fill the lungs quickly but with less volume than normal. To allow more volume to enter the lungs for the given pressure, a lower flow cycle percentage should be set.

46. (18 L/min ÷ 40 L/min) × 100 = 45%

47. 200 mL

48. (5 L/min ÷ 38 L/min) × 100 = 13%

49. 400 mL

50. A. T_I = approximately 0.75 second; B. T_I = approximately 1.25 seconds

51. The flow cycle percentage was lowered, increasing the inspiratory time.

52. A. PEEP +5 cm H_2O; B. peak P_A; C. PIP

53. 35 cm H_2O

54. 500 mL

55. There is +5 cm H_2O PEEP.

56. More pressure is needed to deliver the set volume, so the height of the loop (volume) remains the same but it extends farther to the right and tends to flatten out.

57. Because the pressure remains constant the loop will reach the same pressure but will be shorter because less volume is being delivered to the patient for each breath.

58. Airway resistance increases because of bronchospasm, secretions in the airway, or mucosal edema.

59. Loop A represents a spontaneous breath.

60. Loop A has a clockwise direction because a spontaneous breath is negative on inspiration and becomes positive on exhalation.

61. Loop B represents a patient-triggered mandatory breath.

62. Loop B has a counterclockwise direction because after the initial negative deflection caused by the patient, the ventilator delivers the positive pressure breath (does all the work).

63. 45 L/min = 0.75 L/sec, Raw = P_{TA}/flow; 3 cm H_2O ÷ 0.75 L/sec = 4 cm H_2O/L/sec

64. hysteresis

65. This loop moves in a clockwise direction.

66. Constant flow or rectangular waveform

67. 50 L/min, 55 L/min

68. 425 mL

69. Either a leak in the patient (bronchopleural fistula) or a leak in the patient circuit

70. Air trapping or the presence of auto-PEEP

Answers to Critical Thinking Questions

1. VC-CMV (Constant flow waveforms are associated with volume control. The pressure curves all have peaks, meaning that the pressure is not being maintained.)

2. The patient is not assisting. (No downward deflections below baseline are present on the pressure scalar.)

3. Total cycle time = 1.5 seconds, T_I = 1 second, T_E = 0.5 seconds, set rate = 40 breaths/min

4. The PIP is increasing with each breath.

5. The exhaled volume is decreasing with every breath; inspiration is beginning before all the volume is exhaled.

6. Each breath begins before exhalation is completed. Exhalation should return to zero on the x axis before the beginning of the next breath.

7. Rising PIP, dropping exhaled V_T, inspiration beginning before the completion of exhalation, and an inverse I:E ratio mean air is being trapped in the lungs. In this case it is caused by the rapid set rate.

8. Decrease the set rate to allow for adequate expiratory time.

Answers to Case Studies

Case Study #1

1. This loop is wider because of the increased airway resistance associated with COPD. The axis of the loop is more upright, which is a result of an increase in static compliance in the patient's lungs.

2. Yes, the patient is triggering the ventilator. The small loop to the left of the volume axis on the pressure scale represents patient effort to trigger the ventilator.

3. Approximately 650 mL

4. Approximately 23 cm H_2O

5. The patient has a combined alkalosis from acute alveolar hyperventilation superimposed on chronic hypercapneic respiratory failure. The current V_T setting is 12 mL/kg. This is too high and should be reduced to deliver 8 mL/kg, which would give a volume of 435 mL.

Case Study #2

1. Spontaneous breath

2. inspiration

3. expiration

4. Clockwise

5. There is no set pressure support. If pressure support were present, the loop would be shifted to the positive side of the x axis.

6. VC-CMV (or the mechanical breath during VC-SIMV). A pressure-controlled breath would have a flatter top.

7. Yes, the patient is triggering the breath. A negative deflection is present along the x axis, or pressure axis.

8. Adjust the ventilator sensitivity to be more sensitive to the patient.

9. The type of flow waveform (constant), the peak inspiratory flow (50 L/min), the peak expiratory flow (50 L/min), and the V_T (650 mL)

10. The current loop has a scooped-out appearance on the flow side.

11. This is caused by increased airway resistance. The most likely cause in this case is bronchospasm or increased airway secretions.

12. Aerosolized bronchodilator and tracheobronchial suctioning

Answers to NBRC-Style Questions

1. a	5. c	9. d
2. c	6. b	10. b
3. c	7. a	
4. b	8. c	

Chapter 11, Noninvasive Assessment of Respiratory Function
Answers to Key Terms Crossword Puzzle

Crossword answers include: OCCLUSION, SIDESTREAM, ANATOMIC, RESISTANCE, PLATEAU, PULSEOXIMETRY, COLORIMETRIC, SPECTROPHOTOMETRY, FUNCTIONAL, BILIRUBIN

Answers to Review Questions

1. Pulse oximetry; capnography; transcutaneous monitoring of blood gases; indirect calorimetry; bedside lung function testing

2. Apnea; airway obstruction; equipment failure or disconnection; incorrect gas flow settings.

3. Over a finger, an ear lobe, the forehead, and the bridge of the nose.

4. Spectrophotometry, optical plethysmography

5. The Beer-Lambert law states that the concentration of light-absorbing material in a sample is a logarithmic function of the amount of light absorbed by the sample.

6. A pulse oximeter will shine two wavelengths of light (660 and 940 nm) through the sample site. At a wavelength of 660 nm (red light) deoxygenated hemoglobin absorbs more light than oxyhemoglobin. Conversely, at 940 nm (infrared light) oxyhemoglobin absorbs more light than does deoxyhemoglobin.

7. Because blood volume changes during ventricular systole and diastole, these cyclical changes in volume can be related to light transmission. As local blood volume increases during systole, light absorbancy increases and transmitted light decreases. In contrast, during ventricular diastole blood volume and absorbancy decrease and transmitted light increases.

8. Accuracy ultimately depends on the device's calibration.

9. The minimum saturation at which a pulse oximeter is accurate is 80%.

10. Low perfusion states; the presence of dysfunctional hemoglobin and dyes; variations in patients' skin pigmentation; ambient light interference

11. Administration of peripheral vasoconstrictors; hypothermia; heart-lung bypass.

12. Deoxygenated hemoglobin; oxyhemoglobin; carboxyhemoglobin; methemoglobin

13. Fractional hemoglobin saturation is the percentage of oxyhemoglobin compared with all four types of hemoglobin. The functional hemoglobin saturation compares oxyhemoglobin with only the total amount of hemoglobin capable of carrying oxygen (oxyhemoglobin and deoxygenated hemoglobin).

14. overestimated (or erroneously high)

15. Benzocaine and dapsone

16. When methemoglobin is present, the SpO_2 will either be overestimated or underestimated depending on whether the actual SaO_2 is less than or greater than 85%.

17. Nail polish may affect pulse oximetry values by causing the shunting of light around the finger periphery. This is known as optical shunting.

18. Dark skin pigmentation can lead to an erroneously high SpO_2.

19. Disparities will be determined by running arterial blood through a CO-oximeter.

20. capnogram

21. A colorimetric detector is useful to detect the presence of an ET in the lungs. If the ET is in the stomach, no exhaled carbon dioxide will be detected.

22. The presence of other gases during CO_2 measurements will cause pressure broadening and therefore erroneously high CO_2 readings.

23. One method of sampling is known as *sidestream*. With this method gas from the airway is extracted through a narrow plastic tube to the sample measuring chamber, which is located in a separate console. The other is known as *mainstream*. With this method the sampling chamber attaches directly to the ET and analysis is performed at the airway.

24. 4.5% to 5.5%

25. A. *Phase 1:* initial exhaled gas from conducting airways which is low in CO_2; B. *phase 2:* exhalation with CO_2 from alveoli mixing with gas from airways; C. *phase 3:* alveolar plateau contains CO_2 from the alveoli; D. end-tidal PCO_2 or $PetCO_2$, which is influenced by CO_2 production and the effectiveness of ventilation; E. *phase 4:* inspiration showing the concentration of CO_2 falling to zero

26. Metabolic rate determines CO_2 production. An increased metabolic rate will increase CO_2 production, and a decreased metabolic rate will decrease CO_2 production.

27. Factors that increase metabolic rate include fever, sepsis, hyperthyroidism, and seizures. Factors that decrease metabolic rate include hypothermia, starvation, and sedation.

28. Normally the $P_{ET}CO_2$ is 4 to 6 mm Hg lower than the $PaCO_2$.

29. Elevated $P_{ET}CO_2$ from decreased ventilation relative to perfusion can be caused by respiratory center depression, muscular paralysis, and COPD.

30. The lowest $P_{ET}CO_2$ would be found in the anatomical dead space.

31. Decreased $P_{ET}CO_2$ from decreased perfusion relative to ventilation can be caused by pulmonary embolism, excessive PEEP (added or intrinsic), or any disorder in which pulmonary hypoperfusion is present.

32. Increases in dead space ventilation; hyperventilation; hypoventilation; apnea or periodic breathing; inadequate neuromuscular blockade in pharmacologically paralyzed patients; the presence of CO_2 rebreathing

33. A. A normal capnogram waveform; B. low $P_{ET}CO_2$ because of hyperventilation with a low $PaCO_2$; C. elevated $P_{ET}CO_2$ because of hypoventilation with an elevated $PaCO_2$

34. Low perfusion of the lungs is associated with low $P_{ET}CO_2$ and should not be confused with esophageal intubation.

35. Gastric PCO_2 may be increased after mouth-to-mouth breathing or if the patient recently ingested a carbonated beverage. This could give false-positive colorimetric readings after intubation.

36. maximum expired PCO_2

37. 4 to 6 mm Hg

38. The x axis is exhaled V_T and the y axis is exhaled CO_2.

39. A. Phase 1 is the part of the tracing that represents the gas exhaled from the anatomical dead space. No CO_2 is present in this gas. B. Phase 2 is the transition between dead space from the airways and alveolar gas. A rapid rise is present in this part of the curve. C. Phase 3 represents the gas exhaled from the alveoli. It slopes slightly upwards because alveoli empty at different rates because of anatomy and time constants.

40.

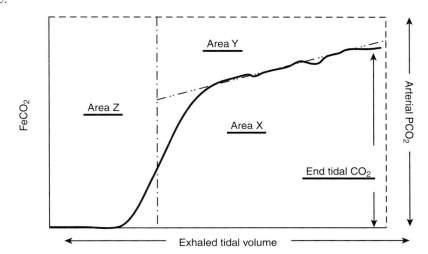

41. Area X represents the actual amount of CO_2 exhaled in a single breath, assuming that no exhaled air is rebreathed. Area Y represents the amount of CO_2 that is not eliminated because of alveolar dead space. Area Z represents the amount of CO_2 that was not eliminated because of anatomical dead space.

42. CO_2 production; circulation; diffusion; ventilation.

43. Trending $\dot{V}CO_2$ during a spontaneous breathing trial can help determine if the patient's increase in respiratory rate is caused by an increase in metabolic rate. An increased metabolic rate would increase the work the respiratory muscles would need to do. Trending the $\dot{V}CO_2$ could also pick up changes in dead space that will affect the patient's ability to wean.

44. Clark electrode

45. The transcutaneous oxygen monitor is heated to between 42° and 45° C to produce capillary vasodilation below the surface of the electrode. This improves the diffusion of gases across the skin because heat increases local blood flow at the site of the electrode.

46. Neonates

47. States of hypoperfusion, including (1) septic shock, (2) hemorrhage, and (3) heart failure, and states of increased vascular resistance, including (4) hypothermia, and (5) pharmacological responses.

48. Stowe-Severinghaus electrode

49. Heating the $PtcCO_2$ probe to 42° to 45° C increases the metabolic rate of the tissues at the site, causing the reading to be slightly higher than that of the $PaCO_2$.

50. Transcutaneous electrodes and the sensor's membrane should be changed weekly or when a signal drift is present during calibration.

51. Before placing the electrode, the skin should be cleansed with an alcohol swab and shaved when hair is present. When attaching the electrode to the patient, place a drop of electrolyte gel or deionized water on the electrode surface to enhance gas diffusion between the skin and the electrode.

52. room air (PO_2 approximately 150 mm Hg), electronic zero

53. 5% CO_2 calibration gas, 10% CO_2 calibration gas

54. Documentation of transcutaneous monitoring should include date and time of measurement, patient's activity level and body position, the site of electrode placement, the electrode temperature, F_IO_2 and type of equipment, assessment of peripheral perfusion (e.g., skin temperature, pallor, capillary refill), and the invasive ABG results when available.

55. A sensor should be repositioned every 4 to 6 hours and more often for a neonate.

56. Open-circuit gas exchange monitor, often referred to as a metabolic cart

57. The major components of indirect calorimetry include oxygen analyzer (polarographic or zirconium oxide); carbon dioxide analyzer (nondispersive, infrared analyzer); flow sensor to measure volume and flow (pneumotachometer, turbine flow meter, or ultrasonic vortex flow meter); and temperature-sensitive integrated circuit transducers to measure barometric pressure and expired gas temperature.

58. The patient should be at rest and in a supine position for at least 30 minutes before making the measurement.

59. $20°$ C, $25°$ C

60. UN is necessary because it is one of the end products of protein metabolism. The number of grams of nitrogen excreted in the urine is directly related to the amount of protein used by the individual.

61. 1500 to 3000 kcal/day, or approximately 30 to 40 kcal/hr/m^2

62. greater than 120%, less than 80%

63. Hypermetabolic states are caused by pancreatitis, hyperthyroidism, pregnancy, stimulants, hyperthermia, seizures, and burns. Hypometabolic states are caused by starvation, hypothyroidism, anesthesia, sedation, and hypothermia.

64. 0.8 to 0.85

65. 1.0, 0.7

66. The RQ will increase.

67. If a mechanically ventilated patient is only being given IV glucose the patient's RQ will be close to 1, meaning that the patient's CO_2 production is elevated. With a limited ventilatory reserve, a patient being weaned will most likely not be able to handle the increased CO_2 load. This type of failure to wean can be avoided by switching the diet to one that has a higher fat-to-carbohydrate ratio.

68. electromechanical transducers

69. PIP and static or plateau pressure

70. Add an inspiratory hold or plateau of 1 to 2 seconds to allow for pressure equilibrium to occur across the airway.

71. Factors that influence plateau pressure include V_T, lung and thoracic compliance, circuit elastance, and the total measured PEEP.

72. Vortex ultrasonic flowmeters, variable orifice pneumotachometers, and turbine flowmeters

73. A variable orifice pneumotachometer can measure bidirectional flow.

74. Bronchospasm, increased mucus, mucus plugging, clogged HME, and water in ventilator tubing

75. $\bar{P}aw = [1/2(PIP - PEEP)\,(T_I/TCT)] + PEEP$

76. $= [1/2(30 - 5)(1\ sec/5\ sec)] + 5 = [(1/2)(25)(1/5)] + 5 = 7.5\ cm\ H_2O$

77. $C_D = V_T - [(PIP - PEEP) \times C_T]/(PIP - PEEP)$
    $= 550\ mL - [(30 - 5) \times 2.5]/(30 - 5)$
    $= [550 - (25 \times 2.5)]/25$
    $= (550 - 62.5)/25$
    $= 487.5/25 = 19.5\ mL/cm\ H_2O$

78. $C_S = \dot{V}_T - [(P_{plateau} - PEEP) \times C_T]/(P_{plateau} - PEEP)$
    $= 400\ mL - [(28 - 10) \times 2]/(28 - 10)$
    $= (400 - 36)/(28 - 10)$
    $= 364/18 = 20.2\ cm\ H_2O$

79. $Raw = (PIP - P_{plateau})/$flow rate (L/sec); 50 L/min = 50 L/60 sec = 0.83 L/sec
    $= (35 - 25)/0.83$ L/sec
    $= 10\ cm\ H_2O \div 0.83$ L/sec
    $= 12\ cm\ H_2O/L/sec$

80. intrinsic work

81. ET; machine sensitivity; demand valve systems; humidifying device; the patient circuit

82. $W = (PIP - 0.5 \times P_{plateau})/100 \times V_T$

83. An increase in airway resistance, such as what happens during bronchospasm, will make inhalation and exhalation more difficult for a patient. This will increase the amount of work a patient must maintain to breathe.

84. A decrease in C_S implies that the $P_{plateau}$ has increased. Increases in $P_{plateau}$ occur when more pressure is needed to overcome elastance. The patient's WOB must increase to accommodate this change. (Note that increases in $P_{plateau}$ will result in higher PIP as well.) Mathematically, this will increase the numerator of the WOB formula, thereby increasing the calculated WOB.

85. Pulmonary interstitial fibrosis; pleural effusion; hyperinflation; consolidation; respiratory distress syndrome; pulmonary vascular engorgement

86. Congestive heart failure is associated with a decrease in both static and dynamic compliance.

87. Increases in airway resistance may be caused by retention of secretions, peribronchiolar edema, bronchoconstriction, and dynamic compression of the airways.

88. Transdiaphragmatic pressure is a measure of the forcefulness of diaphragmatic contractions obtained by simultaneously measuring gastric and esophageal pressures during the respiratory cycle. The electronic difference between these two pressures is the transdiaphragmatic pressure.

89. The pressure-time product is a graph of the transdiaphragmatic pressure plotted over time.

90. Occlusion pressure is the pressure measured by occluding the airway during the first 100 msec of a patient's spontaneous inspiration. It may be a useful index of ventilatory drive and may be used as a predictor of weaning success.

Answers to Critical Thinking Questions

1. COHb and MetHb are unable to carry oxygen but are actually part of fractional hemoglobin saturation. Pulse oximetry values include functional hemoglobin saturation, which is the percentage of oxygenated hemoglobin as a percentage of functional hemoglobin. This will cause SpO_2 values to appear normal when dysfunctional hemoglobins are elevated. Therefore, when dysfunctional hemoglobins are suspected, blood should be drawn for analyzing in a CO-oximeter.

2. The finger sensor may be misaligned by inserting the patient's finger too far into the probe. This is easily fixed by reapplying the finger probe correctly. There may be hypoperfusion to the site. Before applying the finger probe the RT should have performed a capillary refill test. If the test failed, another site should be chosen. The RT may try warming the finger by rubbing it for 20 to 30 seconds.

3. During cardiac arrest blood flow is not occurring. Therefore CO_2 is not being returned to the pulmonary system to be eliminated during exhalation. When using a colorimetric detector, this situation would produce a reading of less than 0.5% end-tidal CO_2. During decreased cardiac output, blood flow to the lungs is decreased and will also produce a low end-tidal CO_2 reading.

4. Use the Harris-Benedict equation for women to predict the patient's basal energy expenditure. $EE = 655.1 + (9.563 \times weight) + (1.85 \times height) - (4.676 \times age)$. The estimated EE for this patient $= 655.1 + (9.563 \times 170) + (1.85 \times 67) - (4.676 \times 48)$. $EE = 655.1 + 1625.71 + 123.95 - 224.45 = 2404.76 - 224.45 = 2180.31$ kcal. Because no urea nitrogen value is given, use the modified deWier equation to calculate resting energy expenditure for this patient. $EE = [(3.9 \times \dot{V}O_2) + (1.1 \times \dot{V}CO_2)] \times 1.44$. The actual energy expenditure for this patient $= [(3.9 \times 420) + (1.1 \times 380)] \times 1.44 = (1638 + 418) \times 1.44 = 2056 \times 1.44 = 2960.64$ kcal. The measured energy expenditure is greater than the predicted energy expenditure for this patient. $(2960.64 \div 2180.31) \times 100 = 135.79\%$ of predicted. This means that the patient is in a hypermetabolic state.

Answers to Case Studies

Case Study #1

1. The accuracy of the pulse oximeter should be questioned. Only pulse oximeter saturations greater than 80% are accurate.

2. An ABG analysis including CO-oximetry is appropriate at this time.

Case Study #2

1. The pulse oximeter is not accurate because it can only evaluate functional hemoglobin.

2. The ABG results for the oxygen saturation will not be accurate because it is a calculated value and does not take into account the COHb.

3. In this situation arterial blood must be analyzed with a CO-oximeter because it measures all four types of hemoglobin and will provide a measured SaO_2.

Case Study #3

1. The capnogram shows a rising $P_{ET}CO_2$. A represents the tracing over several minutes, whereas B shows only two breaths.

2. The gradual increase in the $P_{ET}CO_2$ may be caused by hypoventilation or increased CO_2 production.

3. The increased accessory muscle use along with the increasing respiratory rate and decreasing V_T show that the patient is unable to handle the newly imposed WOB. These clinical findings are reinforced by the $P_{ET}CO_2$ tracing, which is most likely caused by hypoventilation and increasing CO_2 production.

4. Pressure support should be added to decrease the extrinsic WOB.

Case Study #4

1. The patient's physiological dead space is likely increased. This would account for the increase in $P(a\text{-}et)CO_2$.

2. When physiological dead space is increased, the $SBCO_2$ curve will shift to the right. This means that less CO_2 is being eliminated (decreased $\dot{V}CO_2$) and more CO_2 is being retained in the blood (increased $PaCO_2$).

Answers to NBRC-Style Questions

1. d	6. c	11. d
2. c	7. d	12. c
3. b	8. a	13. c
4. c	9. a	14. a
5. c	10. c	15. c

Chapter 12, Hemodynamic Monitoring
Answers to Key Terms Crossword Puzzle

Crossword answers: RELAXATION, DIASTOLE, EJECTION FRACTION, STROKE INDEX, SVR, ISOVOLUMETRIC, PULSE PRESSURE, TRICUSPID, CONTRACTILITY, WHEATSTONE, STROKE WORK, ATRIAL KICK, BRADYCARDIA, V WAVE, MITRAL, Y DESCENT, RETROGRADE, PRELOAD, CENTRAL VENOUS, SWAN-GANZ, AFTERLOAD, RETROGRADE

Answers to Review Questions

1. systemic arterial pressure; central venous pressure; PAP; ABG; mixed venous blood gas; cardiac output

2. (90 beats/min)/60 seconds = 1.5 seconds

3. P wave

4. atrial systole

5. 20% to 40%

6. Atrial systole, ventricular isovolumetric contraction, rapid ventricular ejection, reduced ventricular ejection, ventricular isovolumetric relaxation, rapid ventricular filling, reduced ventricular filling (diastasis)

7. During atrial systole, the AV valves (tricuspid and mitral valves) are open and the aortic and pulmonic valves are closed.

8. Ventricular systole begins with isovolumetric contraction.

9. The first heart sound, S_1, is produced by the closure of the mitral and tricuspid valves at the beginning of ventricular systole.

10. The second heart sounds, S_2, are produced by the closure of the semilunar, aortic, and pulmonic valves.

11.

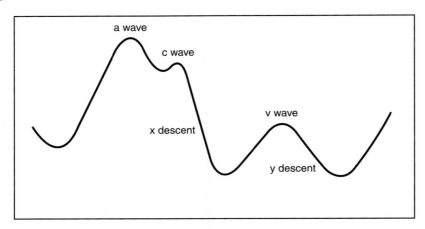

The *a wave* is caused by atrial contraction. The *c wave* is caused by the bulging of the AV valves back into the atrial chambers. The *x descent* is caused by atrial relaxation. The *v wave* is caused by the rise in atrial pressure before atrial systole. The *y descent* is caused by atrial emptying as blood enters the ventricle.

12. Heart rate; preload; contractility; afterload.

13. *Preload* is the filling pressure of the ventricle at the end of ventricular diastole.

14. Ventricular systole begins with isovolumetric contraction. During this period of contraction the left ventricular pressure increases from 0 to 80 mm Hg and the right ventricular pressure increases from 0 to 12 mm Hg. Rapid ejection of blood occurs when the left ventricular pressure exceeds the aortic diastolic pressure of approximately 80 mm Hg and the right ventricular pressure exceeds the diastolic PAP of 12 mm Hg. The peak systolic pressures of the ventricles are 120 mm Hg for the left and 25 mm Hg for the right.

15. RVEDP is estimated by RAP or CVP, and LVEDP is estimated by PAWP.

16. Systemic vascular resistance reflects the afterload of the left ventricle. PVR reflects the afterload of the right ventricle.

17. The major components of a hemodynamic monitoring system include pressure bag with flush solution, flush device, pressure tubing, transducer, cable and pressure monitor, and catheter with a heparinized solution of saline.

18. epistatic, zero-balance

19. Proper positioning of the transducer is important for accurate measurement. If the transducer is lower than the catheter tip, the monitor will read erroneously higher than the actual pressure. If the transducer is higher than the catheter tip, the monitor will read an erroneously low pressure reading.

20. Aseptically assemble, flush, and test tubing and catheter. Perform an Allen test to ensure an ulnar artery refill time of 5 to 10 seconds. Prep and drape the area of insertion by using sterile technique. Inject lidocaine around the insertion site. Percutaneously insert the catheter at an approximately 30-degree angle. Advance the catheter into the artery while holding the needle secure. Remove the needle and secure the catheter. Attach tubing for drip solution and observe monitor for proper waveform.

21. Problems with an arterial catheter line include infection at the site, clot formation, and distal extremity ischemia.

22. A bag of 0.9% NaCl containing 1 to 2 U of heparin per milliliter of normal saline at 2 to 3 mL/hr

23. The use of a surgical cutdown for insertion of the arterial line, cannulation for more than 4 days, and altered host defense all increase the risk of infection.

24. It can lead to overhydration.

25. CVP lines are used to administer fluids, drugs, and nutritional solutions and to monitor right heart pressures.

26. CVP measurement at the end of ventricular diastole can estimate the filling pressure or the preload of the right ventricle or RVEDP.

27. internal jugular, medial basilica, or lateral cephalic veins

28. CVP should be measured during exhalation with the patient in the supine position.

29. pneumothorax, hemothorax, vessel damage, infection, thrombosis, and bleeding

30. 2 to 6 mm Hg

31. Pediatric sizes are 4 and 5 Fr and are 60 cm long. Adult sizes are 7 and 8 Fr and 110 cm long. All are marked in 10-cm increments.

32. Clots are avoided in the PA catheter by having a pressurized flush solution running through the catheter at a rate of 1 to 5 mL/hr, except during pressure measurements.

33.

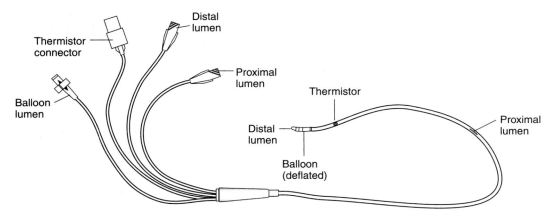

(From Hess DR, MacIntyre NR, Mishoe SC, et al: *Repiratory care: principles and practice,* Philadelphia, 2002, WB Saunders.)

34. Percutaneous sites: internal jugular, external jugular, and femoral; surgical cutdown sites: subclavian and antecubital vein

35. *Cardiac arrhythmias:* caused by irritation of a heart valve or the endocardium; *infection:* caused by nonsterile technique or irritation of the wound; *pneumothorax:* caused by air entering the pleural space during insertion; *air embolism:* caused by air entering a vessel during insertion or balloon rupture; *access vessel thrombosis or phlebitis:* caused by irritation of the vessel by the catheter or nonsterile technique; *PA rupture or perforation:* caused by overinflation of the balloon; *pulmonary infarction:* caused by overinflation of balloon, prolonged wedging, and clots formed in or near the catheter or the catheter advancement into a smaller artery; *catheter knotting:* caused by excessive catheter movement; *damped waveform:* caused by air or kinks in the line, clot in the system, catheter tip against the vessel wall, overwedging, or blood on the transducer; *catheter whip or fling:* caused by high cardiac output or abnormal vessel diameter

36. Fluoroscopy (in the catheterization laboratory) or pressure tracings (in the critical care setting)

37. Internal jugular vein to the superior vena cava where the balloon is inflated. The balloon then floats through the right atrium and right ventricle. It is advanced until it wedges in a small pulmonary artery in West's zone 3 of the lungs.

38. The PA catheter needs to be in zone 3 because this zone accurately reflects the pulmonary venous pressure. If the PA catheter is placed in zone 1 or 2 in the lung the balloon will collapse when inflated because the P_A exceeds the pulmonary venous pressure.

39.

Zone	Pressure Relation
1	$P_A > P_a > P_v$
2	$P_a > P_A > P_v$
3	$P_a > P_v > P_A$

40. 1.5 mL, 15 to 30

41. A. right atrium; B. right ventricle; C. pulmonary artery; D. pulmonary artery wedge

42. a. *Ventricular arrhythmias:* careful ECG monitoring during catheter placement; b. *pulmonary artery infarction:* prevent thrombus by using continuous flushed solution containing heparin and ensure balloon deflation after wedge pressure measurements; c. *pulmonary artery rupture:* ensure catheter balloon is deflated after wedge pressure measurements are made and inflate for only 15 to 30 seconds; d. *balloon rupture:* do not overinflate, maximum balloon volume in adult catheters is 1.5 mL

43. When heart rates are that rapid, a decrease in diastolic filling time occurs.

44. Diastolic pressure will increase.

45. SV, arterial compliance

46. PAP is read at the end of expiration.

47. PEEP or auto-PEEP at levels greater than 15 cm H_2O will produce erroneously high PAWP.

48. Pulmonary hypertension; pulmonary embolus; CHF

49. NO selectively dilates the pulmonary vasculature and decreases PVR and therefore PAP.

50. During spontaneous breathing the PAP falls on inspiration and rises during expiration. In contrast, during mechanical ventilation the PAP rises during inspiration and falls during expiration.

51.

Parameter	Normal Value
Arterial blood pressure	90 to 140/60 to 90 mm Hg
MAP	70 to 100 mm Hg
Pulse pressure	40 mm Hg
CVP	2 to 6 mm Hg
PAP	15 to 35/5 to 15 mm Hg
Mean PAP	10 to 20 mm Hg
PAWP	5 to 12 mm Hg

52.

Calculate Value	Formula	Normal Values
Cardiac output	SV × heart rate	4 to 8 L/min
Cardiac index	C.O./BSA	2.5 to 4.0 L/min/m²
Stroke index	SV/BSA	35 to 55 mL/beat/m²
Arterial oxygen content	(Hb × %sat × 1.34) + (PaO_2 × 0.00031)	20 vol%
Mixed venous oxygen content	(Hb × %sat × 1.34) + ($P\overline{v}O_2$ × 0.00031)	15 vol%
Systemic vascular resistance	(MAP − [CVP/C.O.]) × 80	900 to 1500 dyne × sec × m⁻⁵
PVR	($\overline{P}$AP − [PAWP/C.O.]) × 80	100 to 250 dyne × sec × m⁻⁵

53.

Factor	Effect on Cardiac Output
Tachycardia	Increases C.O.
β-Adrenergic blockade	Decreases C.O.
Increased parasympathetic tone	Decreases C.O.
Increased preload and contractility	Increases C.O.
Bradyarrhythmias	Decreases C.O.
Decreased parasympathetic tone	Increases C.O.

54. $CaO_2 = (SaO_2 \times 1.34 \times Hb) + (PaO_2 \times 0.00031)$
$= (0.75 \times 1.34 \times 10) + (43 \times 0.00031) = 10.06$ vol%

55. $CaO_2 = (SaO_2 \times 1.34 \times Hb) + (PaO_2 \times 0.00031)$
$= (0.94 \times 1.34 \times 13) + 64 \times 0.00031) = 16.39$ vol%

56. $C\overline{v}O_2 = (S\overline{v}O_2 \times 1.34 \times Hb) + (P_{\overline{v}}O_2 \times 0.00031)$
$= (0.75 \times 1.34 \times 15) + (40 \times 0.00031) = 15.09$ vol%

57. $C\overline{v}O_2 = (S\overline{v}O_2 \times 1.34 \times Hb) + (P_{\overline{v}}O_2 \times 0.00031)$
$= (0.85 \times 1.34 \times 16) + (70 \times 0.00031) = 18.24$ vol%

58. When cardiac output is reduced, the blood flows slower through the vessels, giving the tissues more time to extract oxygen from the blood.

59. The caliber of the blood vessels and the viscosity of the blood are the two factors. Vasoconstriction and polycythemia increase SVR.

60. Both alveolar hypoxia and high intraP$_A$ cause PVR to increase.

61. SV, ejection fraction, stroke work, and stroke work index

Answers to Critical Thinking Questions

1. The appropriate place for a PA catheter is resting with the balloon deflated in zone 3 in the lung. When wedge pressure is measured the balloon is inflated. The catheter tip then reads the pressure in front of the catheter. This reflects the pressure in the left atrium. During early ventricular diastole the mitral valve is open and the left atrium is passively empty into the left ventricle. This is when the PAWP reflects the LVEDP. LVEDP is an index of LVEDP and is used to evaluate left ventricular function.

2. Cardiogenic pulmonary edema occurs when left ventricular function decreases to the point at which the left heart is unable to maintain left ventricular SV adequately. When this occurs blood backs up into the lungs and increases the pulmonary capillary hydrostatic pressure. Pulmonary capillary hydrostatic pressure is the primary determinant of fluid shift from the capillaries into the lung tissue. Therefore, with cardiogenic pulmonary edema, the PAWP will be elevated, usually more than 18 mm Hg. In noncardiogenic pulmonary edema, fluid leaks into the alveoli, not because of left ventricular failure but because of fluid and protein leak caused by a disruption of the pulmonary capillary membrane.

3. C aortic valve closing   B aortic valve opening
   A mitral valve closing   D mitral valve opening
   line 1 ventricular ejection   line 3 ventricular filling
   line 4 isovolumetric   line 2 isovolumetric
       contraction   relaxation

4. Pulse pressure is the difference between the systolic blood pressure and diastolic blood pressure. The pulse pressure can increase by either an increase in systolic pressure or a decrease in diastolic pressure. Causes of an increase in pulse pressure include hypervolemia, arteriosclerosis (noncompliant blood vessels), and bradycardia (lowers diastolic pressure). The pulse pressure can decrease by either decreasing systolic pressure or increasing diastolic pressure. The causes of a decreased pulse pressure include hypovolemia, shock, and tachycardia (increases diastolic pressure).

Answer to Case Study Questions
Case Study #1

1. Pulse pressure = systolic BP − diastolic BP = 145 − 68 = **77 mm Hg** ↑

2. SV = C.O./HR = (5.1 L/min)/(92 breaths/min) = **55.4 mL** ↓

3. Stroke index = SV/BSA = 55.43 mL/2.1 m^2 = **26.4 mL/beat/m^2** ↓

4. Cardiac index = C.O./BSA = (5.1 L/min)/2.1 m^2 = **2.4 L/min/m^2** ↓

5. MAP = [145 + 2(68)]/3 = **93.7 mm Hg** WNL

6. mean PAP = [38 + 2(20)]/3 = **26 mm Hg** ↑

7. SVR = [(MAP − CVP)/C.O.] × 80 = [(93.7 − 12)/5.1] × 80 = **1281.6 dyn•s/cm^5** WNL

8. PVR = [($\overline{\text{PAP}}$ − PAWP)/C.O.] × 80 = [(26 − 10)/5.1] × 80 = **251 dyn•s/cm^5** ↑ slightly

9. CaO$_2$ = [(1.34 × SaO$_2$ × Hb) + (PaO$_2$ × 0.0031)] = [(1.34 × 0.99 × 12.6) + (100 × 0.0031)] = **17 vol%** ↓

10. C$\overline{\text{v}}$O$_2$ = [(1.34 × 0.75 × 12.6) + (40 × 0.0031)] = **12.8 vol%** ↓

11. C(a-$\overline{\text{v}}$)O$_2$ = CaO$_2$ − C$\overline{\text{v}}$O$_2$ = 17 − 12.8 = **4.2 vol%** WNL

12. DO$_2$ = C.O. × CaO$_2$ = 5.1 L/min/m^2 × 170 mL/L = **867 mL/min** WNL

13. VO$_2$ = C.O. × C(a-$\overline{\text{v}}$)O$_2$ = 5.1 L/min/m^2 × 42 mL/L = **214.2 mL/min** WNL

14. RVSW = $\overline{\text{PAP}}$ × SV × 0.0136 = 26 × 55.4 × 0.0136 = **19.6 g•m** WNL

15. RVSWI = RVSW/BSA = 19.6 g•m/2.1 m^2 = **9.3 g•m/m^2** WNL

16. LVSW = MAP × SV × 0.0136 = 93.7 × 55.4 × 0.0136 = **70.6 g•m** WNL

17. LVSWI = LVSW/BSA = 70.6 g•m/m^2/2.1 m^2 = **33.6 g•m/m^2** ↓

18. The patient's hemoglobin is low, which decreases the blood's oxygen-carrying capacity. Both PAP and CVP are elevated and may be caused by the slightly high PVR. Given the patient's history of present illness he may be developing ARDS.

Case Study #2

1. Hemodynamic monitoring of PAP and PCWP would most likely be useful for this patient.

2. Right-sided pneumothorax

3. The pneumothorax is most likely caused by the insertion of the PA catheter.

4. The elevated PAWP is indicative of cardiogenic pulmonary edema from left heart failure.

Answers to NBRC-Style Questions

1. c	6. a	11. a
2. d	7. d	12. d
3. b	8. b	13. b
4. d	9. d	14. a
5. a	10. b	15. c

Chapter 13, Methods to Improve Ventilation and Other Techniques in Patient-Ventilator Management

Answers to Key Terms Crossword Puzzle

Across/down answers appearing in the grid:

DYSSYNCHRONY · INSPIRATORY TIME · OLIGURIA · TRANSPYLORIC · ACETYLCYSTEINE · HYPERTHYROIDISM · ALVEOLAR · HYPERVENTILATION · DEAD SPACE · BRONCHOSCOPY · POLYURIA · DOUGLAS · FULL · HYPEROXYGENATE · KETOACIDOSIS · CARBON DIOXIDE · ATROPINE · HYPEROSMOLAR · EXUDATE · PERMISSIVE HYPERCAPNIA

Answers to Review Questions

1. Desired V_T = (known $PaCO_2$ × known V_T)/desired $PaCO_2$

   = (55 × 500)/40

   = (27,500)/40

   Desired V_T = 687.5, or 688 mL

2. Desired f = (known $PaCO_2$ × known f)/desired $PaCO_2$

   Desired f = (65 × 12)/50

   Desired f = (780)/50

   Desired f = 15.6, or 16

3. total ventilation; dead space; CO_2 production

4. pH; $PaCO_2$; bicarbonate

5. decreased, decrease

6. E. Parenchymal lung problem   A. Asthma

   A. Airway disease   B. Drug overdose

   D. Pleural abnormalities   C. Myasthenia gravis

   B. CNS problems   D. Effusions

   C. Neuromuscular disorders   E. Pneumonia

7. decrease, increase

8. 8 to 12 mL/kg

9. 30 cm H_2O

10. Increase set inspiratory pressure; increase inspiratory time

11. less than, greater than, increase

12. Hypoxia; parenchymal lung disease; medications (salicylate, xanthines, analeptics); mechanical ventilation; CNS disorders (meningitis, encephalitis, head trauma); anxiety; metabolic disorders (sepsis, hepatic disease)

13. Desired f = (known $PaCO_2$ × known f)/desired $PaCO_2$

    Desired f = (25 × 18)/40

    Desired f = (25 × 18)/40

    Desired f = 11

14. Changing the frequency is more important. Decreasing the set V_T to less than 10 mL/kg may result in atelectasis from a low V_T.

15. No. As long as the patient continues to trigger breaths, reducing the set frequency will have no effect.

16. SIMV and PSV

17. Hypoxemia; pain; anxiety; fever; agitation; patient-ventilator asynchrony

18. The body will try to compensate for the metabolic acidosis by increasing alveolar ventilation (hyperventilation), which results in a decreased $PaCO_2$.

19. Ketoacidosis (alcoholism, diabetes, starvation); uremic acidosis (renal failure to excrete acid); loss of bicarbonate (diarrhea); renal loss of base after administration of carbonic anhydrase inhibitors (Diamox); overproduction of acid (lactic acidosis); ingested toxins (salicylate, ethylene glycol, methanol)

20. p 7.45 to 7.70, 26 to 48 mEq/L

21. Loss of gastric fluid and stomach acid; acid loss in urine; acid shift into the cells; lactate, acetate, or citrate administration; excessive bicarbonate loads

22. The increase in physiological dead space will result in a decrease in pulmonary perfusion. $PaCO_2$ will increase, which causes pH to decrease.

23. Pulmonary embolism; low cardiac output

24. a. normal $V_D/V_T = 0.2$ to 0.4
    b. $V_D = V_T (PaCO_2 - P_{\bar{E}}CO_2)/PaCO_2$
    $V_D = 800(45 - 36)/45$
    $V_D = (7200)/45$
    $V_D = 160$ mL
    $V_D/V_T = 160/800 = 0.2$

25. Fever; burns; multiple trauma; sepsis; hyperthyroidism; muscle tremors or seizures; agitation; multiple surgical procedures

26. reduces, constriction, decreased

27. *Permissive hypercapnia* is the deliberate limitation of ventilatory support designed to reduce the risk of lung injury from high pressures and volumes.

28. contraindicated, absolutely contraindicated

29.
Ventilatory Data		**Hemodynamic Data**	
b.	Adult	a.	−60 to −100 mm Hg
c.	Child	b.	−100 to −120 mm Hg
a.	Infant	c.	−80 to −100 mm Hg

30. 15 seconds, intermittently

31. ET size × 3/2 − 9.5 × 3/2 = 14.25. The appropriate size is 14 Fr.

32. Coarse breath sounds; inability to generate an effective spontaneous cough; changes in monitored flow/pressure graphs; increased PIP in volume ventilation; a decrease in V_T with pressure ventilation; visible secretions in the airway; radiographic changes consistent with retained secretions

33. When suctioning is indicated, there is no contraindication.

34. g. Hypoxemia/hypoxia
    a. Tracheal/mucosal trauma
    f. Cardiac/respiratory arrest
    e. Cardiac arrhythmias
    b. Atelectasis
    h. Bronchospasm
    d. Infection
    c. Bleeding

35. a. 100% O_2 for 30 seconds; b. 100% O_2 for 1 minute

36.
Advantages	**Disadvantages**
Decreased likelihood of hypoxia and alveolar collapse, decreased risk of airway contamination. decreased risk of airway contamination to caregiver, reduced incidence of VAP	Increased tension on ET, high cost, catheter can migrate into the airway and affect V_T delivery during pressure ventilation, decrease in pressure during procedure can trigger ventilator, saline may may enter airway when rinsing catheter

37. Unstable patients who are ventilated, such as in acute lung injury or ARDS, and have high ventilator requirements, including high PEEP 10 cm H_2O or greater, high mean airway pressure 20 cm H_2O or greater, long inspiratory time of 1.5 seconds or higher, and a high F_IO_2 of 0.6 or greater; patients who become hemodynamically unstable during suctioning with an open system and ventilator disconnection; patients who desaturate significantly (drop in SpO_2) during suctioning with an open system and ventilator disconnection; patients with contagious infections, such as active tuberculosis, where open suctioning and ventilator disconnect may contaminate health care workers; ventilated patients who require frequent suctioning, such as more than six times a day; patients receiving inhaled gas mixtures, such as NO or heliox therapy, who cannot be interrupted by ventilator disconnection

38. Injury to mucosa during intubation and manipulation of tube after insertion; interference with normal cough reflex; aspiration of contaminated secretions that pool above ET cuff; development of a contaminated biofilm around the ET

39. Large ET cuffs can develop longitudinal folds when inflated. Despite increasing cuff pressures, liquid pharyngeal secretions leak past these folds and lead to VAP.

40. The Hi-Lo Evac ET has a suction port just above the cuff on the dorsal side of the tube and is designed to provide the continuous aspiration of subglottic secretions.

41. It can reduce the incidence of nosocomial pneumonia or VAP.

42. | **Advantages** | **Disadvantages** |
| --- | --- |
| Facilitate suctioning by loosening thick secretions, may stimulatea cough and have patient mobilize secretions | Increase risk of dislodging bacteria into the airway, may increase volume of secretions, increase risk of infection, reduce oxygenation, may result in bronchospasm |

43. Acetylcysteine and 2% sodium bicarbonate

44. Improved breath sounds, decrease in PIP, increased V_T during pressure-limited ventilation, improved ABGs or SpO_2

45. Breath sounds, SpO_2, respiratory rate and pattern, pulse rate, blood pressure, ECG (if available), sputum (color, volume, consistency, odor), PIP (with VC) or volume delivered (with PC), ABGs, cough effort, ICP (if indicated and available)

46. a. (1) bronchodilators, (2) corticosteroids, (3) antibiotics, (4) mucolytics, (5) surfactants; b. MDIs and small-volume nebulizers

47. Although MDIs and SVNs are used to deliver bronchodilators and corticosteroids, SVNs can also deliver mucolytics, antibiotics, prostaglandins, and surfactants.

48. ET size; nebulizer placement; aerosol delivery, continuous or intermittent; nebulizer type; fill volume; duration of nebulization; use of humidification device; inspiratory time; brand of ventilator

49. Expiratory monitors will be inaccurate because of added gas flow; increased volume and pressure delivery; patient may have difficulty triggering a breath; various alarms may not function correctly; F_IO_2 will be altered

50. SVNs should be removed from the circuit after each treatment, disassembled, rinsed with sterile solution, air dried, and stored aseptically.

51. Nebulizer is placed closest to the patient (between leak port and face mask); high inspiratory pressure (20 cm H_2O); low expiratory pressure (5 cm H_2O)

52. measurement of lung mechanics (compliance, resistance, PIP); breath sounds; evaluating vital signs and SpO_2; monitoring ventilator graphics (pressure-time curves, flow-volume and pressure-volume loops)

53. PIP, reduced; P_{TA}, reduced; PEFR, increased

54. The goal of chest physiotherapy is to help clear airway secretions and improve the distribution of ventilation.

55. Postural drainage; percussion of the chest wall

56. Supine; 45-degree rotation prone with left side up; 45-degree rotation prone with right side up; return to supine

57. Accidental extubation; loss, stretching, and kinking of catheters; patient discomfort

58. light-transmitting channel to illuminate the airway; visualizing channel to transmit an image of the airway to an eyepiece; open channel for tissue sampling and oxygen administration; suction channel to clear the airway

59. | **Indications** | **Contraindications** |
| --- | --- |
| Evaluate persistent atelectasis; assess patency of upper airway; investigate presence of hemoptysis, persistent or unexplained cough, or stridor; positive sputum cytology results; need to obtain cell washings, secretions, and biopsies; determine the location and extent of toxic inhalation; aid in difficult intubations; remove abnormal tissue or foreign material; retrieve foreign bodies | Coagulopathy that cannot be corrected, severe obstructive airway disease, severe refractory hypoxemia, unstable hemodynamic status including dysrhythmias, recent myocardial infarction, partial tracheal obstruction, moderate to severe hypoxemia, pulmonary hypertension, lung abscess, respiratory failure |

60. prevent atelectasis; prevent hypoxemia; reduce the risk of skin breakdown

61. to decrease shunt and improve oxygenation (increase PaO_2)

62. blood redistributed to better-ventilated areas; blood redistribution may improve alveolar recruitment; redistribution of fluid and gas improves ventilation perfusion ratio; position of the heart no longer puts weight on underlying lung tissue; improved distribution of pleural pressure may improve alveolar recruitment; change in regional diaphragm motion

63. b. hemodynamic instability
    b. arrhythmias
    c. thoracic and abdominal surgery
    a. spinal cord instability

64. a. (1) tip the patient to the side, (2) unhook ECG leads, (3) turn the patient prone, (4) turn the patient's head toward the ventilator, (5) reattach ECG leads; b. (1) check all lines, (2) check ventilator pressure and volume, (3) monitor vital signs, and (4) reposition and recalibrate pressure transducers

65. Accidental extubation; loss of IV lines or urinary catheters; facial and eyelid edema; hemodynamic instability; oxygen desaturation; decreased chest wall compliance

66. Independent lung ventilation; place the patient in a lateral position with the nonaffected lung in the dependent position ("good" lung in the down position)

67. Limit the occurrence of nosocomial infections; ensure that the circuit is physically intact and functioning properly; provide a clean circuit; minimize risks to patients and health care workers

68.

Characteristic	Potential Cause
g. Yellow	a. Old blood
d. Green, thick	b. *Klebsiella* infection
e. Green, foul smelling	c. Pulmonary edema
f. Pink-tinged	d. Sputum has been in airway for long period of time
h. Fresh blood	e. *Pseudomonas* infection
a. Brown	f. May indicate fresh blood or occur after treatment with aerosolized epinephrine or racemic epinephrine
b. Rust	g. Presence of pus (WBCs) and possible infection
c. Pink, copious, and frothy	h. Airway trauma, pneumonia, pulmonary infarction, or emboli

69. a. *Oliguria* is a urine output of less than 400 mL/day or less than 20 mL/hr. b. *Polyuria* is a urine output of more than 2400 mL/day or 100 mL/hr.

70. Decreased fluid intake and low plasma volume; decreased cardiac output, venous return, and an increase in antidiuretic hormone caused by PPV, heart failure, and hypovolemia from dehydration, shock, or hemorrhage; decreased renal perfusion; renal malfunction; obstruction or extravasation from the urethra, bladder, ureters, or pelvis; blocked Foley catheter

71. decrease, increase

72. The goal of patient-centered mechanical ventilation is to improve patient comfort by periodic adjustment of ventilator settings such as flow rate, flow waveform, sensitivity level, pressure target, flow-cycle criteria in PSV, or by switching modes.

73. a. Emergency airway management supplies, stethoscope, manual resuscitator bag and mask, pulse oximeter, ECG and heart rate monitor, sphygmomanometer, hand-held spirometer. b. Sufficient portable power (battery and gas) for the duration of transport; independent control of V_T and rate; CMV or SIMV mode capability; PEEP capability; disconnect, high pressure, and low power (battery) alarms; provision of F_IO_2 (up to 100%)

74. Inability to provide adequate oxygenation and ventilation; inability to maintain acceptable hemodynamic stability; inability to monitor cardiopulmonary status; inability to maintain a patent airway

75. Hyperventilation during manual ventilation; loss of PEEP/CPAP resulting in hypoxemia; position changes resulting in hypotension, hypercarbia, and hypoxemia; tachycardia and other arrhythmias; equipment failure resulting in loss of monitoring ability; accidental disconnection of IV access for drug administration, resulting in hemodynamic instability; disconnection from ventilatory support; accidental extubation; accidental removal of vascular access; VAP resulting from transport

Answers to Critical Thinking Questions

1. In a volume-control mode of ventilation, increasing either V_T or frequency can reduce $PaCO_2$. Increasing V_T is not an option because of high $P_{plateau}$, so the frequency needs to be increased.
   Desired f = (Known $PaCO_2$ × Known f)/Desired $PaCO_2$
   Desired f = (known 60 × 10)/40
   Desired f = 15

2. An increase in metabolism can be found in the presence of fever, multiple trauma, and multiple surgical procedures. This increase in metabolism results in an increase in $\dot{V}CO_2$. In the presence of this increase in CO_2 production, the high $\dot{V}_E$ (20.0 L/min) is required to maintain the $PaCO_2$ within normal range.

3. PPV and PEEP can result in a decrease in cardiac output. If the cardiac output increases when the inspiratory pressure level or PEEP is decreased, the problem is most likely caused by an increase in ($\overline{P}aw$)

Answers to Case Studies

Case Study #1

1. Decreasing the rate had no effect because the patient was triggering breaths above the set rate. Lowering the V_T may be effective in reducing ventilation, but in this case the patient responded by triggering additional breaths. The increase in ventilation is a response to the hypoxemia. Once the hypoxemia is corrected, the patient will no longer need to maintain a high $\dot{V}_A$.

Case Study #2

1. Because the V_T is less than 12 mL/kg, maintaining the f and increasing the V_T by increasing the set pressure is appropriate.

2. Desired V_T = (known $PaCO_2$ × known V_T)/desired $PaCO_2$

   Desired V_T = (65 × 550)/45

   Desired V_T = 795 mL

   Because an inspiratory pressure of 20 cm H_2O results in a V_T of 550 mL, a pressure of 30 cm H_2O will achieve a V_T of 795 mL.

   $C_S = V_T/\Delta P$, $C_S = 550/20$, $C_S = 27.5$ mL/cm H_2O

   Desired P = desired V_T/C_S

   Desired P = 795 mL/27.5 mL/cm H_2O

   Desired P = 30 cm H_2O

Case Study #3

1. When the patient was disconnected from the ventilator PEEP decreased and suctioning further reduced lung volume. The hypoxemia that occurred resulted in the decrease in O_2 saturation and increased heart rate.

2. With a closed suction catheter (in-line suction catheter) disconnecting the patient from the ventilator is not necessary. PEEP levels can be maintained, decreasing the likelihood of hypoxia and alveolar collapse.

Answers to NBRC-Style Questions

1. c	5. a	9. d
2. a	6. c	10. a
3. d	7. c	
4. d	8. b	

Chapter 14, Improving Oxygenation and Management of ARDS

Answers to Key Terms Crossword Puzzle

RECRUITMENT
HYPOVOLEMIC
EXUDATIVE
DEFLATION
ASCINI
DEPENDENT
OPTIMUM
CARDIOGENIC
ATELECTASIS
DUCK
LIP
BAROTRAUMA
FIBROSING
CEPHALAD
SHUNT
HISTOTOXIC

Answers to Review Questions

1. F_IO_2; CaO_2; cardiac output

2. Calculating oxygen delivery provides information about how much oxygen is available to the tissues and oxygen consumption.

3. Oxygen consumption = Cardiac output × O_2 content − Mixed venous O_2 content: $VO_2 = QT \times C_{a-\bar{v}}O_2$

4. The F_IO_2 should be monitored at least every 24 hours in adults and continuously in infants and neonates.

5. An ABG can be drawn within 15 minutes.

6. below 0.4 to 0.5

7. Breathing 100% O_2 can lead to absorption atelectasis and increase intrapulmonary shunting.

8. 60 to 90 mm Hg, 20 mL/dL

9. The cardiopulmonary status must remain fairly constant (minute ventilation, cardiac output, shunt, and ventilation-perfusion mismatching must not change significantly).

10. PaO_2 (known)/F_IO_2 (known) = PaO_2 (desired)/F_IO_2 (desired) or F_IO_2 (desired) = [PaO_2 (desired) × F_IO_2 (known)]/PaO_2 (known)

11. F_IO_2 (desired) = (60 × 75)/50 = 45/50 = F_IO_2 0.90

12. The shunt equation is used to calculate the portion of the cardiac output not taking part in gas exchange.

13.
$$\frac{\dot{Q}_S}{\dot{Q}_T} = \frac{Cc'O_2 - CaO_2}{Cc'O_2 - C\overline{v}O_2}$$

$\dot{Q}_S/\dot{Q}_T$: physiological shunt to total perfusion ratio (percent)

$Cc'O_2$: end-capillary oxygen content (percent)

CaO_2: arterial oxygen content (percent)

$C\overline{v}O_2$: mixed venous oxygen content (percent)

14. $Cc'O_2 = 20.4$ vol%

$CaO_2 = 19.8$ vol%

$C\overline{v}O_2 = 13.4$ vol%

$$\frac{\dot{Q}_s}{\dot{Q}_T} = \frac{CcO_2 - CaO_2}{CcO_2 - \overline{C}O_2}$$

$$= \frac{20.4 - 19.8}{20.4 - 13.4}$$

$$= \frac{0.6}{7}$$

15. $\overline{P}aw$ is the average pressure above baseline during a total respiratory cycle (I + E).

16. PIP, total PEEP (auto-PEEP + set-PEEP), I:E ratios, respiratory rate, and inspiratory flow pattern

17. Increasing mP_{aw} affects mean P_A and alveolar recruitment. As collapsed and partially collapsed alveoli reexpand, PaO_2 increases.

18. PEEP, HFOV, and APRV

19. Prevention or reversal of alveolar and small airway collapse

20. CPAP is positive pressure maintained above ambient pressure during spontaneous breathing. PEEP is the end-expiratory pressure that is above 0 cm H_2O during mechanical ventilatory support.

21. When PEEP is applied during mechanical ventilation, an expiratory valve closes when the expiratory pressure drops to the preset level. The pressure and volume trapped in the lungs prevent or reverse alveolar collapse.

22. Mask CPAP, nasal CPAP, endotracheal or tracheostomy tubes, flow and threshold resistors

23. Full face mask, nasal mask, nasal prongs

24. Maintain a normal $PaCO_2$ without excessive ventilatory effort, they must be able to protect the lower airways from aspiration, have cardiovascular stability, PaO_2/F_IO_2 ratio greater than 200 mm Hg

25. Vomiting and aspiration, CO_2 retention, increased WOB, skin necrosis and/or discomfort from the mask

26. Cerebral hemorrhage at high CPAP pressures in infants; gastric distention; pressure necrosis; swelling of nasal mucosa; abrasion of the posterior pharynx

27. The patient must generate an inspiratory force to obtain an inspiratory flow from the device. The less patient effort required to trigger the flow, the less WOB is required.

28. Positive expiratory pressure therapy achieves expiratory pressure by creating a resistance to gas flow when the patient exhales through a fixed orifice.

29. The positive pressure recruits and distends collapsed alveoli, which increases lung volume and compliance. This results in less pressure change (WOB) required to move the same volume of air per breath.

30. sleep disorders (OSA)

31. Improve tissue oxygenation and maintain a PaO_2 above 60 mm Hg, a saturation greater than 90% with a normal pH on an F_IO_2 less than 0.40 to 0.50 with normal cardiovascular function

32. The level of PEEP that provides optimal oxygen transport and compliance without cardiopulmonary side effects at an F_IO_2 less than 0.40

33. static

34. less than 30 mm Hg

35. a. Increased oxygen transport, increased FRC, improved compliance, decreased shunt; b. Decreased venous return, decreased cardiac output, decreased blood pressure, increased shunting, increased V_D/V_T ratio

36. PaO_2 less than 60 mm Hg on an F_IO_2 of 0.8; $P(A\text{-}a)O_2$ greater than 300 on F_IO_2 of 1.0; refractory hypoxemia: PaO_2 increases less than 10 mm Hg with an F_IO_2 increase of 0.2; shunt of greater than 30%; recurrent atelectasis with low FRC; reduced C_L; PaO_2/F_IO_2 ratio less than 200

37. PEEP should be initiated as soon as possible to avoid lung damage from high ventilating pressures and oxygen toxicity.

38. ALI/ARDS; cardiogenic pulmonary edema; bilateral, diffuse pneumonia

39. Low or minimum PEEP (less than 5 cm H_2O); therapeutic PEEP (more than 5 cm H_2O)

40. Low or minimum PEEP: maintain the FRC in an intubated patient; therapeutic PEEP: treat refractory hypoxemia

41. 3 to 5 cm H_2O, 2 to 3 cm H_2O

42. Patients who require high ventilating pressures and F_IO_2 values of 0.5 or greater

43. PaO_2 of 60 to 100 mm Hg on an F_IO_2 of less than 0.4; optimal O_2 transport (normal = 1000 mL/min O_2); shunt less than 15%; adequate BP, decrease of less than 20% in CO, acceptable pulmonary vascular pressures; improving C_L and lung aeration; PaO_2/F_IO_2 ratio greater than 300; point of minimal arterial to end-tidal $PaCO_2$ gradient; and optimal mixed venous oxygen values

44. blood pressure

45. **Ventilatory Data** **Hemodynamic Data**
$P_{plateau}$, C_S, PIP, $PaCO_2$, BP, PaO_2 ($F_IO_2 = 1.0$), V_E, $V_{Tspontaneous}$/ CaO_2, $P(A-a)O_2$, $V_{Tventilator}$, $f_{spontaneous}$/ $C_{a-\bar{v}}O_2$, $CO \times CaO_2$, $f_{ventilator}$, $PaCO_2$ – $S\bar{v}O_2$, CO, PCWP, PAP $P_{ET}CO_2$, pH

46. To evaluate changes in lung compliance and airway resistance

47. 15 to 20 cm H_2O

48. The optimal PEEP level is +11 cm H_2O. The PaO_2 is acceptable; CO is at its best value with the best O_2 delivery and static compliance.

49. When hyperinflation is present, PEEP may further distend alveoli, which leads to compression of the capillaries and results in increased shunting and hypoxemia.

50. When auto-PEEP is present, the application of mechanical PEEP aids the patient in triggering mechanical breaths.

51. PEEP can reduce CO and blood pressure.

52. Positive pressure will further increase the air present in the intrapleural space and may lead to death.

53. No. An increase in PIP is normal with an increase in the PEEP level because the FRC is increased.

54. Lung recruitment occurred at this level, shunt was reduced, and an increased in PaO_2 resulted.

55. Congestive heart failure (reduces venous return, which reduces myocardial work); mask CPAP (helps prevent postoperative atelectasis and improve PaO_2); OSA (functions as a pneumatic splint to prevent pharyngeal obstruction); cystic fibrosis (application of EPAP aids in secretion removal); airway suctioning (PEEP aids in the loss of lung volume and reduced C_S)

56. An acceptable PaO_2 on an F_IO_2 of less than 0.40; hemodynamic stability; C_S less than 25 mL/cm H_2O; nonseptic; PaO_2/F_IO_2 ratio greater than 250

57. ARDS is a syndrome of severe lung injury accompanied by severe hypoxemia refractory to O_2 therapy, decreased compliance, and lung volumes.

58. ALI is defined by a P/F ratio less than 300, whereas ARDS is defined as a PaO_2/F_IO_2 ratio of less than 200.

59. increased, protein-rich plasma, interstitial space, alveolar space

60. The release of cytokines and other inflammatory and thrombotic mediators into the bloodstream can affect other organs and lead to multisystem organ failure.

61. The pulmonary edema in CHF is caused by the backup of blood in the pulmonary circulation from left-sided heart failure. The pulmonary edema in ARDS is caused by an increase in capillary permeability.

62. ALI and ARDS both produce a decrease in compliance and a reduction in lung volumes.

63. Exudative phase: characterized by inflammation; subacute phase: characterized by fibrosing alveolitis

64. In primary ARDS (direct) the lungs are mostly consolidated. In secondary ARDS (indirect) alveolar collapse is predominant.

65. ARDS is a heterogeneous disorder (not all areas of the lung are affected). If normal V_T is used, a small area receives most of the ventilation, resulting in overdistention and lung injury.

66. Avoid VILI from excessive pressure, volume, and O_2 toxicity

67. V_T 4 to 6 mL/kg; PEEP to prevent alveolar edema and avoid shear stress injury; PaO_2 is not a reliable indicator of an appropriate level; PEEP needs to be applied early and kept 3 to 4 cm H_2O above the lower inflection point; if difficult to maintain low pressures during volume ventilation, change to pressure-controlled ventilation and monitor V_T; maintain $P_{plateau}$ less than 30 cm H_2O; permissive hypercapnia

68. An inflation maneuver to open up as much lung as possible; a deflation maneuver to establish the upper inflection point during deflation; a second inflation maneuver to reopen the lung

69. A significant increase in thoracic pressure; a decrease in CO and blood pressure; uneven distribution of pressure

70. Untreated pneumothorax; hypovolemia; unilateral lung disease

71. Sustained high pressures in the CPAP mode; pressure-controlled ventilation with a single high PEEP level; pressure-controlled ventilation with progressive increases in PEEP levels; sigh maneuvers

72. Increase the PEEP in increments of 5 cm H_2O and remain at each level for 2 to 5 minutes. Observe the pressure-volume loop for a "duck bill" appearance. When the "duck bill" appears the lungs are overinflated. At that point reverse the process by decreasing the PEEP in increments of 2.5 cm H_2O. Remain at each level for 5 minutes and measure static compliance. Observe the PEEP level at which the static compliance drops dramatically. This is the point where a significant amount of lung units collapse, known as the deflation point. Set the PEEP level to 2 to 4 cm H_2O above the deflation point.

73. 0925 hours, PEEP 15 cm H_2O, and C_S 28 mL/cm H_2O

74. The appropriate PEEP level is 17 to 19 cm H_2O.

Answers to Critical Thinking Questions

1. a. point A: PIP; point B: upper inflection point; point C: lower inflection point
   b. The lower inflection point (C) identifies the level of PEEP where the lung is most compliant (also referred to as the critical opening pressure).
   c. The upper inflection point (B) indicates where the lung becomes less compliant and illustrates where overdistention starts to occur. The overdistention can lead to $\dot{V}/\dot{Q}$ mismatch and an increase in $PaCO_2$.

2. a. The PIP is approximately 95 to 100 cm H_2O.
   b. The exhaled V_T is approximately 500 mL.
   c. The cause of the increased airway pressure cannot be determined by observing the pressure-volume curve. If an inspiratory hold or pause is instituted, a $P_{plateau}$ can be obtained. By analyzing the PIP and $P_{plateau}$, whether the cause of the high ventilating pressures is an increase in airway resistance or a decrease in compliance can be determined.

3. In a volume-controlled mode, an inverse I:E ratio may be achieved by (1) using a descending waveform, (2) decreasing peak inspiratory flow rates, and (3) adding an inspiratory pause.

Answers to Case Studies
Case Study #1

1. The opacification of the right lung is caused by the aspiration pneumonia. Because one lung (left) appears normal, the patient has unilateral lung disease. The hypoxemia could be caused by the effects of PEEP on normal lung tissue. Overdistention of normal alveoli results in $\dot{V}/\dot{Q}$ mismatch.

2. Unilateral lung disorders are a relative contraindication to PEEP and are better managed with a double-lumen ET and independent lung ventilation.

Case Study #2

1. The blood gas is normal with severe hypoxemia.

2. A PIP of 55 cm H_2O with a $P_{plateau}$ of 48 cm H_2O is an indication of noncompliant lungs. The chest radiograph revealing bilateral fluffy infiltrates, refractory hypoxemia (PaO_2 of 44 mm Hg on an F_1O_2 of 1.0), and a severe reduction in compliance are all indications that the patient has ARDS secondary to his heroin overdose.

3. Initiating PEEP will help recruit and distend collapsed alveoli, which will improve compliance and increase PaO_2 by decreasing shunt. High ventilating pressures can be minimized by the use of a lower V_T or change to a pressure-controlled mode of ventilation.

Answers to NBRC-Style Questions

1. c	5. c	9. b
2. d	6. d	10. c
3. a	7. c	
4. b	8. d	

Chapter 15, Frequently Used Pharmacological Agents in Ventilated Patients: Sedatives, Analgesics, and Paralytics

Answers to Key Terms Crossword Puzzle

FLUMAZENIL

DIAZEPAM

SUCCINYLCHOLINE

MORPHINE

GABA

PANCURONIUM

PARALYSIS

NEUROLEPTIC

ANTEROGRADE

DEPOLARIZING

(Down answers include: DELIRIUM, NONDEPENDENT, KAPPA, SEDATATIVE, MORPHALONE, PROPOFOL, KRAZEPAM, TRINFUSION, OFFOUNG, FENTANYL, PROLONGED, GABRIZINGS, RASAYSCALE)

Answers to Review Questions

1. Sedatives reduce anxiety and agitation and promote the normalization of sleep.

2. Paralysis is used to facilitate invasive procedures, such as intubation, to ensure the stability of an airway and to decrease mP_{aw} during discoordinated or uncontrolled mechanical ventilation.

3. Benzodiazepines (diazepam, midazolam, and lorazepam); opioids (morphine, fentanyl); neuroleptics (haloperidol); anesthetic agents (propofol)

4. Sedation is often required for high-frequency ventilation, inverse I:E ventilation, and permissive hypercapnia.

5. The four levels of sedation are minimal, moderate, deep, and anesthesia.

6.

Sedation Level	Patient Response	Ventilatory Function	Cardiovascular Function
minimal	positive to verbal commands; cognitive function may be impaired	unaffected	unaffected
moderate	positive to verbal commands; may require tactile stimulation	maintained	maintained
deep	not easily aroused; positive to painful stimuli	inadequate spontaneous ventilation and patent airway	maintained
anesthesia	not able to be aroused even with painful stimuli	requires ventilatory assistance with artificial airway and PPV	may be impaired

7. When a patient is "fighting" the ventilator, moderate levels of sedation may be required.

8. During weaning from mechanical ventilation minimal levels of sedation should be maintained.

9. Ramsay scale

10. A score of 2 to 4 on the Ramsay scale indicates adequate sedation.

11. A score of 1 indicates the need for sedation.

12. Scores of 5 to 6 indicate oversedation for an ICU patient.

13. Benzodiazepines are the drugs of choice for anxiety because of their ability to produce anxiolytic, hypnotic, muscle relaxing, anticonvulsant, and anterograde amnesic effects.

14. Benzodiazepines depress the CNS by binding to receptors in the GABA receptor complex on neurons in the brain. This increases the chloride permeability of the neuron, which in turn hyperpolarizes the neuron, making it less likely to depolarize.

15. Factors that influence the duration of action of benzodiazepines include age, underlying pathology, and concurrent drug therapy.

16. Hepatic and renal insufficiencies prolong the recovery from benzodiazepines.

17. Diazepam has a rapid onset of action because of its high lipid solubility and ability to traverse the blood-brain barrier relatively quickly. Onset is 3 to 5 minutes when administered IV.

18. IV bolus at the start of infusion, followed by a series of smaller boluses with close titration to produce the desired plasma concentration of the drug

19. Acutely agitated patients are best treated with midazolam (Versed) because it has a rapid onset and a short half-life.

20. Prolonged sedation with midazolam can occur from accumulation of the drug and its metabolites in the peripheral tissues when it is used for longer than 48 hours.

21. Lorazepam (Ativan) is the drug of choice for use with ventilated patients for longer than 24 hours.

22. Flumazenil (Romazicon) reverses the effects of benzodiazepines.

23. lactic acidosis, hyperosmolar coma, and a reversible nephrotoxicity

24. morphine and fentanyl

25. Relieve pain, sedate, and relieve anxiety.

26. Their effects are mediated through μ and κ receptors. μ Receptors are responsible for analgesia and the κ receptors mediate the sedative effects.

27. Serious side effects of opioids include nausea, vomiting, reduced gastrointestinal motility, respiratory depression, bradycardia, hypotension, myoclonus, convulsions, histamine release, immunosuppression, and addiction.

28. The severity of the side effects of opioids depends on the severity of the patient's illness and organ function.

29. naloxone hydrochloride (Narcan)

30. Morphine's effects on the CNS include reduction of cerebral blood flow, intracranial pressure, and cerebral metabolic activity as well as drowsiness, lethargy, dilation of the pupils, and suppression of the cough reflex.

31. Morphine lowers esophageal sphincter tone, increases pyloric sphincter tone, and reduces the propulsive peristaltic activity of the intestines, delaying the passage of contents through the gastrointestinal tract.

32. Morphine decreases systemic vascular resistance directly or by causing decreases in sympathetic tone and increases in vagal tone.

33. Fentanyl should be used for a patient with an unstable hemodynamic status.

34.

Drug	Natural or Synthetic	Lipid Solubility	Blood-Brain Barrier	Onset of Action	Duration of Action	Administration
Morphine	natural	low	slow transit time	slow	prolonged	IV bolus or continual transfusion
Fentanyl	synthetic	high	rapid transit time	rapid	short	IV loading dose followed by continual transfusion

35. neuroleptics

36. haloperidol

37. anticholinergic effects on the heart; lower the seizure threshold; causes muscle rigidity, drowsiness, and lethargy

38. propofol (Diprivan)

39. Propofol (Diprivan) causes a reduction in systemic vascular resistance with a concomitant fall in blood pressure and bradycardia during the initial induction phase; it also reduces cerebral blood flow and ICP.

40.

Advantages

Rapid onset, short duration of action (makes rapid awakening possible for neurological assessment), decreased ICP, and clearance unaffected by renal or hepatic dysfunction.

Disadvantages

Hypotension, dysrhythmias, bradycardia, and elevated pancreatic enzymes. Prolonged use has been associated with lactic acidosis and lipidemia in pediatric patients.

41. Morphine and propofol (Diprivan)

42. NMBAs

43. Depolarizing NMBAs bind to acetylcholine receptors, causing prolonged depolarization of the motor end plate. Nondepolarizing NMBAs cause paralysis by competitively inhibiting the action of acetylcholine at the neuromuscular junction.

44. Paralyzing agents (NMBAs) are used to facilitate intubation and facilitate ventilation.

45. Train-of-four is an electronic technique used to assess a patient's depth of paralysis.

46. An electrical current consisting of four impulses is applied to a peripheral nerve over a 2-second period and the mechanical response of the innervated muscle is assessed.

47. One to two twitches when performing the train-of-four indicate that an adequate amount of NMBA is being used.

48. Patients receiving an NMBA must also be given sedation because NMBAs do **not** sedate the patients. Lack of sedation may lead to hypertension, tachycardia, or diaphoresis.

49. succinylcholine (Anectine)

50. Succinylcholine's onset is approximately 1 minute and its duration of action is between 5 and 10 minutes.

51. Succinylcholine is used most often to facilitate endotracheal intubation.

52. The most common side effects associated with succinylcholine include transient hyperkalemia; cardiac dysrhythmias; anaphylactic reactions; prolonged apnea; postoperative myalgias; increase intragastric, intracranial, and intraocular pressures; myoglobinuria; and sustained skeletal muscle contraction. It may also precipitate malignant hyperthermia in susceptible individuals.

53. pancuronium (Pavulon)

54. Vecuronium bromide (Norcuron), atracurium besylate (Tracrium), and cisatracurium besylate (Nimbex) are intermediate-duration nondepolarizing NMBAs.

55. Pancuronium should not be used with hemodynamically unstable patients because its side effects include tachycardia, increased cardiac output, elevated MAP, and pulmonary vasoconstriction.

56. Atracurium besylate (Tracrium)

57. Atracurium besylate (Tracrium)

58. Atracurium besylate (Tracrium) and cisatracurium besylate (Nimbex)

59. cisatracurium besylate (Nimbex)

60. Tolerance, which may necessitate increasing the dosage, and muscle weakness

Answers to Critical Thinking Questions

1. When using an NMBA in a mechanically ventilated patient, the apnea alarm, low inspiratory pressure alarm, low exhaled V_T alarm, and low exhaled minute volume alarm should be set and active. If a pulse oximeter is being continually used, the low SpO_2 alarm should be used.

2. Fentanyl (Sublimaze), a synthetic opioid, is best used with asthma because it does not cause histamine release as morphine does. Morphine is not recommended in asthma because of its mast cell–mediated histamine release, which potentially worsens bronchoconstriction.

Answers to Case Study Questions
Case Study #1

1. A sedative such as a benzodiazepine (e.g., diazepam)

2. an NMBA

3. The RT should switch the patient to full ventilatory support before the administration of an NMBA because the patient's diaphragm and accessory muscles will be paralyzed.

Answers to NBRC-Style Questions

1. b	5. c	9. d
2. a	6. b	10. a
3. c	7. c	
4. d	8. a	

Chapter 16, Effects of Positive Pressure Ventilation on the Cardiovascular, Cerebral, Renal, and Other Organ Systems

Answers to Key Terms Crossword Puzzle

Answers to Review Questions

1. Cardiovascular function; pulmonary function; neurological function; renal function; gastrointestinal function

2. The amount of pressure applied to the airways; the patient's cardiopulmonary status

3. The negative intrapleural pressures that occur during spontaneous inspiration are transmitted to the intrathoracic vessels. A drop in pressure in the vena cava increases the pressure gradient back to the heart, and venous return increases.

4. Right ventricular preload is increased during inspiration because more blood is returning to the right heart.

5. Left ventricular preload is decreased during passive expiration. When intrapleural pressure becomes less negative, venous return is decreased and right ventricular SV is decreased, which causes a decrease in left ventricular preload.

6. Increases the pressure gradient

7. Diagram A represents the largest gradient.

8. Diagram C represents the smallest gradient.

9. Diagram A represents the system with the largest venous return.

10. Because the pulmonary capillaries are interlaced with the alveoli, when the alveoli are overdistended the pulmonary capillaries are stretched and narrowed. As a result, resistance to blood flow through the pulmonary circulation increases. The increased PVR increases right ventricular afterload.

11. High levels of positive pressure (more than 15 cm H_2O) and a volume-depleted patient

12. The reduction in cardiac output created by decreased venous return will reduce coronary artery perfusion pressure gradient for both sides of the heart. This, plus the direct effect of compression of the coronary vessels caused by increases in intrathoracic pressure, can ultimately lead to myocardial ischemia.

13. Increase in sympathetic tone; increase in systemic vascular resistance; increase in peripheral venous pressure from arterial and venous constriction; peripheral shunting of blood away from the kidneys and lower extremities

14. Sympathetic blockade, spinal anesthesia, moderate levels of general anesthesia, spinal cord transaction, or severe polyneuritis

15. The RT should measure blood pressure soon after PPV is initiated.

16. more than 15 cm H_2O

17. The presence or absence of the normal compensatory mechanism for maintaining arterial blood pressure; the lung and chest wall compliance and airway resistance; the duration and magnitude of the positive pressure

18. PPV can reduce venous return and therefore reduce preload to the heart. This will improve length-tension relations within the heart and improve SV.

19. mP_{aw}

20. $mP_{aw} = \frac{1}{2}[PIP \times (T_I/TCT)]$; TCT = 60/12 = 5
    $= \frac{1}{2}[25 \times (1 \text{ sec}/5 \text{ sec})]$
    $= \frac{1}{2}(5)$
    $= 2.5$ cm H_2O

21. $mP_{aw} = \frac{1}{2}[(PIP - PEEP) \times (T_I/TCT)] + PEEP$
    $= \frac{1}{2}[(35 - 10) \times (1/5)] + 10$
    $= \frac{1}{2}[25 \times (1/5)] + 10$
    $= \frac{1}{2}(5) + 10$
    $= 12.5$ cm H_2O

22. Adding a 1-second inspiratory hold will increase the T_I to 2 seconds, so that
    $mP_{aw} = \frac{1}{2}[(35 - 10) \times (2/5)] + 10$
    $= \frac{1}{2}(25) + 10$
    $= 12.5 + 10$
    $= 22.5$ cm H_2O

23. High inspiratory flow rates are likely to cause uneven ventilation.

24. 1:2 to 1:4 or smaller

25. A longer expiratory time

26. The severity of a patient's lung disease

27. Inspiratory gas flow and pattern; I:E ratio; inflation hold; PEEP; ventilator mode

28. Rapid flow rates deliver the desired V_T is in a shorter time. The faster the flow, the shorter the inspiratory time, the lower the mP_{aw}.

29. To affect cardiac output, the PEEP must transmit its pressure to the intrathoracic space and intrathoracic vessels. If this occurs, PEEP will cause a decrease in cardiac output.

30. High levels of PEEP would **not** cause a decrease in cardiac output when the patient has "stiff" lungs. This situation could exist because the stiff lungs do not allow the transmission of pressure to the intrathoracic space and intrathoracic vessels.

31. CPP = MABP − ICP; 85 mm Hg − 18 mm Hg = 67 mm Hg

32. PPV can increase CVP, making it harder for blood to return to the right heart from the head. This will cause a backup of pressure into the head, increasing ICP.

33. Jugular vein distention is a clinical sign of increased ICP.

34. Hyperventilation lowers $PaCO_2$, which constricts cerebral vessels and reduces ICP.

35. The kidneys respond to hemodynamic changes resulting from a high intrathoracic pressure; humoral responses, including antidiuretic hormone, atrial natriuretic factor changes occur with PPV; abnormal pH, $PaCO_2$, and PaO_2 abnormalities affect the kidneys.

36. Urinary output will become severely reduced when the glomerular capillary pressure falls below 75 mm Hg.

37. This redistribution of blood flow within the kidney will cause less urine, creatinine, and sodium to be excreted.

38. Antidiuretic hormone; atrial natriuretic factor; renin-angiotensin-aldosterone

39. Blood pressure changes from PPV precipitate the release of ADH, which will cause oliguria. PPV and PEEP can reduce atrial filling pressure by reducing atrial stretch, which leads to decreased secretion of atrial natriuretic factor, causing water and sodium retention. Plasma renin activity is increased during PPV, which activates the renin-angiotensin-aldosterone cascade and results in retention of both sodium and water.

40. Decreased PaO_2 values in patients with respiratory failure cause reduction in renal function and a decrease in urine flow. Severe hypoxemia (PaO_2 less than 40 mm Hg) dramatically interferes with normal renal function. $PaCO_2$ level greater than 65 mm Hg can also severely impair renal function.

41. Many drugs, such as sedatives and NMBAs, and their metabolites are excreted by the kidneys. The altered renal function, created by PPV, can prolong the effects of these drugs and affect patient care.

42. PPV and PEEP cause an elevation of serum bilirubin (more than 2.5 mg/100 mL) even when no evidence of preexisting liver disease is present. Several factors may lead to this effect of the liver. The drop in cardiac output, downward movement of the diaphragm against the liver, decrease in portal venous flow, and increase in splanchnic resistance may all lead to liver ischemia and other factors that impair liver function.

43. Gastric distention during PPV can result from swallowing air that leaks around ET cuffs. A gastric tube can remove this air and decompress the stomach.

44. Seriously ill patients are at risk of malnutrition because of a combination of inadequate intake of food and hypermetabolism associated with fever and wound healing.

45. Altered ability to effectively respond to infection; impaired wound healing; severely reduces ability to maintain spontaneous ventilation from weakened respiratory muscles

46. Overfeeding can lead to increased oxygen consumption, increased CO_2 production, and the need for increased minute ventilation, resulting in increased WOB.

47. Actual versus predicted body weight; fat versus lean muscle mass; creatinine/height index; serum albumin (less than 3.5 g/dL = visceral protein malnutrition); transferrin (less than 300 mg = visceral protein malnutrition)

48. Complications can be reduced through early recognition of the signs and symptoms of the problems associated with PPV, followed by appropriate intervention.

Answers to Critical Thinking Question

1. Arrow A represents decreased venous return caused by the increase in intrapleural pressure. Arrow B represents the septal shifting that occurs when high levels of positive pressure are used and the patient is volume depleted. When this happens LVEDV is encroached upon and LV SV may decrease because its ability to fill is limited. Arrow C represents compression of the heart between the expanding lungs. The transmission of positive pressure to the heart from the lungs exerts a cardiac tamponade effect. Arrow D represents the stretch and narrowing of the alveoli and pulmonary capillaries. As a result, resistance to blood flow through the pulmonary circulation increases PVR, which will decrease right ventricular output.

Answers to Case Study

Case Study #1

1. $MAP = \frac{1}{2}[(PIP - PEEP) \times (T_I/TCT)] + PEEP$

   $T_I = V_T/\text{flow rate} = 0.56\ L \div 1.4\ L/sec\ (84\ L/min = 1.4\ L/sec)$

   $MAP = \frac{1}{2}[(30 - 10) \times (0.4/5)] + 10$

   $ = \frac{1}{2}[20 \times (0.4/5)] + 10$

   $MAP = 0.8 + 10 = 10.8\ cm\ H_2O$

2. The acid base status is within normal limits. However, the patient still has mild hypoxemia with an F_IO_2 of 50% and PEEP +10 cm H_2O. The patient's C_S is 43 mL/cm H_2O. Therefore his lungs are not stiff.

3. Because the patient does not have stiff lungs, an increase in PEEP is not appropriate at this time. According to the patient's ventilator settings, inspiratory time is only 0.4 second. This is not sufficient time for oxygenation. Inspiratory time should be at least 0.5 second. Therefore the most appropriate ventilator change would be to decrease the set flow rate to increase inspiratory time. This will increase the mP_{aw} and improve oxygenation. Decreasing the flow to 60 L/min (1 L/sec) will increase mP_{aw} to 12 cm H_2O.

Answers to NBRC-Style Questions

1. b	5. c	9. d
2. a	6. b	10. b
3. c	7. d	
4. c	8. b	

Chapter 17, Effects of Positive Pressure Ventilation on the Pulmonary System
Answers to Key Terms Crossword Puzzle

Crossword answers include:
ABSORPTION, VOLUTRAUMA, PVR, CARDIAC TAMPONADE, PLATEAU, HYPOVENTILATION, ENDOGENOUS, EXOGENOUS, DYSSYNCHRONY, DEEP SULCUS SIGN, VAP

Answers to Review Questions

1. *Volutrauma* is lung injury caused by excessive volume in the lungs. *Biotrauma* is caused by the release of inflammatory mediators that cause problems in other organs of the body. *Atelectrauma* is the term used for shear stress injury and loss of surfactant in the lungs.

2. VILI is a form of lung injury that occurs at the alveolar level and resembles ARDS. VALI includes injury from extraalveolar gas, patient ventilator dyssynchrony, air trapping, and VAP.

3. High peak airway pressures with low end-expiratory pressures; presence of bullae; high levels of PEEP with high V_T; aspiration of gastric acid; necrotizing pneumonias. This answer is also correct: ALI/ARDS.

4. Subcutaneous emphysema

5. a pneumothorax

6. Treatment for a pneumothorax involves placing a 14-gauge needle into the anterior second to third intercostal space on the affected side in the midclavicular line over the top of the rib with the patient in the upright position.

7. The patient should be manually ventilated with a resuscitation bag on 100% O_2 with a manometer in-line to monitor pressure.

8. Absent breath sounds on the affected side; tracheal deviation away from the affected side; tympanic percussion note over the affected side; neck vein distention

9. The chest radiograph would have one diaphragm more depressed than the other and may display a deep sulcus sign with air appearing adjacent to the depressed diaphragm.

10. pneumoperitoneum

11. 30 to 35 cm H_2O

12. The lungs are very stiff and the pleural pressure is near normal; the lungs are normal, but there is a right mainstem intubation with a large V_T; both lungs are overdistended inside a normal chest wall.

13. Volutrauma, or damage from overdistention, occurs because of regional differences in lung compliance. The more compliant lung areas will fill more easily and expand to accommodate large volumes, whereas the noncompliant areas do not. The overdistention causes alveolar injury and the formation of pulmonary edema by both increased permeability and filtration mechanisms. The excess stretching of the alveolar cells leads to the release of chemical mediators, which cause inflammation.

14. Placing the patient in the prone position will restrict the chest wall movement and minimize lung injury from overdistention.

15. Managing a patient with ALI/ARDS with low V_T and inadequate levels of PEEP

16. Shear stress; surfactant alteration; microvascular injury

17. Cytokines and TNF (others include platelet activating factor, thromboxane B_2, interleukin-1β)

18. Overdistention causes chemical mediator release, which can leak into the blood vessels. The circulation then carries these substances to other areas of the body and causes inflammatory reactions in other organs such as the kidneys, gut, and liver.

19. Multiple organ dysfunction syndrome can be avoided during mechanical ventilation by using lung-protective strategies such as low V_T and therapeutic PEEP.

20. Ventilation and perfusion are best matched in the dependent lung areas near the back.

21. The diaphragm is most displaced in the nondependent regions of the lung; therefore gas flows easily to this area, whereas blood flow to this area is decreased. Alveolar collapse is most likely to occur in the dependent areas of the lung where perfusion is greatest.

22. The cause of increased PVR in most patients is severe hypoxemia.

23. Nasotracheal tube or ET; IV lines; central venous lines; arterial monitors; PA catheters; intracranial pressure monitors; indwelling urinary catheters

24. Severity of illness; increased length of stay; increased age and disability; previous or current use of antibiotics; use of invasive devices (ET, IV catheters); major surgery; supine position; presence of COPD; immunosuppression

25. VAP refers to pneumonia acquired 48 hours after intubation in a patient receiving mechanical ventilation.

26. Microaspiration or silent aspiration is the main reason for VAP.

27. *Pseudomonas aeruginosa*, *Klebsiella pneumoniae*, and *Escherichia coli* (others include *Enterobacter* spp., *Serratia marcescens*, *Acinetobacter calcoaceticus*, *Proteus mirabilis* and *Haemophilus influenzae*)

28. *Staphylococcus aureus* and *Streptococcus pneumoniae*

29. Early-onset VAP is often associated with community-acquired bacteria that are susceptible to antibiotic therapy. Late-onset VAP is typically caused by an antibiotic-resistant nosocomial organism.

30. Fever greater than 38.2° C; WBC greater than 10,000/mL; purulent secretions aspirate (more than 25 neutrophils/hpf by Gram stain); new infiltrates on chest radiograph

31. Gram stain and culture of endotracheal aspirates may be helpful in diagnosing the presence of VAP.

32. VAP develops in the presence of chronic microaspiration of subglottic secretions from the oropharynx or stomach. These secretions contain the infecting organism. When the organism reaches the alveolar level the host defenses are overwhelmed either by the virulence of the organism or by the inoculum's size.

33. Endogenous sources of microorganisms include bacterial colonies in the nose, mouth, oropharynx and trachea; sinusitis; gastric colonization; and hematogenous spread.

34. Exogenous sources of microorganisms include biofilm of the tracheal tube, ventilator circuits, nebulizers, humidifiers, and health care workers.

35. Noninvasive ventilation has a lower rate of nosocomial pneumonia than does invasive mechanical ventilation.

36. The semirecumbent position, if tolerated by the patient, has been shown to be a useful, low-cost, low-risk procedure that is effective in reducing the aspiration of gastric contents when compared with the supine position.

37. As the acidity of gastric contents decreases, gastric colonization by potentially pathogenic organisms increases.

38. VAP risk increases when intracuff pressures are less than 20 cm H_2O.

39. Before deflating the cuff, suction and clear secretions above it.

40. The caregiver should be wearing a gown and using aseptic technique.

41. Continuous aspiration of subglottic secretions (CASS) reduces the number of gram-positive cocci and *Haemophilus influenzae* organisms and demonstrates an approximately 50% reduction in VAP.

42. Ventilator circuits should be changed when they are nonfunctional or if they are visibly soiled with secretions or blood.

43. The SVN should be disinfected, rinsed with sterile water, and air dried.

44. Having a dedicated person or group take ownership of the process; having a mechanism for tracking the rates of nosocomial infections; distributing the information obtained; developing a plan for dealing with ways to improve care

45. Acidosis causes a right shift in the oxyhemoglobin dissociation curve and reduces the ability of the hemoglobin to bind and carry oxygen in the lung. Alkalosis causes a left shift in the oxygen dissociation curve, which enhances the ability of hemoglobin to pick up oxygen in the lungs but makes it less available at the tissue level.

46. At the tissue level, acidosis facilitates the unloading of oxygen.

47. Hypoventilation leads to elevated hydrogen ion concentrations, which in turn increase serum potassium levels. Hyperkalemia can lead to cardiac dysrhythmias.

48. Sensitivity or flow may be inadequate.

49. Hypoxemia; pain and anxiety syndromes; circulatory failure; airway inflammation

50. Prolonged periods of hyperventilation while receiving mechanical ventilation stop respiratory muscle activity, which leads to respiratory muscle atrophy.

51. Hyperventilation causes respiratory alkalosis, which leads to the diffusion of CO_2 out of the CSF because of the low blood CO_2 levels. Accordingly, the H^+ concentration in the CSF decreases and respirations are not stimulated.

52. In the presence of life-threatening hyperkalemia either caused by or associated with metabolic acidosis and in the presence of toxin excretion, such as salicylate toxicity

53. HCO_3^- required = [(wt. kg ÷ 3) × BE]/2

54. Vomiting; administration of diuretics; bicarbonate; lactate; acetate; citrate

55. Administration of carbonic anhydrase inhibitors, infusion of ammonium chloride or potassium chloride, or low sodium dialysis

56. Direct measurement of auto-PEEP, observing flow-time waveform, through measurement of PAWP

57. 3 to 4 time constants

58. *Dynamic hyperinflation* is the failure of lung volume to return to passive FRC during exhalation by the time the next inspiration begins.

59. Mechanical ventilatory settings that increase risk of auto-PEEP include (1) minute ventilation more than 10 to 20 L/min, (2) high respiratory frequency, (3) short expiratory time, and (4) high V_T.

60. Increased risk of auto-PEEP occurs with patients who (1) have COPD; (2) are older than 60 years; (3) have increased airway resistance from a small ET, bronchospasm, increased secretions, or mucosal edema; and (4) have increased lung compliance (longer time constants).

61. Auto-PEEP slows the beginning of gas flow during inspiration because flow delivery will not start until P_M exceeds P_A, which is now higher than ambient pressure at the end of exhalation. Auto-PEEP also makes it more difficult for spontaneously breathing patients to trigger a ventilator breath even when sensitivity settings are appropriate.

62. $C_S = V_T/[P_{plateau} - (PEEP + auto\text{-}PEEP)]$
$= 525 \text{ mL}/[30 \text{ cm } H_2O - (12 \text{ cm } H_2O + 5 \text{ cm } H_2O)]$
$= 525/[30 - 17]$
$= 525/13 = 40.4 \text{ mL/cm } H_2O$

63. Shorten inspiratory time and allow for longer expiratory time by increasing the inspiratory flow rate; use a smaller V_T and low respiratory rates to increase expiratory time; use low-resistance exhalation valves; use large ETs to reduce air trapping.

64. SIMV; pressure support; CPAP; APRV

65. Oxygen becomes a potential hazard when concentrations of more than 60% are administered for more than 48 hours in an adult and if the F_IO_2 provides a PaO_2 of more than 80 mm Hg in a newborn or premature infant.

66. VC will decrease; compliance will decrease; diffusing capacity will decrease; alveolar to arterial PO_2 difference will increase

67. Normal inspiratory WOB is approximately 0.5 J/L or 0.05 kg·m/L.

68. 1.5 J/L (or 15 J/L/min)

69. A high spontaneous respiratory rate and use of accessory muscles

70. $\text{Work} = [PIP - (0.5 \times P_{plateau})]/(100 \times V_T \text{ in liters})$
$= [45 - (0.5 \times 33)]/(100 \times 0.475)$
$= 28.5/47.5$
$= 0.6 \text{ J/L}$

71. Use the largest possible ET; use pressure support when appropriate; use PEEP; use automatic tube compensation

72. Use of accessory muscles; tachypnea; retractions; chest-abdominal paradox

73. *Trigger dyssynchrony* occurs when the ventilator sensitivity setting is not appropriate for the patient. Adjusting the trigger setting appropriately or switching to flow triggering, which in older ventilators has a faster response time, may alleviate this problem.

74. 80 L/min

75. Pressure-targeted breaths, such as with PCV and PSV, because the ventilator rapidly provides a high flow to achieve and maintain the set pressure. As long as the set pressure is adequate, the flow to the patient will be adequate.

76. *Cycle dyssynchrony* occurs when the patient begins to exhale before the completion of a ventilator breath (inspiration). This may occur when inspiratory time is set too long by a control itself, or as a result of a combination of rate, flow, and volume settings.

77. During full ventilatory support either the flow rate can be increased to shorten T_I or the set T_I may be reduced. During spontaneous breaths the flow cycle percentage can be changed.

78. VC-SIMV with pressure support

79. Water traps; temperature probes; oxygen analyzers; humidification systems; or capnographs in the circuit.

80. Hypothermia; underhydration and impaction of mucous secretions; hypoventilation or alveolar gas trapping caused by mucus plugging of airways; possible increased resistive WOB caused by mucus plugging of airways; possible increased resistive WOB through the HME; possible hypoventilation caused by increased dead space; ineffective low-pressure alarm during disconnection because of resistance through HME.

Answers to Critical Thinking Questions

1. The patient-triggered breath displays inadequate ventilator flow, which causes the pressure-time curve to take on a concave shape.

2. Increasing the ventilator flow setting should alleviate this problem.

3. This scalar shows cycle dyssynchrony. The patient is actively trying to exhale before the end of the breath, as noted by the rise in pressure toward end inspiration.

4. The problem can be corrected by increasing the flow cycle percentage. This will end inspiration at a higher flow rate and shorten the inspiratory time.

Answers to Case Studies

Case Study #1

1. The most outstanding problem noted on the ventilator flow sheet is the fact that the arterial PCO_2 did not fall with incremental increases in the delivered minute ventilation.

2. Increasing PCO_2 in this patient cannot be caused by an increase in CO_2 production because the patient is unresponsive. The cause of this increase can only be accounted for by a progressive increase in dead space. The increased dead space is caused by auto-PEEP.

3. Barotrauma (subcutaneous emphysema, pneumothorax, pneumomediastinum); atelectrauma (shear stress, surfactant alteration, biotrauma); multiple organ dysfunction syndrome; increased WOB; ineffective triggering of the ventilator leading to respiratory muscle fatigue

4. The respiratory rate is set too high and is not allowing enough time for exhalation. This is causing the auto-PEEP. At 1400 hours with a respiratory rate of 40 breaths/min, the C_{STAT} is 8.4 mL/cm H_2O because the lungs are overinflated.

Case Study #2

1. Intubation; coma; leukocytosis (elevated WBC); nasogastric tube feedings; antibiotic therapy

2. Protected tracheal aspiration and protected tracheal specimen brush through fiberoptic bronchoscopy

Answers to NBRC-Style Questions

1. c	5. a	9. a
2. c	6. a	10. b
3. d	7. b	
4. d	8. c	

Chapter 18, Troubleshooting and Problem Solving
Answers to Key Terms Crossword Puzzle

ELECTROMAGNETIC
PULMONARY EDEMA
PNEUMOTHORAX
INNOMINATE
TACHYCARDIA
DYSSYNCHRONY
RINGING
ASYNCHRONY
TROUBLESHOOTING
ASCITES
BRONCHOSPASM
THROMBOLYTIC

Answers to Review Questions

1. A *problem* is a situation in which a person finds discord or in which a person is uncomfortable and does not have an immediate solution.

2. *Troubleshooting*, in the context of mechanical ventilation, is the identification and resolution of technical malfunctions in the patient ventilator system. It involves purposefully resolving inappropriate and potentially dangerous situations.

3. Patient safety is the RT's first priority. The RT needs to be sure that the patient is adequately ventilated and oxygenated.

4. Immediate steps to assess the patient include type of alarm, patient's level of consciousness, color, use of accessory muscles, chest wall movement, breath sounds, pulse oximeter reading, and pulse.

5. The RT should disconnect the patient from the ventilator and begin manual ventilation with a resuscitation bag.

6.

Advantages	Disadvantages
Ensuring the patient is being ventilated, assessing (feeling) the patient's lung compliance and airway resistance, and determining if the problem lies with the patient or the ventilator.	Increased risk of barotrauma from inappropriate patterns of ventilation and excessive pressures; derecruitment of the lungs when PEEP is lost, leading to desaturation; and increased risk of VAP from contamination of the airways. Therefore manual ventilation should be reserved for situations in which the patient is not being adequately ventilated or oxygenated.

7. Retraction of the suprasternal, supraclavicular, and intercostal spaces; accessory muscle use; nasal flaring; hypotension; arrhythmias; tachycardia; diaphoresis; abnormal movement of thorax and abdomen; tachypnea; and abnormal breath sounds

8. Bronchospasm; secretions; pulmonary edema; pulmonary embolus; dynamic hyperinflation; pneumothorax

9. Artificial airway problems; abnormal respiratory drive; alteration in body posture; drug-induced problems; abdominal distention; anxiety

10. Patient-ventilator dyssynchrony may be caused by (1) inappropriate ventilatory support mode, (2) inappropriate trigger sensitivity, (3) inappropriate inspiratory flow setting, (4) inappropriate cycle variable, (5) inappropriate PEEP setting, and (6) problems with closed-loop ventilation.

11. System leaks, circuit malfunctions or disconnections, and inadequate F_IO_2

12. When the patient is in severe distress, disconnecting the patient from the ventilator and manually ventilating the patient allows the RT to distinguish the cause of the distress. If the patient's distress immediately ends, the problem is with the ventilator. If the distress does not subside, the problem is with the patient.

13. Remove the patient from the ventilator; initiate manual ventilation with a self-inflating resuscitation bag with 80% to 100% supplemental oxygen and maintain normal ventilating pressures; manually evaluate compliance and resistance through bag ventilation; perform a rapid physical examination and assess monitored indexes and alarms; check patency of the airway by passing a suction catheter; if death appears imminent, consider and treat most likely causes: pneumothorax or airway obstruction; once the patient is stabilized, perform a more detailed assessment and management

14. Measured at the teeth, an ET should measure between 22 and 24 cm for men and 20 to 22 for women.

15. A patient with a pneumothorax will exhibit use of accessory muscles, uneven chest wall movement, absence of breath sounds on the affected side, hyperresonant percussion on the affected side, tracheal deviation away from the affected side, and an increase in plateau and peak pressures.

16. A 14- or 16-gauge needle should be inserted into the second intercostal space at the midclavicular line over the top of the rib on the affected side.

17. Bronchospasm should be suspected when a patient exhibits dyspnea; wheezing; accessory muscle use; paradoxical chest and abdominal movement; retractions of the suprasternal, supraclavicular, and intercostal spaces; and an increase in PIP and $P_{plateau}$.

18. Secretion problems may be avoided by providing warmed and humidified gas to the patient and suctioning when indicated. Bronchial hygiene, including postural drainage, percussion, and therapeutic bronchoscopy, may be performed.

19. Cardiogenic pulmonary edema can occur suddenly. Noncardiogenic pulmonary edema or ARDS usually develops over a day or two and is not a sudden-onset problem.

20. Pain, anxiety, increased peripheral sensory receptor stimulation, medications, increased ventilatory needs, and inappropriate ventilator settings

21. These are the clinical manifestations of a pulmonary embolism. Pulmonary embolism can be confirmed with a pulmonary angiogram and treated with thrombolytic therapy.

22. Leaks are often present around the ET cuff, at junctions in the patient circuit where connections exist, including water traps, HME or humidifiers, in-line suction catheters, temperature probes, in-line metered dose inhaler chambers, proximal airway pressure lines, capnography sensors, and exhalation valves.

23. Patient disconnection, leaks in the ventilator circuit, airway leaks, or chest tube leaks.

24. High Pressure alarm situations may be caused by airway-related problems such as secretions or mucus, coughing, patient biting the tube, or the tube migrating into the right mainstem. Lung conditions that may lead to high pressure alarm situations include increased airway resistance from bronchospasm, mucosal edema, or secretions; decreased compliance from a pneumothorax or pleural effusion; and patient-ventilator asynchrony. Other causes of high pressure alarms situations include accumulation of water condensate in the patient circuit, kinking of the inspiratory circuit, or malfunction of the inspiratory or expiratory valves.

25. PIP = 30 cm H_2O, low pressure alarm setting = 20 – 25 cm H_2O, and high pressure alarm setting = 40 cm H_2O.

26. A leak in the circuit that is not being compensated for by the ventilator, or active inspiration by the patient that drops the pressure below the alarm threshold

27. Patient apnea, patient disconnect, system leaks, inadequate machine sensitivity, or inappropriately set apnea parameters.

28. Disconnected high-pressure line and source gas failure

29. Loss of power and not connected to an emergency power outlet during a power test

30. A "vent inop" alarm will be triggered by an internal malfunction usually detected by the ventilator's self-testing systems.

31. A leak in a patient ventilator system may cause low pressure, low volume, low minute volume, and apnea alarms to ring. On a volume-time scalar the volume would not go down to zero at the end of the breath. On a volume-pressure loop and flow-volume loop the volume would not return to zero.

32. Simultaneously looks at the flow-time and pressure-time scalars can alert the RT to inadequate flow. The flow curve will be constant and the pressure-time graphic will be concave when inadequate flow is present.

33. Auto-PEEP may be detected when the expiratory flow on a flow-time scalar does not return to zero before the next mandatory breath. It may also be detected on a flow-volume loop when the loop is not closed between expiration and inspiration.

34. ringing, spiking, or overshooting

35. The gas flow and pressure delivery at the beginning of the breath can be adjusted with the inspiratory rise time parameter.

36. Air trapping; an active exhalation; a flow sensor out of calibration

37. An externally powered nebulizer can (1) cause the accumulation of residue on the expiratory valve, (2) block the machine's ability to sense a patient's inspiratory effort, (3) increase V_T delivery, and (4) cause auto-PEEP. (It can also cause a leak if it becomes disconnected.)

38. Turning a ventilated patient may cause accidental extubation, kinking of the patient circuit, changes in oxygenation level, or dislodging of a clot that may lead to a pulmonary embolus.

39. ET cuff leak may cause low pressure, low PEEP/CPAP, low V_T, or low minute volume alarms to be activated.

40.

Clinical Findings	Right Mainstem Intubations	Left-Sided Pneumothorax	Right-Sided Pneumothorax
PIP	increased	increased	increased
$P_{plateau}$	increased	increased	increased
breath sounds	decreased over the left lung	decreased over the left lung	decreased over the right lung
chest movement	asymmetrical, increased on right	asymmetrical, increased on right	asymmetrical, increased on left
percussion	resonance over right, decreased resonance over left	hyperresonance (tympanic) over left	hyperresonance (tympanic) over right
tracheal shift	none	toward the right	toward the left

41. The presence of a pulmonary embolus should be suspected when the end-tidal CO_2 value is decreased when compared with previous values. A widening of the arterial-to–end-tidal partial pressure CO_2 gradient will also be present.

42. The reduced volume delivery while in pressure control is most likely from a decrease in lung compliance or an increase in airway resistance.

43. In addition to the PIP, the RT needs to measure the $P_{plateau}$. An increase in P_{TA} is indicative of an increase in airway resistance, whereas an increase in both PIP and $P_{plateau}$, with a constant P_{TA}, is evidence of decreasing lung compliance.

44. Cycle dyssynchrony

45. A slight elevation of pressure would occur at the end of inspiration of a pressure-time scalar. This is actually active exhalation.

46. An intermittent high pressure alarm may be activated by patient coughing or biting the ET.

47. The ET could be completely blocked with mucus or the patient could be biting the ET. For a completely blocked ET, the ET must be changed. If the patient is biting the ET, a bite block needs to be inserted.

48. Suction the airway, administer bronchodilator therapy, allow more time for exhalation by increasing flow rate or decreasing inspiratory time, decrease minute ventilation, or increase the ET size if appropriate

49. The I:E ratio indicator and alarm are activated when I:E is greater than 1:1. This may be caused by an increased airway resistance, decreased lung compliance, or an inadequate flow setting for the desired V_T delivery.

50. The ventilator could be auto-triggering, the patient's metabolism could have increased, the alarm may be set inappropriately, or the patient could be hypoxemic.

Answers to Critical Thinking Questions

1. Check the ET position and try to pass the suction catheter into the tube to assess the patency of the artificial airway. If the ET is obstructed and cannot be cleared the ET needs to be changed.

2. Total or partial occlusion of the artificial airway by secretions, patient biting the ET, ET slipped into the right mainstem (also patient circuit obstructed, pneumothorax, patient-ventilator dyssynchrony)

3. Change the artificial airway if totally occluded, suction out secretions if necessary, insert a bite block if patient is biting, or reposition the artificial airway if it is in the right mainstem (also drain condensate and check for kinks, put in chest tube, check mode and settings for dyssynchrony)

4. When the high pressure alarm threshold is reached the ventilator will alarm, limit the pressure, and prematurely cycle to exhalation. This can severely decrease the delivered V_T and therefore trigger the low exhaled V_T alarm. After several seconds of the low V_T alarm, the low exhaled minute volume alarm will begin ringing if the high pressure threshold is still being met.

5. The patient may not be ready to handle all the spontaneous breathing, or auto-PEEP may be present, making it very difficult for the patient to trigger spontaneous breaths. Both situations could cause the apnea alarm.

6. Place the patient back on a mode of ventilation that provides more support for the patient; if auto-PEEP is suspected, decrease the pressure support and/or the CPAP level

Answers to Case Studies

Case Study #1

1. The flow-volume loop shows increased airway resistance.

2. This patient needs an aerosolized $\beta2$ adrenergic bronchodilator.

Case Study #2

1. The patient should be disconnected from the ventilator and manually ventilated to see if this will relieve the patient's distress. Pass a catheter to check the patency of the ET.

2. Increasing the F_IO_2 as well as the PEEP did not relieve the patient's oxygen status. The capnography reads low on the $P_{ET}CO_2$. The most likely cause of this patient's distress is a pulmonary embolism.

Case Study #3

1. An increase in P_{TA} with a stable plateau pressure means that the rising PIP is caused by an increase in airway resistance.

2. Increased secretions, bronchospasm, mucosal edema, and high inspiratory flow rates

3. Suction the ET, auscultate lungs, if bronchospasm is likely give aerosolized $\beta2$ adrenergic bronchodilator, adjust inspiratory flow rate if necessary

Answers to NBRC-Style Questions

1. c	5. b	9. c
2. a	6. c	10. b
3. c	7. d	11. b
4. c	8. b	12. c

Chapter 19, Basic Concepts of Noninvasive Positive Pressure Ventilation
Answers to Key Terms Crossword Puzzle

Crossword answers (words formed in the grid):

- CPAP
- IRON LUNG
- IPPB
- CENTRAL
- FATIGUE
- RAMP
- SIMETHICONE
- PASSOVER
- CAP
- IAPV
- VELCRO
- ORONASAL
- PNEUMOBE (PNEUMOBELT)
- CARDIOGENIC
- OBSTRUCTIVE
- CHESTCUIRASS
- PPV
- COMPLIANCE
- NPV
- SECONDARY
- PRESSURESUPPORT
- DELAY
- EPAP
- IPAP
- PNEUMAP
- NCPAP
- CONSENSUS
- PISSIST (PISSISTAT)
- VELCRO
- ROCKING

Answers to Review Questions

1. The delivery of mechanical ventilation to the lungs by techniques that do not require an endotracheal airway

2. NPVs operate by intermittently applying negative pressure to the entire body region below the neck or upper region of the chest. This negative pressure is transmitted across the chest wall, into the pleural space, and finally into the alveolar space. The result is an increase in transpulmonary pressure, which causes air to enter the lungs. Exhalation is passive and depends on the elastic recoil of the lungs and chest wall.

3. iron lung and chest cuirass

4. An IAPV moves the abdominal contents and the diaphragm to facilitate breathing.

5. A pneumobelt contains a motorized inflatable bladder that fits like a corset over the abdomen. The motor inflates the bladder, which pushes the diaphragm upwards, facilitating exhalation. The bladder deflates during inspiration, returning the diaphragm to its resting position during a passive inhalation. The device can only assist spontaneous breathing while a patient is standing or sitting.

6. rocking bed

7. NPPV operates with the use of small pressure- and volume-targeted ventilators that are lightweight, easy to operate, and have variable interfaces.

8. Decreases need for intubation; decreases rate of nosocomial pneumonia; decreases length of ICU stay; decreases length of hospital stay; decreases mortality rate; preserves airway defenses; improves patient comfort; decreases need for sedation

9. Alleviates symptoms of chronic hypoventilation; improves duration and quality of sleep; improves functional capacity; prolongs survival

10. The avoidance of intubation and invasive ventilation are the two most significant benefits.

11. NPPV in ARF improves gas exchange by resting the respiratory muscles and increasing alveolar ventilation.

12. NPPV by facemask for ARF from COPD significantly reduces the need for intubation, decreases the duration of mechanical ventilation, decreases the length of stay in the ICU, decreases complications, and reduces mortality rate.

13. Mask CPAP (10 to 12 cm H_2O), and if the patient remains hypercapnic and dyspneic with CPAP, then a trial of NPPV by mask with PSV plus PEEP has been found to be effective for the treatment of cardiogenic pulmonary edema.

14. Chronic hypoventilation, nocturnal desaturation, respiratory muscle fatigue, and poor sleep quality

15. Fatigue; morning headache; daytime hypersomnolence; cognitive dysfunction; dyspnea

16. 4 to 6 hours

17. Nocturnal or intermittent daytime NPPV shows improvement in daytime gas exchange and respiratory muscle strength and alleviates symptoms of hypoventilation for patients with neuromuscular disorders.

18. Patients with chronic, stable COPD may benefit from NPPV if they have severe daytime CO_2 retention (CO_2 52 mm Hg or greater) and nocturnal hypoventilation despite the administration of nocturnal oxygen therapy.

19. NPPV could help support a patient with advanced CF while the patient awaits lung transplantation.

20. OSA that does not respond to CPAP is an indication for NPPV.

21. Decreasing the number of days a patient spends receiving invasive mechanical ventilation decreases the risk of infection and other complications, lowers mortality rate, and lowers health care costs.

22. After extubation NPPV can reduce WOB and maintain adequate gas exchange for patients who exhibit fatigue.

23. NPPV may provide relief from severe dyspnea and preserve patient comfort. NPPV may also reverse the acute process in disorders such as COPD or pulmonary edema and give the patient more time to live.

24. 1. acute exacerbation of COPD; 2. acute asthma; 3. hypoxemic respiratory failure; 4. community-acquired pneumonia; 5. cardiogenic pulmonary edema; 6. immunocompromised patients; 7. postoperative patients; 8. postextubation (weaning); 9. do not intubate

25. Moderate to severe dyspnea is indicated by a respiratory rate greater than 24 breaths/min, accessory muscle use, and paradoxical breathing.

26. Physiological criteria for NPPV are either (1) $PaCO_2$ more than 45 mm Hg and pH less than 7.35, or (2) PaO_2/F_IO_2 less than 200.

27. Respiratory arrest or the need for immediate intubation; hemodynamic instability; inability to protect the airway; excessive secretions; agitation and confusion; facial deformities or conditions that prevent mask fit; uncooperative or unmotivated patient; brain injury with unstable respiratory drive

28. NPPV is recommended for these patients when $PaCO_2$ is 45 mm Hg or more or when sustained nocturnal desaturation occurs as evidenced by an SpO_2 less than 88% for more than 5 consecutive minutes, MIP is less than 60 cm H_2O, and FVC is less than 50% predicted.

29. $PaCO_2$ greater than 55 mm Hg; $PaCO_2$ 50 to 54 with SpO_2 less than 88% for 5 consecutive minutes; $PaCO_2$ 50 to 54 with recurrent hospitalizations for hypercapneic respiratory failure (more than 2 hospitalizations in a 12-month period)

30. Polysomnographic evidence of OSA not responsive to CPAP

31. Pressure-targeted ventilators have a single-circuit gas delivery system that uses an intentional leak port for patient exhalation instead of a true exhalation valve.

32. These ventilators are flow and time triggered, pressure limited, and flow and time cycled.

33. IPAP and EPAP

34. IPAP 2 to 30 cm H_2O and EPAP 2 to 20 cm H_2O

35. CPAP, assist mode, assist/control, and control (timed) mode

36. The patient's delivered V_T depends on the gradient between the IPAP level and the EPAP level, the inspiratory time, patient inspiratory effort, and the patient's lung characteristics.

37. The source for unintentional leaks is around the patient interface (e.g., mask).

38. Flow triggering is made easier by the PTV's ability to compensate for leaks.

39. inspiratory and expiratory sensitivity controls

40. 1. oxygen flow rate; 2. type of leak port in the system; 3. site where oxygen is bled into the circuit; 4. IPAP and EPAP pressure levels

41. An inadequate continuous flow will prevent exhaled gases from being flushed from the system, causing the patient to rebreathe exhale CO_2.

42. It depends on the EPAP setting and the patient's I:E ratio.

43. An EPAP level of 4 cm H_2O or more will keep the continuous gas flow high enough to avoid CO_2 rebreathing.

44. The newer portable volume ventilators are designed to be used for either invasive or noninvasive ventilation. This will facilitate a seamless transition from the extended care facility to the home.

45.

Advantages	Disadvantages
Availability of more ventilatory support options, more alrms, precise F_1O_2 levels, more monitoring features than portable PTVs	Prolonged inspiratory phase caused by leaks with no compensation, increased WOB from active exhalation, impaired ability to flow trigger because of increased flow in circuit

46. The patient would be most comfortable in the PC-CMV during NPPV because cycling to exhalation will be a function of time instead of a function of flow. This may provide better synchronization with the ventilator and less patient respiratory effort.

47. Heated humidity reduces drying of the nasal mucosa that may lead to nasal congestion and increased nasal resistance. Mucosal drying will lead to patient discomfort and noncompliance.

48. A heated passover humidifier should be used.

49. The nasal mask is the most widely used interface for administration of CPAP and NPPV.

50. The nasal mask is easier to fit and secure to the patient's face. It is more tolerable for those who are claustrophobic. The nasal mask allows the patient to cough and clear secretions, speak, and possibly eat; less mechanical dead space is also present, which reduces the potential for rebreathing CO_2.

51. Air leaks and skin irritations

52. When large leaks occur through the mouth the oronasal mask may be used.

53. Disadvantages to face masks with NPPV include the risk for aspiration from vomit; asphyxia if the ventilator malfunctions; increased dead space, leading to CO_2 retention; the inability of the patient to eat, communicate, cough, and expectorate secretions; and claustrophobia.

54. Mouthpieces and lip seals do not allow leaks from the mouth and they minimize CO_2 rebreathing.

55. (1) Patient should be sitting upright; NPPV procedure, goals, and potential complications should be explained. (2) Size the patient for a properly fitted mask. (3) Attach mask and circuit to ventilator. Turn ventilator on and set EPAP to 4 to 5 cm H_2O and IPAP to 8 to 10 cm H_2O. (4) Allow the patient to hold the mask to the face. Encourage proper breathing techniques. (5) Monitor pulse oximetry and adjust F_1O_2 to maintain saturation greater than 90%. (6) Secure the mask to the patient while avoiding excessive tightening of the straps. (7) Titrate IPAP and EPAP levels to achieve patient comfort, adequate exhaled V_T, and synchrony with the ventilator. Avoid peak pressures greater than 20 cm H_2O. (8) Check for leaks and readjust straps if necessary. (9) Monitor respiratory rate, pulse, level of dyspnea, pulse oximetry, minute ventilation, and exhaled V_T. (10) Obtain a blood gas reading within 1 hour.

56. Clinical indicators that demonstrate improved patient comfort include a decrease in respiratory rate, a decrease in inspiratory muscle activity, and synchronization with the ventilator.

57. When the patient is not comfortable with NPPV, corrective measures include refitting or changing the mask to decrease air leaks, encouraging and coaching the patient in the proper breathing pattern, and adjusting the ventilator settings.

58. 5 to 7 mL/kg or greater

59. Worsening pH and $PaCO_2$, tachypnea (more than 30 beats/min), decreased level of consciousness, hemodynamic instability, SpO_2 less than 90%, inability to clear secretions, and inability to tolerate interfaces

60. 4 to 6 hours per 24 hours

61. Lack of motivation and compliance because of discomfort, advanced age, or the existence of comorbidities; cognitive defects or the need for additional therapeutic efforts

62. Mask discomfort; air pressures; flows

63. Eye irritation is usually a result of air leaks from around the mask. The mask should be refitted or resized and changed.

64. The straps may be too tight because of the mask being too large. The mask should be refitted or resized and changed to a different style (e.g., nasal pillows, nasal seal, nasal gel masks). Forehead spacers or wound care dressing should be applied to alleviate pressure on the nasal bridge.

65. Nose clips may alleviate this problem.

66. It is a common occurrence that may be diminished with the administration of simethicone agents.

67. Aspiration pneumonia; mucus plugging; hypoxemia; hypotension; respiratory arrest

68. Increasing periods of time off NPPV

Answers to Critical Thinking Questions

1. When both IPAP and EPAP are equal or set at the same setting, the ventilator will not deliver a timed or spontaneously triggered breath. The pressure will remain constant in the circuit at the set pressure supplying CPAP.

2. Issues such as drying of the nasal mucosa can be avoided with a heated humidifier, improper interfaces leading to leakage can be avoided by ensuring that the mask is not too large, and skin irritations from tight straps can be avoided by minimizing headgear tension as much as possible and using forehead spacers.

3. Portable PTVs use a leak port for patient exhalation instead of a true exhalation valve. The leak port allows a continuous flow of gas through it to help maintain pressure levels and flush exhaled gases from the circuit. If this port and the oxygen bleed-in are located in the same area, the oxygen bled into the circuit would be lost through the leak port. Therefore, to achieve the highest oxygen concentrations, the leak port and oxygen bleed-in must be located as far apart as possible (e.g., leak port in the circuit and oxygen bled into the patient mask).

Answers to Case Studies

Case Study #1

1. Yes, the patient is demonstrating signs of moderate to severe dyspnea as evidenced by a respiratory rate greater than 24 breaths/min (28 breaths/min) and accessory muscle use with a $PaCO_2$ greater than 45 mm Hg (49 mm Hg), pH less than 7.35 (7.31), and PaO_2/F_1O_2 less than 200 (53 ÷ approximately 0.7 = 76).

2. NPPV beginning with IPAP/EPAP 10/5 cm H_2O to start by nasal mask if tolerated by patient. Bleed in oxygen to titrate SpO_2 to between 90% and 92%. Titrate the IPAP until V_T is at least 5 to 7 mL/kg.

3. This patient is demonstrating criteria for the termination of NPPV. The patient should be intubated and placed on invasive mechanical ventilation.

Case Study #2

1. Acute hypercapnic respiratory failure superimposed on chronic respiratory failure is seen in the ABG; bronchospasm is evidenced by the wheezing; hypoxemia is evidenced by the ABG and the presence of cyanosis; retained secretions are evidenced by the productive sputum; upper respiratory tract infection is evidenced by the elevated WBC and green purulent sputum

2. Aerosolized albuterol 2.5 mg and ipratropium bromide 0.5 mg, air entrainment mask with 24% oxygen (or 28%), repeat ABG (IV antibiotics and a sputum culture and sensitivity)

3. NPPV

Answers to NBRC-Style Questions

1. a	5. d	9. c
2. b	6. a	10. c
3. b	7. d	
4. c	8. a	

Chapter 20, Discontinuation of and Weaning from Mechanical Ventilation
Answers to Key Terms Crossword Puzzle

Crossword solution (across answers): PRESSURE SUPPORT, PARADOXICAL, STRIDOR, RESPIRATORY ALTERNANS, RACEMIC, CROP, SLUG, ATC, EXTUBATION, GLOTTIC EDEMA. Down/partial answers include: NEUROMUSCULAR, SBT, WEAN, CANNING, SPINKLE, etc.

Answers to Review Questions

1. The gradual reduction of ventilatory support from a patient who is improving

2. Recovery from anesthesia; treatment of uncomplicated drug overdose; exacerbations of asthma

3. VILI; nosocomial pneumonia; airway trauma from the ET; unnecessary sedation

4. Ventilatory muscle fatigue; compromised gas exchange; loss of airway protection; higher mortality rate

5. SIMV; PSV; T-piece

6. SIMV

7. improvement or reversal of the condition that required mechanical ventilation

8. The patient's respiratory muscles work during spontaneous breathing intervals and rest during mandatory mechanical breaths.

9. Pressure support should be added to reduce the patient's WOB during spontaneous breaths and prevent excessive fatigue.

10. patient-, pressure-, flow-

11. The patient controls the rate, time, and depth of each breath.

12. The pressure level that accomplishes a reasonable ventilatory pattern for a given patient

13. A respiratory rate of 15 to 25 breaths/min and a V_T of 300 to 600 mL

14. Tachycardia, hypertension, tachypnea, diaphoresis, paradoxical breathing, respiratory alternans, and excessive accessory muscle use

15. 5 cm H_2O

16. A time schedule that progressively increases the length of time the patient is removed from ventilatory support

17. This method requires constant monitoring by a clinician.

18. a. CPAP; b. provides continuous monitoring of the patient and backup ventilator modes in case of apnea

19. Patients with (1) severe underlying heart disease, (2) severe muscle weakness, (3) psychological problems, or (4) preexisting chronic lung conditions

20. Automatic tube compensation; volume-targeted pressure support ventilation (e.g., volume support); mandatory minute ventilation; adaptive support ventilation; knowledge-based system

21. | **Weaning mode** | **Description** |
|---|---|
| C ATC | A. patient breathes spontaneously between mechanical breaths |
| F Volume support | B. similar to a T-piece with alarm capability |
| G MMV | C. compensates for increased resistance and WOB through an ET |
| F ASV | D. adjusts the PS level or mode based on measured parameters |
| D KBS | E. the patient controls the rate, time, and depth of each breath |
| A SIMV | F. provides pressure-limited breaths that target a specific volume and rate |
| E PSV | G. maintains a consistent, minimum $\dot{V}_E$ |
| B CPAP | H. delivers a set V_T in a pressure mode of ventilation |

22. Use of accessory muscles; asynchronous breathing; nasal flaring; diaphoresis; anxiety; tachypnea; substernal and intercostal retractions; patient asynchronous with ventilator; more than 1.8 kg·m/min (measured WOB) or more than 0.8 J/L; O_2 consumption 15% or more of total $\dot{V}O_2$

23. An increase in respiratory rate greater than 30 to 35 breaths/min; V_T decreases below 250 to 300 mL; a significant change in blood pressure (drop of 20 mm Hg systolic, a rise of 30 mm Hg systolic, systolic values greater than 180 mm Hg, a change of 10 mm Hg diastolic); a rise in HR more than 20% or above 140 beats/min; sudden onset of PVCs; diaphoresis; deterioration of ABG values and SpO_2

24. Search for all causes that may be contributing to ventilator dependence

25. Evidence of some reversal of underlying cause of respiratory failure; PaO_2 60 mm Hg or more on F_IO_2 0.4 or less, PaO_2/F_IO_2 ratio 150 to 200 mm Hg or more, PEEP 5 to 8 cm H_2O or less, F_IO_2 0.4 to 0.5 or less, pH 7.25 or more; hemodynamic stability (absence of hypotension and requiring no vasopressors); patient able to initiate an inspiratory effort

26. Fear; anxiety; delirium; ICU psychosis; depression; anger; fear of shortness of breath; fear of being left alone

27. a. Underfeeding results in muscle wasting (diaphragm, heart, and other organs). Malnutrition can also lead to a reduced central response to hypoxemia, hypercapnia, and an impaired immune response. b. Overfeeding may result in increased $\dot{V}O_2$, increased $\dot{V}CO_2$, and increased $\dot{V}_E$.

28. The patient is disconnected from the ventilator, the cuff is deflated, and the ET or tracheostomy tube is obstructed.

29. A leak of less than 110 mL may indicate the presence of subglottic edema and a high risk of postextubation stridor.

30. Because the test requires patient cooperation

31. The drive to breathe is established by measuring airway occlusion pressure.

32. ventilatory muscle strength

33. high, increased

34. a. CROP index; b. Compliance, respiratory rate, oxygenation, inspiratory pressure

35. a. CROP = $[C_D \times MIP \times (PaO_2/P_AO_2)] \div f$
    CROP = $[20 \times 25 \times (70 \div 1000)] \div 18$
    $= [500 \times 0.7] \div 18$
    $= 19.4$

    b. Yes. CROP values greater than 13 may indicate the likelihood of success in ventilator withdrawal.

36. 30 to 120 min

37. a. The RSBI is calculated by dividing respiratory frequency (breaths/min) by the V_T in liters. b. RSBI = $f \div V_T$; $26 \div 0.6 = 43.3$ c. Values less than 105 (range, 60 to 105) indicate successful weaning is more likely.

38. Patient's ability to protect the airway; airway patency

39. Ability to mobilize secretions; has a peritubular leak on cuff deflation; strong cough; no excessive secretions

40. Upper airway burns; a weak cough; large amounts of secretions

41. VAP; VILI; damage to the airway

42. a. Heliox is a low-density gas that may decrease the WOB by relieving the effects of partial airway obstruction and temporarily supporting gas exchange. This may provide time for medical treatment (e.g., racemic epinephrine and steroid administration). b. nonrebreathing mask

43. Use of muscle relaxants; the presence of a gastric tube; the presence of abnormal periglottic sensations; the ability to mechanically close the glottis; excessive amounts of secretions; the inability to effectively clear secretions

44. Patients who no longer need an artificial airway but require additional ventilatory support after extubation.

45. Improves survival; lowers mortality rate; reduces the risk of nosocomial pneumonia; lowers the incidence of septic shock; shortens the length of ICU and hospital stay

46. Resolution of problems leading to respiratory failure; ability to tolerate a spontaneous breathing trial for 10 to 15 minutes; strong cough reflex; hemodynamically stable; minimal airway secretions; low F_IO_2 requirements; functioning gastrointestinal tract; optimal nutritional status

47. Sedatives; narcotics; tranquilizers; hypnotic agents

48. These ventilator modes guarantee a certain breath rate and minute ventilation and are ideally suited for patients with unreliable respiratory drives.

49. Therapist-driven protocols shorten the time required for ventilatory support, result in a lower rate of extubation failures, and help reduce hospital costs.

50. who require high levels of sedation to tolerate ETs; who have marginal respiratory mechanics; who may gain psychological benefit from the ability to eat orally, communicate by speech, and experience greater mobility; whose increased mobility may aid physical therapy efforts

51. Less facial discomfort; decreased WOB; less dead space; better secretion removal; opportunity for oral feeding

52. The most important outcome from a tracheostomy is the facilitation of the discontinuation from mechanical ventilatory support.

53. Regional weaning centers; noninvasive respiratory care units; long-term acute care facilities; extended care facilities; long-term ventilator units in acute-care hospitals; home

54. Reduce the amount of ventilatory support; decrease the invasiveness of support; increase independence from mechanical devices; preserve or improve current function; maintain medical stability

Answers to Critical Thinking Questions

1. A leak of less than 80 mL may indicate the presence of subglottic edema and a high risk of postextubation stridor.

2. Treatment with steroids or racemic epinephrine before extubation.

3. Because the patient did not respond to the aerosolized racemic epinephrine, immediate reintubation is indicated.

Answers to Case Studies

Case Study #1

1. No reversal or significant improvement in the disease process or condition required ventilatory support.

2. The patient should be returned to full ventilatory support and reassessed.

Case Study #2

1. Because the patient has periods of apnea, a closed-loop mode of ventilation (mandatory minute ventilation, adaptive support ventilation) would be appropriate. A closed-loop system monitors the patient's $\dot{V}_E$ and automatically increases the level of support if a patient's spontaneous ventilation decreases, maintaining a consistent minimum $\dot{V}_E$.

Case Study #3

1. The patient does not have the muscle strength to generate an adequate V_T. The V_T of 185 mL is mostly dead space, resulting in little or no gas exchange. The patient is trying to compensate for the low V_T by increasing his respiratory rate.

2. Adding pressure support will augment the patient's spontaneous V_T, which will enhance ventilatory muscle conditioning without causing fatigue.

Answers to NBRC-Style Questions

1. d	5. b	9. d
2. a	6. b	10. d
3. c	7. c	
4. b	8. b	

Chapter 21, Long-Term Ventilation

Answers to Key Terms Crossword Puzzle

```
U S E R F R I E N D L Y               O
  E                 I                 O
  S         E S O P H A G U S         A       G
  P             C   N           A             G
  I             H   E                         L
  T             A   U                         O
  E             R   M           F             S
    J   P       G   O       I L E U S         O
D E C A N N U L A T E   B           N         O
  J   S   P           E     P       E         P
  U   S   V     V O C A L C O R D S           H
  N   Y         I   U   T   R       T         A
  O   M         N   I       T       R         R
  S   U         E   R   D M E       A         Y
  T   I         G   A       X       T         N
  O   R   V     A   S       M I E   E         G
  M     G A S T R O S T O M Y       D         E
  Y       I                                   A
                                              L
```

Answers to Review Questions

1. Enhance the individual's living potential, improve physical and psychological function, reduce morbidity, reduce hospitalizations, extend life, provide cost-effective care

2. The psychosocial well-being of a patient on long-term ventilation will improve when the patient progresses to the point of maximal activity.

3. Patients requiring mechanical ventilation longer than 7 days who remain unweanable after 4 weeks

4. Patients recovering from acute illness and those with chronic progressive disorders

5. Disease process, clinical stability, and psychosocial factors

6. Respiratory diagnosis, severity of symptoms, recent chest radiograph, pulmonary function tests, ABGs on current ventilator settings, nonrespiratory treatments

7. Factors to be considered include medical and physiological stability to the degree that they are free from any complications for at least 2 weeks before discharge. Medical stability would include stability of the cardiopulmonary and renal systems, no uncontrolled hemorrhage, no coma (or if comatose, prognosis for improvement), acceptable ABG values, freedom from acute respiratory infections and fever, no large fluctuations in F_IO_2 requirements, no high levels of airway pressure or PEEP required, and stable ventilator settings.

8. subacute care unit

9. Patient's diagnosis, age, level of acuity, need for personnel, type of ventilator selected, need for monitoring, supplemental oxygen, medications

10. Intensive care or acute care units, long-term acute care facilities, extended care facilities, the patient's home

11. Reliability, safety, versatility, user-friendly, easy patient cycling

12. **Backup Equipment**

Backup Equipment	Rationale
second mechanical ventilator	mechanical failure of primary ventilator
manual resuscitator	to provide ventilatory support
set backup ventilatory support mode	in case of electrical failure or ventilator malfunction
O_2 cylinder	to provide supplemental oxygen or failure of oxygen concentrator

13. Positive trends in weight gain and growth curve; stamina for periods of play while ventilated; family determined to be suitable candidates as shown by awareness of potential stressors of long-term health care; adequate family support from home nurses, aides, family, and friends

14. The ventilatory requirements of infants and children change because of their growth.

15. Patients unable to maintain adequate spontaneous ventilation for long periods; patients requiring continuous ventilatory support to survive; patients diagnosed as terminally ill, having little prognosis for long-term survival

16. Psychological evaluation of patient and family members, family's ability to provide necessary care, family's financial status, patient's and family's ability to learn necessary skills, availability of other health care providers

17. Size of patient care area to determine if it is adequate for prescribed equipment, adequate area for storage and cleaning of equipment, accessibility in and out of the home and in between rooms, availability of phone service, ability of electrical system to provide adequate amperage for all necessary electrical devices

18. Difficulty performing some procedures (suctioning); intimidated by the ventilator; not enough time for sleep, relaxation, and work

19. Refer to Box 21-7 of text: Respiratory Care Plan Equipment Checklist for Ventilator-Dependent Patients at the Home Site

20. 115- to 120-volt AC outlet, internal battery, 12-volt external battery

21.

Ventilator	Advantages	Disadvantages
Iron lung	Simple to use, noninvasive	Large, no access to patient (bronchial drainage, IV therapy, and physical contact with the patient difficult), lack of mobility, may cause upper airway obstruction
Chest cuirass	More mobility, better tolerated	Least efficient NPV, discomfort and skin abrasions, not adequate for severely compromised patients, may cause upper airway obstruction
Body suit	Best system besides iron lung, patients can sleep in their own beds	Very expensive, hard to seal completely, restricts movement and patient positioning, can result in muscle and joint pain

22. Excessive secretions; decreased pulmonary compliance; increased airway resistance; risk of aspiration

23. Use of the mode imposes an increase in the WOB.

24. The additional oxygen flow may make it more difficult for the ventilator to sense the patient's inspiratory effort. Adding PEEP may increase the patient's WOB if the sensitivity is not properly readjusted.

25. They are more versatile and provide additional features such as pressure-targeted ventilation, continuous-flow SIMV, F_IO_2 and internal PEEP controls, and apnea backup ventilation.

26. Pulmonary; cardiovascular; gastrointestinal

27. The threshold has become dislodged, resulting in a leak and loss of pressure.

28. Damage to gastrointestinal mucosa from stress; swallowing dysfunction and aspiration; constipation and ileus; erosive esophagitis

29. neurologic, ventilator dependence

30. Severity of illness; longevity of illness; multiple medications; sleep disruption; delirium; anxiety, depression

31. They operate by the principle of moving the abdominal contents and diaphragm to aid in breathing.

32. Obese patients; chest wall deformities; intrinsic lung disease

33. Bilateral diaphragmatic paralysis, high spinal cord lesions

34. Diaphragm pacing

35. CPAP

36. hypercapnic, hypoxemic, hypoxemia, alveolar collapse

37. Increase expired lung volumes, decrease inspiratory and expiratory resistance, improve PaO_2, decrease respiratory rate, and prevent air trapping

38. Nasal mask and nasal pillows

39. Pressure transducers regulate the amount of flow into the circuit; no patient access to controls

40. Aerophagia; gastric distention; hypoventilation

41. nasal dryness, congestion, humidification, irrigating nasal passages

42. Good tongue strength, intact gag reflex, absence of a tracheostomy, ability to close nasal passages and larynx, ability to swallow

43. VC of 1.5 L and PCEF of 3 L/sec

44. Assisted coughing; mechanical oscillation; MI-E

45. abdominal thrusts, compressions, expiratory flow

46. MI-E does not cause airway irritation and discomfort.

47. Patients with bullous emphysema and patients predisposed to barotrauma

48. A cuffed nonfenestrated tube

49. A fenestrated or cuffless tube

50. Children with tracheostomies are at risk for delays in communication skills development.

51. Increase inspiratory time or adding PEEP

52. Increase in airway resistance and WOB, hyperinflation, a drop in cardiac output, barotrauma

53. swallow, protect, aspiration

54. Smaller size tubes may increase the WOB; throat dryness; oxygen lines may become disconnected

55. A one-way valve opens on inspiration and closes on expiration, directing air to the larynx.

56. A comatose/unconscious patient, foam cuff in place or cuff must remain inflated, increased or thick secretions, severe upper airway obstruction, increased airway resistance or compliance (which may cause air trapping), ET in place, reduced lung compliance, laryngeal and pharyngeal dysfunction

57. White vinegar mixed with distilled water

58. 30 minutes

59. Suction trachea and pharyngeal area above the cuff; check PIP and VT; deflate cuff; increase VT if needed to maintain adequate ventilation; adjust alarms as necessary; monitor HR, RR, SpO_2, cough, subjective expression of comfort

60. Suctioning and tracheostomy care, ventilator settings, circuit maintenance, infection control, troubleshooting, emergency measures

61. Date and time of visit; patient name, address, and phone number; diagnosis; physician and phone number; prescribed equipment and procedures; assessment (vital signs, breath sounds, sputum evaluation, SpO_2, ventilator parameters, alarm settings, equipment function); caregiver and patient comprehension of equipment and procedures; compliance with care plan; recommendations

Answers to Critical Thinking Questions

1. An air leak around the mask is most likely the cause of both problems. The leak is preventing the patient from receiving the prescribed level of CPAP, and the escaping air is also causing the eye irritation.

2. The RT can readjust the straps to obtain an air-tight seal. If making the mask tighter causes the patient discomfort, another option available to help alleviate the problem would be the use of nasal pillows.

3. Breaths are flow-cycled during PSV. Once the cuff is deflated, the resultant leak prevents the breath from entering the expiratory phase, causing the respiratory distress.

Answers to Case Studies
Case Study #1

1. The patient is hypoventilating because of respiratory muscle weakness, which is resulting in hypercapnia and hypoxemia.

2. NPPV by nasal mask at night

3. NPPV will increase alveolar ventilation and help normalize PaO_2 and $PaCO_2$. The reduction in the WOB at night will result in an increase in respiratory muscle strength during the day.

4. Patient's subjective improvement in symptoms and an increase in the ability to perform activities of daily living

Case Study #2

1. Similar to a hospital setting, a frequent cause of patient illness is poor infection control techniques. The RT should review hand washing, suctioning, tracheostomy care, and all equipment and disinfection procedures with all persons involved in the care of the patient.

Answers to NBRC-Style Questions

1. d	5. c	9. c
2. c	6. d	10. a
3. b	7. d	
4. a	8. c	

Chapter 22, Neonatal and Pediatric Mechanical Ventilation

Answers to Key Terms Crossword Puzzle

(Crossword grid — answers include:) RDS, BPD, MECONIUM, FISTULA, BRONCHOMALACIA, CONGENITAL, CLEFT PALATE, DIAPHRAGMATIC HERNIA, CPAP, HFPV, DUCTUS ARTERIOSUS, HFOV, AOP, FETAL

Answers to Review Questions

1. CPAP devices, BiPAP units, and mechanical ventilators

2. The goals of mechanical ventilatory support for newborn and pediatric patients are to (1) provide adequate ventilation and oxygenation, (2) achieve adequate lung volume, and (3) improve lung compliance.

3. The goal for these patients is to prevent periods of apnea until pharmacological therapy can take effect.

4. PaO_2 less than 50 mm Hg or $PaCO_2$ greater than 55 mm Hg

5. 7.20

6. The potential risks of endotracheal intubation and VILI must be weighed against the fact that infants tolerate moderate hypoxemia and acidosis better than their adult and older pediatric counterparts.

7. PaO_2 less than 70 mm Hg or $PaCO_2$ more than 50 to 60 mm Hg

8. Tissue oxygenation can be assessed by observing the color of the skin and mucous membranes. A newborn with a dark complexion will be difficult to assess. A newborn with a light complexion should have a pinkish hue to the skin. The mucous membranes should be pink in all well-oxygenated patients. A blue or pale color of the skin or mucosa indicates hypoxemia.

9. Oxygen delivery and tissue oxygenation may be evaluated by using capillary refill and looking at the patient's hematocrit level. The hematocrit should be maintained above 40% in infants and children with respiratory disease.

10. Fetal hemoglobin has an increased affinity for oxygen, which causes a left shift in the oxyhemoglobin dissociation curve. Therefore this type of hemoglobin does not readily give up oxygen to the cells.

11. In pediatric patients the most common uses for CPAP are (1) to avoid endotracheal intubation and (2) to provide a transition from mechanical ventilation to extubation.

12. CPAP is usually used for patients with adequate alveolar ventilation who are hypoxemic in spite of receiving F_IO_2 values greater than 0.60.

13. Nasal prongs; nasopharyngeal tube; nasal mask.

14. 30% to 40% increase in normal respiratory rate; substernal and suprasternal retractions; grunting; nasal flaring; pale or cyanotic skin color; agitation.

15. inability of the patient with adequate minute ventilation ($PaCO_2 = 50$ mm Hg with pH 7.25 or greater) to maintain PaO_2 more than 50 mm Hg with an F_IO_2 of 0.60

16. The presence of poorly expanded or infiltrated lung fields

17. RDS; pulmonary edema; atelectasis; apnea of prematurity; recent extubation; tracheal malacia or other similar abnormality of the lower airways; transient tachypnea of the newborn

18. Prophylactic use of CPAP is indicated for very low birth weight infants at risk for developing RDS.

19. Cardiac defects that increase pulmonary blood flow, such as ventricular septal defects, arterial septal defects, atrioventricular canal, and patent ductus arteriosus can cause decrease in lung compliance and FRC. The creation of positive intrathoracic pressure by CPAP serves to reduce pulmonary blood flow mechanically while restoring FRC.

20. Contraindications to CPAP include nasal obstruction or severe upper airway malformation such as choanal atresia, cleft palate, or tracheoesophageal fistula, and untreated congenital diaphragmatic hernia.

21. a snug-fitting set of nasal prongs

22. that they be fitted correctly so that no leak occurs and no injury is caused

23. Headgear consisting of a bonnet, cap, and/or straps is used to stabilize the CPAP apparatus.

24. Assurance of effective CPAP delivery should be made frequently. The patient's nose should be checked for signs of pressure necrosis from the nose mask, and the prongs should be checked routinely for patency.

25. Either a commercially available nasopharyngeal tube or an appropriately trimmed ET may be used. The tip of the tube is lubricated with a water-soluble lubricant and passed into either nasal passage. After advancement of the tube the clinician inserts a finger into the infant's mouth toward the posterior oropharynx and gently feels for the tip of the tube behind the soft palate. When the tube is felt, it is then pulled back 0.5 to 1 cm and stabilized. The posterior oropharynx can be viewed with a laryngoscope to confirm placement.

26. Skin irritation; pressure necrosis; nasal irritation; septal distortion.

27. Improvised CPAP systems are assembled by using flowmeters, tubing, adapters, and valves. They do not have built-in alarm or safety systems in their design as do commercially available, free-standing CPAP devices and mechanical ventilators.

28. Initial pressure setting for CPAP is approximately 4 to 5 cm H_2O, which can be increased in increments of 1 to 2 cm H_2O until a maximum of 10 cm H_2O.

29. Adequate CPAP is considered to be when the required F_IO_2 is 0.60 or less and the PaO_2 is at least 50 mm Hg.

30. Pulmonary overdistention; ventilation perfusion mismatch; decreased pulmonary blood flow; increased PVR; decreased cardiac output; CO_2 retention; abdominal distention and gastric insufflation; aspiration; perforation of the gastrointestinal tract; injury to the nose and nasal mucosa

31. nSIMV is mostly accomplished by external triggering devices.

32.

Disorder	CPAP Application Device
4-year-old with juvenile spinal muscle atrophy (Kugelberg-Welander disease)	nasal mask
1 year-old with progressive spinal muscular atrophy of infants (Werdnig-Hoffmann paralysis)	nasal prongs
10-year-old with OSA	nasal mask
3-year-old with bronchomalacia	tracheostomy tube

33. Indications for mechanical ventilation of the neonate include the following conditions: (1) apnea, (2) respiratory or ventilatory failure despite the use of CPAP and supplemental oxygen, (3) alterations in neurological status that compromise the central drive to breathe, (4) impaired respiratory function resulting in a compromised FRC from decreased lung compliance or increased airways resistance, (5) impaired cardiovascular function, and (6) postoperative state characterized by impaired ventilatory function.

34. Respiratory failure in the neonate is characterized by (1) pH less than 7.20 to 7.25; (2) PaO_2 less than 50 mm Hg; (3) increased WOB as evidenced by grunting, nasal flaring, tachypnea, and sternal and intercostal retractions; and (4) the presence of pale or cyanotic skin and agitation.

35. Neurological problems that can compromise a newborn's central drive to breathe include apnea of prematurity, intracranial hemorrhage, and congenital neuromuscular disorders.

36. Decreased lung compliance and increased airway resistance can be caused by (1) RDS, (2) meconium aspiration syndrome, (3) pneumonia, (4) bronchopulmonary dysplasia, (5) bronchiolitis, (6) congenital diaphragmatic hernia, and (7) sepsis.

37. Impaired cardiovascular function can be caused by (1) persistent pulmonary hypertension of the newborn, (2) postresuscitation status, (3) congenital heart disease, and (4) shock.

38. Indications for respiratory failure in pediatric patients are $PaCO_2$ greater than 50 to 60 mm Hg and PaO_2 less than 70 mm Hg.

39. The neuromuscular and hypotonic disorders that are indications for mechanical ventilation of a pediatric patient are (1) muscular dystrophies, (2) spinal muscular atrophy, (3) Guillain-Barré syndrome, and (4) myasthenia gravis.

40. The essential characteristics of an infant ventilator include (1) continuous flow with TCPL or multimodal capability, (2) visible/audible alarm systems for high and low pressure and volumes, (3) high pressure release to ambient capability, (4) visible/audible alarms for low and high oxygen concentrations, (5) visible/audible alarm for loss of power and gas source, (6) servo-regulated humidifier with low compressible volume water chamber and continuous feed water supply system, (7) low compliance ventilator circuit and/or capability for ventilator to measure and subtract compressible volume from delivered and monitored volume displays, and (8) ability to drain water condensate from circuit or heated inspiratory/expiratory circuit limbs.

41. The nonessential features provide for improved monitoring capabilities and more physiological ventilator parameters.

42. TCPL

43. Flow controllers were less expensive to produce and largely accepted by clinicians.

44. A. O_2 input; B. air input; C. flowmeter; D. timer; E. gas flow direction; F. pop-off valve; G. patient; H. exhalation valve. This figure represents the spontaneous phase of ventilation. The gas is continuously flowing by the patient, who has the opportunity to breathe spontaneously from that gas.

45. When the inspiratory phase begins, the exhalation valve (H) will close and the gas from the ventilator will be diverted to the patient.

46. During the pressure-limiting phase, the exhalation valve (H) will continue to be closed. When the set pressure is reached, the excess pressure will be vented out through the pop-off valve (F). The set pressure will be maintained until inspiration is time cycled.

47. Continuous flow provides a noninterrupted supply of gas and does not require the infant to initiate a breath to begin gas flow. Demand flow provides a low background or bias flow through the circuit at all times. When the infant begins inspiration the flow increases to maintain a baseline pressure.

48. Flow triggering results in better patient-ventilator synchrony and reduces WOB and caloric and sedation requirements.

49. While manually ventilating an infant with an airway pressure manometer, evaluate for bilateral lung aeration and chest movement in-line while noting the average PIP. The PIP level that provides good aeration and optimizes the infant's skin color and oxygen saturation level is a good place to set the ventilator's PIP setting.

50. V_T should be 6 to 10 mL/kg for TCPL.

51. In newborns, PEEP is used to establish FRC and prevent alveolar collapse.

52. The flow setting should be twice the patient's minute ventilation, or approximately 2 to 3 L/min for most patients.

53. Signs of insufficient flow include retractions, ventilator asynchrony, pressure fluctuations on the manometer around the baseline PEEP, and the ability of the ventilator to reach the desired PIP with mandatory breaths.

54. a. Time constant = Raw × C_L = 45 cm H_2O/L/sec × 0.004 L/cm H_2O = 0.18 second; b. T_I should be set at 3 to 5 times the time constant, which is 0.54 second – 0.9 second.

55. a. Time constant = Raw $\times$ C_L = 30 cm H_2O/L/sec $\times$ 0.002 L/cm H_2O = 0.06 second; b. T_I should be set at 3 to 5 times the time constant, which is 0.18 second – 0.3 second.

56. The I:E ratio can be manipulated to extend T_E permitting lung emptying before the next breath.

57. 0.5 seconds $\times$ (4L/min $\div$ 60) = 0.067 L, or 67 mL

58. Percent leak = $[(V_T$inspiratory $-$ $V_T$expiratory)/ V_T inspiratory] $\times$ 100

$$= [(67 \text{ mL} - 55 \text{ mL})/67] \times 100$$
$$= [12 \div 67] \times 100$$
$$= 18\%$$

59. 60 $\div$ 40 breaths/min = 1.5 seconds for inspiration and expiration. I:E is 1:2, I + E = 3, 1.5 seconds $\div$ 3 = 0.5 second for inspiratory time.

60. 12 cm H_2O

61. The major difference between PCV and TPTV is that inspiratory flow can be much greater in PCV, resulting in an almost immediate rise to peak pressure.

62. Mixed-mode ventilation is the combination of pressure-controlled ventilation and pressure-supported spontaneous breaths. The advantage is that it enables the ventilator to be better synchronized to the patient with challenging ventilatory needs, such as with narcotic withdrawal.

63. PaO_2/F_IO_2 less than 100, PIP greater than 35 cm H_2O, and PEEP greater than 8 cm H_2O

64. 4 to 6 mL/kg

65. The term "flow chop" is used to describe the phenomenon produced by a very short inspiratory time in which limitation of inspiratory flow is so great that flow does not decelerate to zero as it normally does during PCV. This means that the inspiratory phase "time limits" and that the delivered V_T is smaller than if the flow had been permitted to taper to zero.

66. When volume ventilation is used, V_T and inspiratory flow determine inspiratory time. $T_I = V_T$/FR

67. VV with SIMV is recommended for infants weighing more than 2 kg who do not have significant lung disease and for infants with bronchopulmonary dysplasia requiring long-term ventilation. Use 5 to 6 mL/kg and PEEP 2 to 3 cm H_2O.

68. VSV targets a preset V_T or minute ventilation whereas PSV does not. When surfactant therapy is given, drastic changes in compliance may occur. The ventilator in the VSV mode could make adjustment in the amount of PIP needed to obtain the target V_T.

69. Weaning is accomplished by reducing PIP until a PIP of 10 to 15 cm H_2O is reached.

70. The lung-protective strategies used to minimize the effects of both VILI and dynamic hyperinflation include using lower V_T, appropriate PEEP levels, and plateau pressures less than 30 cm H_2O; allowing higher $PaCO_2$ levels (permissive hypercapnia); and using short inspiratory times.

71. The most typically used surfactant replacements are extracted from calf washings and contain some proteins plus the major phospholipids.

72. The procedure for administering surfactant includes manual or mechanical ventilation with a rate of at least 30 breaths/min with an F_IO_2 of 1.0 before dosing. After each partial dose the patient is ventilated with these parameters for 30 seconds. Once the full dose has been given, the ventilator is adjusted back to baseline settings. Patient assessment during and after surfactant dosing is important to pick up on any adverse reactions or complications.

73. The recommended therapeutic range for nitric oxide NO concentration is 80 ppm or less.

74. Two types of toxicity reported with inhaled NO include (1) pulmonary tissue toxicity and (2) methemoglobinemia.

75. HFV should be considered for a patient with heterogeneous lung disease for whom mP_{aw} on conventional ventilation exceeds 15 cm H_2O. At lower mP_{aw} levels, the decision to change from conventional ventilation to HFV may be considered if the patient's clinical picture is worsening and settings on the conventional ventilator are escalating.

76. Complications from HFV include (1) lung hyperinflation, (2) impaired cardiac output, and (3) intraventricular hemorrhage.

77.

HFV Type	Definition (Including Frequency)	Uses
HFPPV	modified conventional ventilation with high rates and low V_T values; rates between 60 and 150 breaths/min	low birth weight infants with RDS not responding to conventional methods; pediatric patients with surfactant deficiency syndromes
HFFI	V_T created by a device that interrupts a gas flow or a high-pressure source at frequencies as high as 15 Hz	under investigation
HFPV	therapeutic device administered, by mask or mouthpiece, to internally percuss the chest for secretion removal, mobilization of secretions, or as a continuous mode of ventilation; high-frequency pulsations can be as high as 600 cycles/min (10 Hz)	used continuously with children and has been used as a prophylactic measure to prevent pneumonia and atelectasis in patients with thermal injury
HFOV	oscillations are delivered by an electro-magnetically driven piston pump at frequencies between 8 and 30 Hz (480 to 1800 cycles/min)	patients with air leak syndromes such as pulmonary interstitial emphysema, pneumothorax, or bronchopleural fistula
HFJV	involves the delivery of short jet breaths, or pulsations, of an air-oxygen mixture under considerable pressure through a small lumen located in the trachea at rates between 4 and 11 Hz (240 to 660 breaths/min)	infants with RDS and air leak syndromes

78. Gas transport in HFV does not fully rely on bulk convection. The mechanisms thought to cause gas transport in HFV are theoretical and not completely understood. These mechanisms include pendelluft, streaming, Taylor type of dispersion, and simple molecular diffusion.

79. Preparations that should be completed before HJV include (1) administering of the initial dose of artificial surfactant; (2) repositioning the patient; (3) completing any procedures that could cause agitation; (4) suctioning the ET to avoid interruptions during the initial period; (5) placing the pulse oximeter, ECG leads, BP cuff, and transcutaneous CO_2 monitor; and (6) providing adequate sedation.

80. The goal for all types of HFV is to provide effective gas exchange with the lowest F_IO_2 and mP_{aw} possible.

Critical Thinking Questions

1. This problem is caused by a failure to flow cycle because of an ET leak. The RT should set up a backup time cycle to avoid the excessive inspiratory time.

2. Volume-supported ventilation has the advantage of being able to measure lung compliance and to make automatic adjustments to the PIP. This would help avoid overdistention of the lungs after surfactant therapy.

3. The CPAP is being lost through the open mouth and may be avoided by placing a pacifier in the infant's mouth. This will keep the mouth closed around the pacifier and stop the pressure leak.

Answers to Case Studies

Case Study #1

1. 25 cm H_2O

2. Decrease in compliance

3. Lung hyperinflation

Case Study #2

1. Reduce F_1O_2 to 0.60 and repeat ABG

2. Worsening atelectasis and respiratory distress syndrome

3. Administer another dose of Survanta

Case Study #3

1. 10 cm H_2O

2. 15

3. The pressure at which chest movement is adequate

Answer to NBRC-Style Questions

1.	c	5.	c	9.	b
2.	a	6.	a	10.	c
3.	b	7.	b	11.	a
4.	d	8.	d	12.	a

Chapter 23, Special Techniques in Ventilatory Support

Answers to Key Terms Crossword Puzzle

Crossword answers include: NONDEPENDENT, AMPLITUDE, CHESTWIGGLE, APRV, MAP, BIASFLOW, HELIOX, ILV, DEPENDENT, INERT, PISTAT, SPOTATAPRV, SINERTZ, HERTZ, ECMO, RELEASET (RELEASETIME), SPONTANEOUS, ARDS, MEASE, AMPAW, BITUBE, BILEVEL.

Answers to Review Questions

1. APRV is a mode of ventilatory support designed to provide two levels of CPAP and allow spontaneous breathing at both levels when spontaneous effort is present.

2. a. P_{low} = 4 cm H_2O; b. P_{high} = 20 cm H_2O

3. both time

4. Bi-Vent (on the Servo[i]) and Bi-Level (on the Puritan Bennett 840)

5. APRV physiological and hemodynamic advantages include (1) better oxygenation, (2) less hemodynamic compromise, (3) decreased CVP, (4) reduced physiological dead space, (5) reduction in peak and mP_{aw}, (6) increased cardiac index, (7) reduced need for sedation and paralysis, and (8) improved renal perfusion and function, increasing urine output.

6. The main disadvantages of APRV include (1) CO_2 elimination depends on lung compliance, airway resistance, and spontaneous breathing efforts of the patient; (2) not all ventilators allow patient triggering of breaths from P_{high} to P_{low} and P_{low} to P_{high}; (3) limited staff experience; and (4) lack of sufficient evidence-based application.

7. T_{low} = 0.75 second and T_{high} = 4.75 seconds; T_{low} + T_{high} = TCT, 0.75 + 4.75 = 5.5 seconds, 60 ÷ 5.5 = 11 cycles/min.

8. In APRV, minute volume depends on the patient's spontaneous effort during all time intervals plus the release interval volume change.

9. P_{high} = 15 to 35 cm H_2O

10. P_{low} = 0 to 15 cm H_2O

11. T_{high} = 4 to 15 seconds

12. 0 cm H_2O

13. The T_{low} should be established on the basis of the patient's pulmonary problem. Patients with low lung compliance should have short T_{low} settings. Patients with high airway resistance should have longer T_{low} settings.

14. 0.5 to 1.0 second

15. The three factors that determine ventilation and $PaCO_2$ are (1) release time, (2) volume exchanged during release time, and (3) the patient's spontaneous ventilation.

16. Reduce P_{high} by 2 to 3 cm H_2O at a time and increase T_{high} by 0.5- to 2-second increments. When P_{high} is 14 to 16 cm H_2O and T_{high} is between 12 and 15 seconds the ventilator may be switched to traditional CPAP.

17. 3 to 16 Hz (180 to 900 cycles/min)

18. A reciprocating diaphragm-shaped piston creates the oscillations in the 3100B.

19. A sine waveform is created by the 3100B.

20. The amplitude of the wave set by the power (ΔP) control determines the forward and backward excursion of the piston and therefore the V_T.

21. The appropriateness of the power setting is determined by observing chest wall movement, or "chest wiggle factor." The chest wiggle factor should be visible from the level of the clavicle to the mid-thigh when the amplitude is appropriate.

22. Increasing the frequency will result in decreased ventilation because less volume will be displaced by the piston.

23. Decreasing the frequency will result in increased ventilation because greater volume will be displaced by the piston.

24. $T_I\%$ represents the portion of the respiratory cycle that the piston spends in a forward motion.

25. If the bias flow is set too low, not enough flow will be available to wash out exhaled gas. This will lead to an elevated $PaCO_2$. If the bias flow is set too high, the backward motion of the piston will only remove gas from the circuit. This will also lead to an increased $PaCO_2$ and may also result in auto-PEEP.

26.

Control	Brief Description	Typical/Initial Setting
mP_{aw}	has a direct affect on PaO_2 by changing lung volume; displaces patient's diaphragm downward; good lung expansion checked by chest radiograph should show ninth posterior rib above the level of the diaphragm in the midclavicular line	typical setting 25 to 30 cm H_2O; initial setting 3 to 5 cm H_2O greater than mP_{aw} during conventional ventilation
amplitude	primary control for ventilation; changes the amount of piston displacement; adequate amplitude is checked by observing chest wiggle factor from clavicle to mid-thigh initial	power control range 1 to 10; typical power control setting is 6 to 7 for adults; setting should result in ΔP of approximately $PaCO_2 + 20$ (typically 60 to 70 cm H_2O)
frequency	the time allowed for the piston to move forward and backward; secondary control for ventilation	range of 3 to 15 Hz; initial setting 5 to 6 Hz
$T_I\%$	inspiratory portion of the respiratory cycle or the forward movement of the piston; also controls ventilation	initial setting 33% for adults
bias flow	rate of continuous flow through the patient circuit; generally the first parameter set when starting HFOV; influences mP_{aw} and $PaCO_2$	typical adult range 25 to 40 L/min; initial setting 30 L/min
F_IO_2	maintains target range for PaO_2 or SpO_2.	initial setting 1.0 and titrated according to PaO_2 or SpO_2 by decreasing in increments of 0.1

27. The control valve on the expiratory limb of the circuit provides variable resistance to exhalation and controls mP_{aw}. The dump valve, also located on the expiratory limb of the circuit, opens when the piston is off. The limit valve, located on the inspiratory limb, limits the inspiratory pressure.

28. Patients with ARDS who weigh at least 35 kg who have acute respiratory failure as evidence by unresponsive severe hypoxemia (F_IO_2 more than 0.6, PEEP 10 cm H_2O or more, with a PaO_2 of 65 mm Hg or less) or who have a significant risk of VALI. Additional indications might include air leaks, early interventional technique to recruit the lungs, and where clinical staff is comfortable using the equipment.

29. Patients who require aerosolized medications

30. For the transition from conventional ventilation to HFOV, sedatives, analgesics, and sometimes NMBAs are necessary. Sedation usually includes a combination of benzodiazepines (e.g., midazolam) and a narcotic (e.g., fentanyl). NMBAs include pancuronium, cisatracurium, and vecuronium.

31. mP_{aw} of 20 to 24 cm H_2O; SpO_2 88% or greater on an F_IO_2 less than 0.5

32. PC-CMV and APRV

33. Helium is inert, odorless, colorless, has a low density (0.18 g/L), the lowest melting point, a boiling point close to absolute zero, and a high thermal conductivity.

34. Asthma, bronchiolitis, COPD, dyskinesia, foreign body obstruction, laryngeotracheal bronchitis, postextubation stridor, tracheobronchitis, tumors (laryngeal or mediastinal), viral laryngitis, and vocal cord paralysis

35. Laminar flow occurs somewhere between the third- and eleventh-generation bronchi, depending on the rate of gas flow.

36. Actual flow = Displayed flow $\times$ 1.8; $6 \times 1.8 = 10.8$ L/min

37.
Ventilator	Volume with Heliox
VIASYS Avea	no significant difference in V_T delivered by VC, PC, or PS ventilation with and without heliox, 80:20 and 60:40
Hamilton Veolar and Galileo	V_T del greater than V_T set; the greater the helium concentration the more the V_T del exceeds the V_T set. The exhaled V_T monitor will underestimate the actual V_T.
Puritan Bennett 7200	V_T del less than V_T set when F_IO_2 less than 0.9
Puritan Bennett 840	cannot be use with heliox
Servo 300	works well with heliox in VC-CMV, PC-CMV, and PRVC; V_T exp less than actual V_T del
Servo^i	works with heliox in VC and PC modes. V_T exp less than actual V_T del
Dräger Dura-2	V_T del greater than V_T set; V_T exp reads greater than actual V_T del
Dräger E-4	V_T del greater than V_T set

38. Heliox is connected to a mechanical ventilator by connecting a compressed air inlet hose directly to a 50-psi heliox gas source.

39. Because the heliox mixture replaces compressed air within the ventilator, some ventilators will only be accurate when set at 21% oxygen. With others, such as the Galileo, Veolar FT, Servo 300, and Servo 900C, the actual delivered F_IO_2 is the same as the set F_IO_2. A ventilator's internal oxygen analyzers may alarm and should be disabled. An oxygen analyzer equipped with alarm settings should be put in the ventilator circuit.

40. Pressure during ventilation with heliox is not a problem because pressure is not density dependent. Pressure ventilation is easily accomplished.

41. If the patient's oxygen requirement is greater than 40%, heliox therapy should not be used.

42. *Independent lung ventilation* is a technique that allows the gas flow to each lung to be controlled separately and is accomplished by using a specialized double-lumen ET in which each bronchus receives different volumes and pressures.

43. ILV is used during the following surgical procedures: thoracoabdominal aortic aneurysm repair, thoracic organ transplant, lung volume reduction surgery, pneumonectomy, and video-assisted thoracoscopy.

44. Pulmonary hemorrhage and isolation of infected secretions (any unilateral lung disease)

45. When using two ventilators that are not connected, dyssynchronous ventilation of the lungs can occur. Each ventilator operates independently, and as long as they are not 180 degrees out of phase, this type of ventilation is probably not detrimental. Rate synchronization can be accomplished by linking the rate controller of both ventilators together. One ventilator becomes the master, dictating the rate to the second ventilator.

46. Before use of a slow-flow inflection maneuver, the patient must be sedated to eliminate spontaneous breathing during the procedure. With the double lumen endotracheal tube, the left lung is connected to the ventilator. A single-breath maneuver with 5 to 7 mL/kg IBW is delivered at a very low constant flow rate (e.g., 10 L/min). The pressure and volume information is graphically displayed and evaluated for the first lung. The procedure is then repeated with the ventilator connected to the opposite lung. The loops are then evaluated.

47. The *expiratory inflection point*, also called the deflation or deflection point, is the point on the expiratory limb of a pressure-volume curve where derecruitment or alveolar collapse occurs.

48. Use VC-SIMV or VC-CMV, rate of 4 breaths/min and 5 to 7 mL/kg IBW for one lung and 13 to 15 mL/ kg IBW for both lungs.

49. Once the SFIM is performed on each lung, the LIP and UIP are established for each lung. The PEEP levels are set independently for each lung at a few centimeters of water pressure above the LIP.

50. The IPV-1 can provide internal chest physiotherapy, volume-oriented IPPB, and high-density aerosol delivery.

51. The IPV-1 can deliver 100 to 450 bursts/min with adjustable inspiratory and expiratory times (up to 1:5). Percussive pressures are between 8 and 40 cm H_2O.

52. The use of an IPV-1 during VC-CMV will generate high PIP values and cause the exhaled V_T to read high. An actual increase in V_T occurs, between 25 and 50 mL per machine breath. A pressure relief valve in the ventilator adapter goes in-line with the ventilator circuit on the inspiratory limb. With this relief valve fully open volume will be lost through the adapter. If the valve is fully closed, excessive peak pressures can occur in VC-CMV. This valve needs to be set correctly.

Answers to Critical Thinking Questions

1. P_{high} = 30 cm H_2O, P_{low} = 3 cm H_2O, T_{high} = 5 seconds, T_{low} = 1 second, I:E = 5:1; ventilator rate = 60 ÷ 6 = 10 cycles/min

2. If adequate lung expansion has been achieved, then the diaphragm should be visualized at the ninth posterior rib in the midclavicular line. Because the diaphragm is only at the sixth rib, the mP_{aw} needs to be increased.

3. LIP = 20 cm H_2O and UIP = 42 cm H_2O

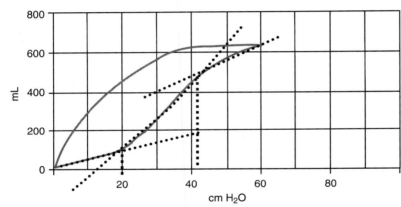

4. PEEP should be set at 22 cm H_2O.

5. A V_T should be used that keeps PIP below the UIP.

Answers to Case Studies

Case Study #1

1. I:E = 4:1; 4 + 1 = TCT = 5. 60 ÷ 5 = 12 cycles/min

2. The P_{high} should be increased.

3. An increase in the P_{high} level will increase the pressure gradient and effectively increase the V_T level.

Case Study #2

1. Increase F_IO_2

2. Because the patient's P_{high} is at the maximum recommended and the F_IO_2 is still relatively low, the F_IO_2 should be increased.

3. Once the P_{high} and F_IO_2 values being used are high, the prone position may provide improvement.

Case Study #3

1. The left lung, because the TAAA procedure requires physical compression and deflation of the left lung to allow more free access to the aorta.

2. 7 mL/kg IBW calculates to $7 \times 81 = 567$ mL for each maneuver.

3. PEEP should be set at a few centimeters of water above the lower inflection point. PEEP for the right lung should be set at 8 cm H_2O and at 20 cm H_2O for the left lung.

Answers to NBRC-Style Questions

1. a	6. a	11. d
2. c	7. d	12. a
3. a	8. c	13. d
4. c	9. a	14. d
5. d	10. b	